Clinical Manual of
PSYCHIATRIC NURSING

Clinical Manual of
PSYCHIATRIC NURSING

Ruth Parmelee Rawlins, R.N., D.S.N., C.S.
Associate Professor
School of Nursing
University of Central Arkansas
Conway, Arkansas

Patricia Evans Heacock, R.N., Ph.D.
Associate Professor
School of Nursing
University of Arkansas for Medical Sciences
Little Rock, Arkansas

SECOND EDITION

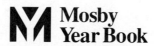
Mosby
Year Book

St. Louis Baltimore Boston Chicago London Philadelphia Sydney Toronto

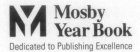
Mosby
Year Book
Dedicated to Publishing Excellence

Executive Editor: Linda L. Duncan
Developmental Editor: Teri Merchant
Project Manager: Karen Edwards
Senior Production Editor: Gail Brower
Designer: Jeanne Wolfgeher
Cover Photo: © David Bishop/PHOTOTAKE, NYC

SECOND EDITION

Printed in the United States of America

Mosby–Year Book, Inc.
11830 Westline Industrial Drive
St. Louis, Missouri 63146

Library of Congress Cataloging in Publication Data

Rawlins, Ruth Parmelee.
    Clinical manual of psychiatric nursing/Ruth Parmelee Rawlins,
Patricia Evans Heacock.—2nd ed.
        p.   cm.
    Includes bibliographical references and index.
    ISBN 0-8016-6333-4
    1. Psychiatric nursing—Handbooks, manuals, etc.   I. Heacock,
Patricia Evans.   II. Title.
    [DNLM: 1. Psychiatric Nursing—handbooks.   WY 39 R259c]
RC440.R35   1993
610.73'68—dc20
DNLM/DLC
for Library of Congress

92-12910
CIP

93 94 95 96 97 GW/VH 9 8 6 5 4 3 2 1

To all my students for their caring
and listening to clients and each other.

To all my clients for sharing of themselves
so that I could learn from them and
share those learnings in helping others.

To Monte whose warm, purring body next to me
helped me persist in completing this project.

Ruth Parmelee Rawlins

To my mentors:

Anna Mae and C. A. Evans

Frances Evans Jackson

Gretta Cain, R.N.

Sarah O'Rielly, R.N.

Sister Ellen Marie, R.N.

Betty Bregg, R.N., M.S.N.

Dorothy Corona, R.N., M.S.N.

Mary Crockett, R.N., D.N.Sc.

Celeste Dye, R.N., Ph.D.

Patricia Evans Heacock

Preface

The focus of this manual is a practical, holistic application of the nursing process for use in the inpatient clinical setting. It is intended to provide guidelines for nursing actions. Supporting principles from the major theories of personality development and behavior are presented to increase the student/practitioner's understanding of behavior.

The manual is designed as a quick reference guide to assist the student/practitioner in assessing problem behavior, as well as in analyzing, planning, implementing, and evaluating care given to a client who exhibits maladaptive behavior. The client in this process is perceived as an active collaborator who maintains autonomy and assumes responsibility for problem resolution. The nursing process is offered as a method of identifying a client's problems, planning solutions, and implementing those plans. While the nursing process is aimed at problem identification and resolution, emphasis is on the client's strengths, which can be identified and used to aid in the process. This manual can be used as an adjunct to the text, *Mental Health—Psychiatric Nursing: A Holistic Life-Cycle Approach.*

Part One represents a comprehensive assessment tool and provides guidelines for obtaining needed data. The tool is detailed and the student/practitioner can select those areas for assessment that are clinically significant to the presenting problem and can identify the client's interest in and commitment to health maintenance.

Part Two addresses specific behaviors commonly seen in a psychiatric setting and often in other clinical settings. In this manual, the holistic approach conceptualizes an individual as having five dimensions—physical, emotional, intellectual, social, and spiritual—and provides the organizing framework. This approach recognizes each aspect of the person as interacting with the environment. Each of the dimensions themselves interact at all times and, consequently, influence the whole person. Certain concepts basic to holism such as health maintenance and prevention are emphasized in many of the nursing actions, and the actions are directed toward prevention of problems and restructuring a lifestyle more conducive to health.

Each section of Part Two begins with a brief description of the identified behavior and related concepts, including the DSM-III-R classification of mental disorders. This is followed by a section on principles. Principles are derived from theories that have had an impact on nursing. They are succinct statements that propose to explain the development and presence of a certain behavior in individuals. The statements are categorized according to their most representative dimension. It is recognized that many statements are applicable to and interact with more than one dimension. The Principles section provides a rationale for nursing diagnoses and implementation of care.

The assessment of each behavior includes client data, an analysis, and sample nursing diagnoses. The fact that individuals are complex and variable limits these sections to factors specifically seen in association with the identified behavior. Nursing diagnoses are written to help the student identify and label the client's maladaptive behavior and to provide a basis for planned nursing interventions. It is recognized that a nursing diagnosis is a summary statement that is made following data collection and analysis. A nursing diagnosis is not ordinarily based on a single piece of datum; therefore because of the variability of human behavior, the full spectrum of possible nursing diagnoses is presented. We hope our approach is helpful to the student.

Nursing diagnoses used in this manual include those accepted by the members of the North American Nursing Diagnoses Association (NANDA) at the 1992 Tenth National Conference on Classification of Nursing Diagnoses. Also included are nursing diagnoses from the Psychiatric Mental Health (PMH) classification system developed by the ANA task force of the Council of Psychiatric Mental Health Nursing. An asterisk (*) indicates nursing diagnoses from the PMH classification system. All others are NANDA nursing diagnoses.

Considerable emphasis is placed on nursing diagnoses to help the student practitioner identify the client's many responses to illness.

Part Two concludes with examples of goals and outcome criteria, nursing actions and rationale, discharge planning, and evaluation. Discharge planning begins on admission and is included as a part of the plan of care; consequently, statements under discharge planning are written in terms of client behaviors. The identified behaviors indicate the client's readiness for discharge. A bibliography specific to the behavior completes this section.

Part Three is composed of case studies with sample care plans. The care plans show the interrelation of all the dimensions.

The use of gender-oriented pronouns is avoided as much as possible. However, when necessary for clarity and simplicity, the nurse is referred to as *she* and the client as *he*.

Efforts have been made to provide student/practitioners with a systematic approach in dealing with a massive and sometimes mystifying amount of data. It is hoped that this manual will assist them in their endeavor to provide quality nursing care to their clients.

Ruth Parmelee Rawlins
Patricia Evans Heacock

Contents

ASSESSMENT

Part One provides a comprehensive holistic assessment tool. Each of the five dimensions of the person—physical, emotional, intellectual, social, and spiritual—are included in the tool. The physical dimension is divided into three sections: history, physical examination, and diagnostic tests. Diagnostic tests are included so that the nurse may become familiar with procedures done for diagnostic purposes and to ensure that possible physical causes for a problem are considered in the holistic assessment. The assessment tool is intended to systematically guide the student or practitioner through the assessment process. Comments and considerations are provided to assist further the student or practitioner in obtaining the necessary data.

The behavioral guidelines presented in this manual are designed primarily for assessing client behaviors in mental health clinics and psychiatric hospitals. The holistic approach is used because of its comprehensive nature and its recognition of the relationships of body, mind, and environment that are essential in providing comprehensive nursing care. It is an effective approach because of the consideration given to individuals as dynamic forces influencing and being influenced by interactions with the body, the mind, each other, and the environment.

The holistic approach to health care recognizes all aspects of a person and promotes a balanced, whole view of the person. In this manual individuals are separated into physical, emotional, intellectual, social, and spiritual dimensions. Although this artificial separation can occur only for purposes of analysis, it is an effective way to assess and implement care for the total client in a systematic and organized manner. In reality, the dimensions are integrated and the person as a whole functioning organism is more than the simple combination of all the dimensions.

A holistic framework for health care then encompasses all aspects of the person as significant and considers how these aspects interact to affect the whole person. All aspects of the person contribute to health and illness. Thus the balance in all the dimensions of a person is valued. No one dimension can be considered in isolation and any attempt to do so results in an incomplete view of the whole person. When people are viewed in such a fragmented manner, the tendency is to interact with them in a fragmented way.

An arbitrary selection of the components for each dimension has been made to help the student and practitioner identify these components. It is, of course, difficult to ascribe certain characteristics to a particular dimension because of the intricate interaction patterns within each person and within the environment. The case studies in Part Three represent the holistic process of putting the client back into perspective as an integrated functioning person.

PHYSICAL DIMENSION

The physical dimension involves everything associated with a person's physical body including diet, sleep, exercise and activity, sexuality, habits (for example, alcohol, smoking, drugs, coffee, tea, and colas), genetics, body image, and physiological functioning. The various aspects of the physical dimension interact constantly with each other. Nutritional status affects a person's physiological and emotional processes. Heredity affects growth and development. Physical activity is an effective way to counteract stress and tension. Socially, it is difficult to have fun and laugh and play when not feeling physically well. A person's level of physical well-being is an indicator of how effectively that person is taking care of the total self.

EMOTIONAL DIMENSION

A major component of the emotional dimension is an individual's affect, the observable feeling or emotional tone of the individual (for example, happy, sad, angry, or anxious). Other components include the client's report of feelings, the congruency of affect with the client's report, and the appropriateness of the affect to the situation. Duration and quality of the person's emotional responses are additional components of the emotional dimension. Reactions to a traumatic situation, as in post-trauma syndrome, are important considerations in this dimension, affecting all other dimensions. The ability to make decisions is influenced by a person's feelings; feelings affect relationships with others, physiological functioning, the ability to make judgments, and the ability to become self-actualized. In some ways the environment contributes to a person's feelings at a given time, and feelings affect the person's interactions with the environment. The way people express their feelings or choose not to is an indication of the degree of their emotional development, maturity, and total well-being.

INTELLECTUAL DIMENSION

Components of the intellectual dimension include perception, cognition, and communication. Perception has particular significance for clients with psychiatric problems, since determinations are made concerning the reality or distortion of the clients' perceptions. Several aspects of cognition are addressed in the intellectual dimension: memory, orientation, fund of information, judgment, insight, ability to think abstractly, and defense mechanisms that provide information about the client's mental status. Lastly, the client's communication is assessed. The manner of speaking, the quality and quantity of speech, and the degree of flexibility in thinking are appraised. As with the other dimensions, the intellectual dimension interacts with and affects all other dimensions. Thoughts affect a person's heart rate. Mental images affect the body; for example, images of danger elicit autonomic nervous system responses, and calming images reduce hyperactive nervous system responses. The effect of a person's intellectual functioning contributes to the ability to acquire, filter, organize, recall, and communicate information through activities such as problem solving and decision-making.

SOCIAL DIMENSION

Aspects of the individual that enable a person to function in society make up the social dimension. A basic component of this dimension is self-concept, and self-esteem is a major component of self-concept. Whereas self-concept involves an individual's beliefs, feelings, and attitudes about the self, which are seemingly intellectual functions, self-concept and its components, self-esteem and self-identity, are placed in the social dimension because of the strong influence society and social relationships have on the formation of the self.

The client's level of trust and the amount of dependence or independence demonstrated add information about interpersonal relationships. Members of the family unit are assessed for relationships, support systems, and communication patterns. Other components of the social dimension include role functioning, cultural factors, and environmental factors. Environmental factors, while seemingly physical, are viewed as social because of their relationship with the individual and their effect on social functioning. The social dimension interacts with and influences each of the other dimensions. Social interactions enable people to meet their physical, emotional, intellectual, social, and spiritual needs. Socialization allows a person to develop communication skills and through these skills permits interactions with the environment. The quality of a person's relationships and the ability to meet needs through relationships with others determine how effectively a person's social self is functioning.

SPIRITUAL DIMENSION

The spiritual dimension allows individuals to experience and understand the reality of their existence in unique ways that go beyond the usual limits. Spirituality encompasses far more than a person's religion; it permeates the person's life and incorporates the whole being. One component of the spiritual dimension is a person's philosophy of life. Life values and beliefs about health and illness provide data for an assessment of this philosophy. Other components of this dimension include the client's concept of deity, religion, religious beliefs, and perception of faith. The client's ability to transcend the rudiments of daily existence and find expression and creativity is a meaningful part of the spiritual dimension. Lastly, an assessment of the client's spiritual fulfillment, as seen in the ability to lead an enriched and self-actualized life, is an important aspect of the spiritual dimension. Abilities to create, to enjoy beauty, and to face one's own mortality provide a foundation for spiritual fulfillment. The spiritual dimension interacts with all dimensions of the person and is affected during a physical illness. Spirituality also affects a person's thoughts and feelings about personal value and life itself.

The interactions of all the dimensions are seen in the diagram on p. 3. In this manual, discharge plans follow goals and outcome criteria. It is believed that planning for the client's discharge begins as soon as treatment plans are made and are included as a component of nursing interventions.

The assessment tool that follows provides a systematic and organized method for a holistic assessment of a client. The student or practitioner is encouraged to select those items appropriate for an assessment of the individual client.

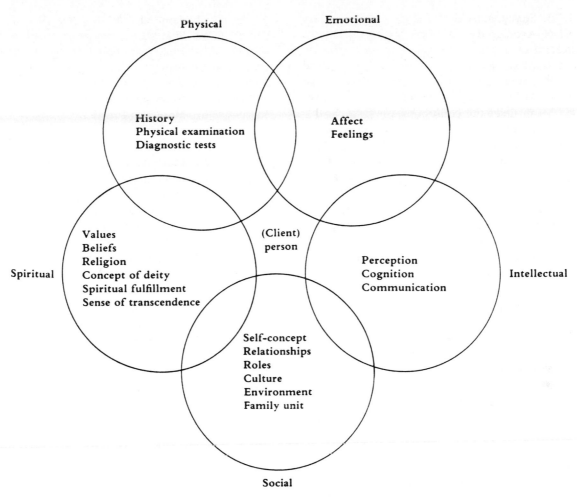

Integration of the Five Dimensions of the Person

Circle labels:

Physical — History / Physical examination / Diagnostic tests

Emotional — Affect / Feelings

Spiritual — Values / Beliefs / Religion / Concept of deity / Spiritual fulfillment / Sense of transcendence

(Client) person

Intellectual — Perception / Cognition / Communication

Social — Self-concept / Relationships / Roles / Culture / Environment / Family unit

ABBREVIATED OUTLINE FOR A HOLISTIC ASSESSMENT

Physical Dimension

I. History

  A. Identifying information
1. Name
2. Address
3. Telephone number
   a. Home
   b. Work
4. Birth date
5. Age
6. Race
7. Ethnic group
8. Sex
9. Marital status
10. Education
11. Occupation
12. Religion
13. Nationality
14. Informant
15. Date of interview

  B. Statement of presenting problem
1. Duration

  C. History of presenting problem
1. Onset
2. Interval history
3. Current status
4. Reason for seeking help at this time

  D. Activities of daily living
1. Nutrition
   a. Appetite
   b. Eating patterns
   c. Weight changes
2. Sleep
3. Recreation, hobbies, and interests
4. Physical activities and limitations

5. Sexual activity
6. Average day
E. Habits
  1. Alcohol
  2. Smoking
  3. Medications and drugs
    a. Over the counter
    b. Prescription
    c. Illegal
  4. Caffeine
    a. Coffee
    b. Tea
    c. Colas
F. Destructive behavior
  1. Aggression
  2. Suicide
G. Health history
  1. Illnesses
  2. Injuries
  3. Allergies
  4. Hospitalizations
  5. Surgeries
  6. Coping skills
H. Family health history
  1. Bipolar disorder
  2. Depression
  3. Suicide
  4. Schizophrenia
  5. Mental retardation
  6. Substance abuse
  7. Stress-related illness
I. Body image
  1. Physical description of self
  2. Thoughts and feelings about body
J. Sexuality
  1. Perception of own sexuality
  2. Ways of expressing self sexually
  3. Satisfaction with sex life
  4. Concerns related to sex life
  5. Sexual partner preference
K. Physical abuse
  1. Incest
  2. Sexual abuse
  3. Child abuse
  4. Spouse abuse
  5. Elderly person abuse
  6. Other trauma
    a. Mugging
    b. Beating
    c. Robbery
    d. Disaster
L. Review of systems

1. General
2. Skin
3. Head
4. Ears
5. Eyes
6. Nose and sinuses
7. Mouth and throat
8. Neck
9. Breasts
10. Cardiovascular
11. Respiratory
12. Gastrointestinal
13. Genitourinary
14. Reproductive
    a. Male
    b. Female
    c. Obstetric history
    d. Methods of contraception
      (1) Male
      (2) Female
15. Musculoskeletal
16. Peripheral vascular
17. Neurological
18. Psychiatric
19. Endocrine
20. Hematological

II. Physical examination
A. General appearance
  1. Height
  2. Weight
  3. Vital signs
  4. Body type and stature
  5. Apparent age
  6. Posture
  7. Gait
  8. Body movements
  9. Hair and hair growth patterns
  10. Odors
  11. Nails
  12. Manner of dress
  13. Personal hygiene
  14. Speech
B. Skin
C. Head
D. Eyes
E. Ears
F. Nose and sinuses
G. Mouth and throat
H. Neck
I. Back
J. Posterior thorax and lungs
K. Breasts, axillae, and epitrochlear nodes

L. Anterior thorax and lungs
M. Heart
N. Carotid pulsations and jugular venous pulses
O. Abdomen
P. Inguinal area
Q. Genitalia
   1. Male
   2. Female
R. Legs
S. Musculoskeletal system
T. Peripheral vascular system
U. Neurological examination
   1. Motor
   2. Sensory
V. Mental status

III. Diagnostic tests—any tests that may aid in the diagnosis or treatment of the problem

Emotional Dimension

1. Affect
2. Client's self-report
3. Congruency of affect with client's self-report
4. Appropriateness of affect to situation
5. Duration
6. Quality
7. Post-trauma response

Intellectual Dimension

1. Perception
2. Cognition
   a. Memory
   b. Orientation
   c. Fund of information
   d. Judgment and insight
   e. Abstract thinking
   f. Thought content
   g. Defense mechanisms
3. Communication
   a. Manner of speaking
   b. Quality
   c. Quantity
   d. Flexibility or rigidity of thinking

Social Dimension

1. Self-concept
   a. Ideal self
   b. Perceived self
   c. Self-esteem
2. Interpersonal relations
   a. Level of trust
   b. Level of dependence or independence
3. Family unit
   a. Relationship
   b. Birth order
   c. Support system
   d. Communication patterns
4. Social role functioning
   a. Conflict
   b. Ambiguity
   c. Incongruity
   d. Overload
   e. Involvement with criminal justice system
5. Cultural factors
   a. Traditions
   b. Customs
   c. Norms
6. Environmental factors
   a. Stressors
   b. Safety factors
   c. Resources

Spiritual Dimension

1. Philosophy of life
   a. Life values
   b. Beliefs about illness
2. Concept of deity
   a. Religion
   b. Spiritual beliefs
   c. Perception of faith
3. Sense of transcendence
   a. Hope or despair
   b. Suicide
4. Self-actualization
   a. Creativity
   b. Aesthetic sense
   c. Beliefs about life and death

DETAILED OUTLINE FOR A HOLISTIC ASSESSMENT

ASSESSMENT	COMMENTS AND CONSIDERATIONS
Physical Dimension	
I. *History:* to obtain biographical data	Consider immediate thoughts, feelings, and impressions of client at first meeting.
A. Identifying information	Collect identifying information first since it is less threatening and is a way to establish trust.
1. Name	
2. Address	Obtain information from records (when available) to avoid repetitious questioning.
3. Telephone number	Under informant include impression of reliability, general attitude, and willingness to communicate.
a. Home	
b. Work	
4. Birth date	
5. Age	
6. Race	
7. Ethnic group	
8. Sex	
9. Marital status	
10. Education	
11. Occupation	
12. Religion	
13. Nationality	
14. Informant	
15. Date of interview	
B. Statement of presenting problem: to elicit the client's perception of the problem	Record client's own words (for example, "I'm depressed," "I'm here for a rest").
	If client has difficulty isolating one problem, ask client to state the problem that led to seeking help at this time.
	Client: "I have two sons, and what is happening to them is killing me. I have diabetes and am losing my eyesight, and last summer I had a heart attack."
	Nurse: "Which of these problems is bothering you the most at this time?"
1. Duration: to determine length of time client has experienced symptoms	"How long have you had these symptoms?"
C. History of presenting problem: to gather further data about the chief complaint	Focus on the chief complaint. Other illnesses and hospitalizations will be dealt with later.
1. Onset	Ask questions that encourage description: "When did you first feel depressed?"
2. Interval history	"What has been going on in your life since that time?"
3. Current status	"How are you feeling now?"
4. Reason for seeking help at this time	"What is the reason you are seeking help now?"
D. Activities of daily living: to develop an understanding of the client as an individual; to determine health habits and life-style; to provide a basis for comparison of usual health habits with changes during illness and progress toward returning health	"What do you want help with?"
1. Nutrition: to determine adequacy of client's diet	"What did you eat for breakfast, lunch, and dinner during the past 24 hours?"
a. Appetite	"What changes have you noticed in your appetite?"
b. Eating patterns	"How many meals do you usually eat each day?"
c. Weight changes	"What changes have you noticed in your weight over the past 3 months?"
2. Sleep: to determine client's sleep patterns	"How many hours do you sleep each night?"
	"What time do you get up, and what time do you go to bed?"
	"How many times do you get up at night?"
3. Recreation, hobbies, and interests: to determine client's skills and use of leisure time to use as a basis for planning therapy	"What do you do in your spare time?"
	"What are your favorite activities?"
	"Rank these in order of preference."
4. Physical activities and limitations: to determine client's ability to participate in physical activities	"What kinds of physical activities do you engage in?"
	"What limits your participation in activities?"

ASSESSMENT	COMMENTS AND CONSIDERATIONS
5. Sexual activity: to elicit from client information about his sexual behavior; to provide an opportunity for client to discuss concerns and problems	Respect the sensitive nature of questions. "In what ways has being ill affected your sexual activity?" "How active are you sexually?" "What are your concerns (problems) about your sexual activity?" "How satisfied are you with your sexual functioning?" Refer client to the physician or a sex therapist when you are uncomfortable or feel inadequate to help client.
6. Average day: to elicit information about client's daily life in terms of productivity and pleasures	"Tell me what your average day is like, beginning with when you get up in the morning and continuing through the day until you go to bed at night." For example, "I get up at 6 AM, shower, drink a cup of coffee, make my lunch, and go to work at 6:45. I work until 4 PM, come home, and cook supper for the kids and me. After supper I clean up around the house, watch TV, and go to bed about 10:30 PM. Maybe once a week I go see my mother."
E. Habits: to elicit information about client's health habits 1. Alcohol: to determine alcohol intake	Refrain from asking, "Do you drink?" because the responses are likely to be what the client thinks you want to hear. "How much do you drink?" "What kinds of alcoholic beverages do you drink?"

2. Smoking: to determine smoking habits
3. Medications and drugs: to determine client's use of drugs and medications
  a. Over the counter
  b. Prescription
  c. Illegal
	"How many cigarettes do you smoke each day?"
	Some clients have an aversion to the word *drugs*. Use *medication* if it seems more appropriate.
	"What medications are you taking currently? What for?"
	
	"How much marijuana do you smoke?"
	"What other drugs do you take?"
	Avoid asking, "Do you smoke pot?" The safe answer is "No."

4. Caffeine (coffee, tea, colas): to determine amount of caffeine client consumes	Be aware that caffeine is a stimulant and interferes with the action of some medications. "How many cups of coffee (tea, colas) do you drink each day?" "How much chocolate candy do you eat?"

F. Destructive behavior: to determine client's potential for harm to self or others
  1. Aggression
  2. Suicide
	"Are you considering hurting someone else?"
	Always ask about suicide when client is depressed.
	"Do you feel hopeless?"
	"Have you considered suicide (killing yourself, harming yourself)?"
	"Do you feel so bad (worthless, so much a burden) that you don't want to live any longer?"
	"What is your plan?"

G. Health history: to elicit client's past health problems 1. Illnesses	"What illnesses have you had in the past (physical, mental, emotional)?"
2. Injuries	"What injuries have you had?" "Have you been molested, raped, or battered?"
3. Allergies	"What are you allergic to (foods, additives, drugs, or airborne allergens)?"
4. Hospitalizations 5. Surgeries 6. Coping skills	"What have you been hospitalized for?" "What operations have you had? When?" "How have you dealt with problems in the past?"

DETAILED OUTLINE FOR A HOLISTIC ASSESSMENT—cont'd

ASSESSMENT	COMMENTS AND CONSIDERATIONS

H. Family health history: to determine family history of psychiatric illnesses
  1. Bipolar disorder
  2. Depression
  3. Suicide
  4. Schizophrenia
  5. Mental retardation
  6. Substance abuse
  7. Stress-related illness
	"Who in your family has been mentally or emotionally ill?"
	"Who in your family has had symptoms similar to yours?"
	"Describe that person's symptoms."

I. Body image: to determine client's perception of his body
  1. Physical description of self
  2. Thoughts and feelings about body
	"Describe yourself physically."
	"What is the most valued aspect of your body?"
	"What do you dislike most about your body?"

J. Sexuality: to elicit information about client's sexuality
 	
  1. Perception of own sexuality
 	
  2. Ways of expressing self sexually
 	
  3. Satisfaction with sex life
  4. Concerns related to sex life
  5. Sexual partner preference
	Consider that sexual practices the client sees as abnormal or disapproved of by the interviewer are often not volunteered.
	"Describe the way you see yourself as male (or female)."
	"How comfortable are you with your maleness (or femaleness)?"
	"Do you hug, kiss, touch, caress your partner?"
	"How often do you have sex?"
	"How often do you masturbate?"
	"How satisfied are you with your sex life?"
	"What are your concerns regarding your sex life?"
	"What is your sexual partner preference—male or female?"

K. Physical abuse: to determine history of abuse in client
  1. Incest
  2. Sexual abuse
 	
  3. Child abuse
 	
  4. Spouse abuse
 	
  5. Elderly person abuse
  6. Other trauma
    a. Mugging
    b. Beating
    c. Robbery
    d. Disaster
	Ask questions matter-of-factly. Victims often feel ashamed and are reluctant to reveal sexual abuse or incest. Awareness on the part of the nurse of his or her own negative feelings toward the perpetrator, victim, or family is essential.
	If a child is the victim, say, "I wonder if someone has done something to your body that has scared or hurt you."
	Direct questions are effective: "Have you been beaten by your husband?"
	Assess memory to validate or invalidate claims of abuse.
	Assess crisis status of the victim:
	  What is the client's perception of the problem?
	  Who is supportive?
	  What are the client's coping skills?

L. Review of systems: to gather information about the past and present health of each of the client's body systems
  1. General
    ___ Weakness
    ___ Fatigue
    ___ Change in weight (# of pounds)
    ___ Change in appetite
    ___ Change in sleep habits
    ___ Malaise
    ___ Fever
    ___ Other
  2. Skin
    ___ Color changes
    ___ Hair changes
    ___ Rash
    ___ Insect bites
    ___ Lumps
    ___ Itching
	Inform client that a number of questions will be asked.
	
	Use a checklist or written reminder of questions to ask to prevent leaving out essential questions.
	If client is acutely ill or uncooperative, wait 1 or 2 days before attempting to collect information.
	Use terms client is likely to understand or define terms in easily understood language.
	Collect data from less threatening systems first (cardiovascular). Conclude with personal information (reproductive) after trust is established and anxiety is reduced.

ASSESSMENT	COMMENTS AND CONSIDERATIONS

___ Lesions
___ Bruises
___ Scars
___ Changes in moles
___ Perspiration
___ Other

Mark location of skin conditions on diagram.

3. Head
___ Headache
___ Head injury
4. Ears
___ Tinnitus
___ Hearing loss
R ___ L ___
___ Aches
___ Discharges
___ Infections
___ Other
5. Eyes
___ Vision loss
R ___ L ___
___ Cataracts
___ Glaucoma
___ Pupils (dilated or constricted)
___ Glasses or contact lenses
___ Itching
___ Burning
___ Pain
___ Redness
___ Other
6. Nose and sinuses
___ Sense of smell
___ Epistaxis
___ Sinus infections
___ Frequent colds
___ Allergies
___ Other
7. Mouth and throat
___ Teeth and gums
___ Sore tongue
___ Hoarseness
___ Sore throats
8. Neck
___ Swollen glands
___ Lumps
9. Breasts
___ Lumps
___ Nipple discharge
___ Self-examination
10. Cardiovascular
___ Chest pain
___ Dyspnea on exertion
___ Tachycardia
___ Bradycardia
___ Edema
___ Palpitation
___ Varicosities
___ Syncope
___ High blood pressure
___ Other

Front   Back

DETAILED OUTLINE FOR A HOLISTIC ASSESSMENT—cont'd

ASSESSMENT	COMMENTS AND CONSIDERATIONS

11. Respiratory
___ Rate
___ Rhythm
___ Cough
___ Shortness of breath
___ Wheezing
___ Bronchitis
___ Recurring respiratory infections
___ Emphysema
___ Tuberculin test
___ Chest x-ray examination
___ Other
12. Gastrointestinal
___ Nausea
___ Vomiting
___ Diarrhea
___ Constipation
___ Heartburn
___ Gas
___ Indigestion
___ Loss of appetite or taste
___ Use of laxatives
___ Normal bowel patterns
___ Other
13. Genitourinary
___ Pain
___ Burning or stinging
___ Urgency
___ Incontinence
___ Nocturia
___ Frequency
___ Hesitancy
___ Infections
___ Other
14. Reproductive
  a. Male
___ Penile discharge
___ Prostate problems
___ Vasectomy
___ Impotence
___ Libido
___ Sexually transmitted disease
___ Hernia
___ Other
  b. Female
___ Last menstrual period
___ Age of menarche
___ Age of menopause
___ Date of last Pap smear
___ Dysmenorrhea
___ Vaginal discharge
___ Premenstrual tension
___ Breast self-examination
___ Libido
___ Sexually transmitted disease
___ Other
  c. Obstetric history
___ Number of living children
___ Abortions
___ Complications of pregnancy
___ Stillbirths	

ASSESSMENT	COMMENTS AND CONSIDERATIONS

d. Methods of contraception
  (1) Male _____
  (2) Female _____
15. Musculoskeletal
  ___ Joint pain
  ___ Muscle pain or cramps
  ___ Muscle tenseness
  ___ Muscle rigidity
  ___ Stiffness
  ___ Deformity
  ___ Back problems
  ___ Arthritis
  ___ Other
16. Peripheral vascular
  ___ Cramps
  ___ Varicose veins
17. Neurological
  ___ Fainting spells or dizziness
  ___ Seizures
  ___ Tingling
  ___ Numbness
  ___ Memory loss
  ___ Nervousness
  ___ Mood changes
  ___ Disorientation
  ___ Pain
  ___ Tremors
  ___ Personality changes
  ___ Other
18. Psychiatric
  ___ Nervousness
  ___ Tension
  ___ Mood
  ___ Depression
19. Endocrine
  ___ Heat intolerance
  ___ Cold intolerance
  ___ Change in hair distribution or texture
  ___ Hypoglycemia
  ___ Hyperglycemia
  ___ Other
20. Hematological
  ___ Anemia
  ___ Easy bruising
  ___ Transfusions
II. *Physical examination:* to determine state of client's physical health
  A. General appearance
    1. Height _____
    2. Weight _____
      Ideal weight _____
    3. Vital signs
      a. Temperature _____
      b. Pulse _____
      c. Respirations _____
      d. Blood pressure _____
    4. Body type and stature
      a. Musculature
      b. Short or stocky
      c. Tall
      d. Thin
	Collaborate with the physician to determine whether the physical examination has been done and, if not, who is responsible for doing it.

DETAILED OUTLINE FOR A HOLISTIC ASSESSMENT—cont'd

ASSESSMENT	COMMENTS AND CONSIDERATIONS

5. Apparent age
6. Posture
7. Gait
   a. Slow or fast
   b. Foot dragging
   c. Unsteady
8. Body movements—tremors
9. Hair and hair growth patterns
10. Odors
   a. Alcohol
   b. Fruity
   c. Bad breath
11. Nails
   a. Cleanliness
   b. Length
   c. Evidence of biting
12. Manner of dress
   a. Cleanliness
   b. Appropriateness (to age and situation)
13. Personal hygiene
   a. Cleanliness
   b. Grooming
14. Speech
   a. Pace
   b. Clarity
   c. Volume
   d. Voice tone and inflection
B. Skin
C. Head
D. Eyes
E. Ears
F. Nose and sinuses
G. Mouth and throat
H. Neck
I. Back
J. Posterior thorax and lungs
K. Breasts, axillae, and epitrochlear nodes
L. Anterior thorax and lungs
M. Heart
N. Carotid pulsations and jugular venous pulses
O. Abdomen
P. Inguinal area
Q. Genitalia
   1. Male
   2. Female
R. Legs
S. Musculoskeletal system
T. Peripheral vascular system
U. Neurological examination
V. Mental status
III. *Diagnostic tests:* to augment or verify the physical examination results; to provide a biochemical database for an analysis of client's state of health or illness; to assess the progress of medication therapy	

Emotional Dimension	
1. Affect: to determine client's observable feeling or emotional tone	Observe the client's predominant feeling (anxious, sad, or angry), affect (flat or blunted), or indifference to feelings (la belle indifference).

ASSESSMENT	COMMENTS AND CONSIDERATIONS
2. Client's self-report: to elicit client's perception of own condition	"What are your feelings at this time?" If client responds with "better," follow up on what client was feeling before or ask what contributed to the better feelings. Ask what client means by "better," that is, what is better (mood, appetite).
3. Congruency of affect with client's self-report: to determine if the client's affect is congruent with the client's reports about his feelings	"You say you're fine, but you look worried (sad, annoyed)."
4. Appropriateness of affect to situation: to determine if client's feelings are appropriate for situation	Considering the situation, are the client's feelings appropriate? For example, is the client crying over her husband's death 12 years ago (inappropriate)?
5. Duration: to determine how long client has had the feelings	"How long have you been feeling this way?"
6. Quality: to determine the depth, intensity, and state of the client's feelings	
a. Shallow and superficial	Do the client's feelings seem shallow and superficial?
b. Intense	Do the client's feelings seem appropriately intense?
c. Immature	Does the client's expression of feelings seem childlike or juvenile (pouting)?
d. Mood swings	Does the client's mood swing from happy to sad (labile) quickly? Is the client's mood reasonably stable?
7. Post-trauma response: to determine any trauma that may contribute to client's emotional response	Consider illness, injuries, rape, disaster, and war experiences.

Intellectual Dimension

ASSESSMENT	COMMENTS AND CONSIDERATIONS
1. Perception: to determine whether client's perceptions are realistic or distorted	Assess for the presence of disturbed thinking such as phobias, obsessions, illusions, or delusions during the course of the interview.
a. Reality based	
b. Distorted	Determine the presence or absence of hallucinations by asking, "Do you ever hear voices that others do not hear or see things others do not see?"
(1) Phobias	
(2) Obsessions	
(3) Delusions	
(4) Hallucinations	
(5) Illusions	
2. Cognition: to determine functioning of client's cognitive abilities	
a. Memory	
(1) Immediate	Assess client's immediate memory (past 24 hours).
(2) Recent	Assess client's recent memory (past 6 weeks).
(3) Remote	Assess client's remote memory (beyond 6 weeks). "Tell me about your childhood."
b. Orientation	Does client know own name, the date, and where he or she is?
(1) Time	
(2) Place	
(3) Person	
c. Fund of information	Ask client to name the last three presidents or state a current news event to ascertain information about general knowledge level.
d. Judgment and insight	Does the client behave in a socially acceptable manner? How well does client manage money? How realistic are client's job expectations? Ask client: "If you found a letter, stamped and addressed, what would you do with it?" Is the client aware that he or she is ill? To what extent does the client recognize own contributions to the problem? How aware is the client of the effects of his behavior on others?

DETAILED OUTLINE FOR A HOLISTIC ASSESSMENT—cont'd

ASSESSMENT	COMMENTS AND CONSIDERATIONS
e. Abstract thinking	Can the client conceptualize, generalize, or come to a conclusion by a logical reasoning process? Does client think concretely? For example, Nurse: "What brought you to the hospital?" Client: "The sheriff." (concrete) Client: "I'm so nervous and uptight I can't think straight anymore." (abstract)
f. Thought content	Be alert for any recurring themes, preoccupations, unrelated topics, or threats.
g. Defense mechanisms	Assess client's use of defense mechanisms.
3. Communications: to determine how client expresses thoughts	
a. Manner of speaking	
(1) Circumstantial	Does the client use circumstantiality (tangentiality) when expressing ideas?
(2) Tangential	
(3) Blocking	Is there evidence of blocking, flight of ideas, or loose associations?
(4) Flight of ideas	
(5) Loose associations	
b. Quality	What kind of words does the client use (highly educated, poorly educated)? What is client's tone of voice (monotone, loud)?
c. Quantity	Is the client's speech excessive, pressured, rapid-fire? Is client verbally active, inactive, mute?
d. Flexibility or rigidity of thinking	Is the client open and able to change when new ideas are presented? Does client's thinking seem rigid and inflexible? What are client's prejudices and stereotypes?
Social Dimension	
1. Self-concept: to elicit the client's overall view of self	
a. Ideal self: to elicit the client's perception of how he or she would like to be	"What kinds of goals and aspirations do you have for yourself?" "In what ways are you reaching your goals and aspirations?" Consider if they are realistic for the client.
b. Perceived self: to elicit client's view of self	"What kind of person would you say you are?" "Describe yourself." "What are your thoughts and feelings about yourself?" "How do you think others view you?" "Do you see yourself with mostly positive or mostly negative characteristics?"
c. Self-esteem: to elicit client's judgment of own worth	"How important are you to yourself? To others?" "Who are you important to?" "Who is important to you?" "How much do you like yourself?" Consider eye contact as a measure of self-esteem with an awareness of cultural influences on eye contact.
2. Interpersonal relations: to elicit information about client's relationships and interactions with others	"How do you get along with your family, friends, people at work (school) and in the community?"
a. Level of trust: to determine client's ability to interact with others with meaningful, positive outcomes	"Do you think most people are basically good and can be trusted?" "Do you think most people are generally reliable?"
(1) Family	"With how much ease or discomfort can you discuss differences with others?"
(2) School	
(3) Work	Consider whether the client's thinking is realistic or distorted.
(4) Community	

ASSESSMENT	COMMENTS AND CONSIDERATIONS
b. Level of dependence or independence: to determine client's ability to function inter-dependently (1) Family (2) School (3) Work (4) Community	Consider client's responses to stressful event and ability to give and receive nurturing. "What do you do when you are sad (mad)?" "Who is supportive of you?" "Who needs your support?" Consider client's school and work record. Consider client's participation in community activities.
3. Family unit: to elicit information about the general health of the client's family; and to identify any illnesses of genetic, familial, or environmental nature that may have implications for the client's problem a. Relationships b. Birth order c. Support system d. Communication patterns	Is client a leader or a follower? How much responsibility for own actions does the client accept? Consider the following members: grandparents, parents, siblings, aunts, uncles, nieces, nephews, spouse, and children. "Where were you in the order of birth (first, second)?" "Who in the family is supportive of you?" "Describe your family communication (who talks to whom, who makes decisions)."
4. Social role functioning: to determine the client's ability to function in social role(s) a. Conflict: to determine conflicts in client's roles b. Ambiguity: to determine problems from unclear role expectations c. Incongruity: to determine changes in attitudes or values required of client to function in role(s) d. Overload: to determine client's ability to cope with demands at home, school, on the job e. Involvement with criminal justice system	"What is your role in the family?" "In what ways is your role satisfying?" "In what ways are you dissatisfied?" "Tell me about your job." "How long have you held it?" "How satisified are you with it?" "How far did you go in school?" "What is the reason you stopped at that time?" "What are the pressures and conflicts in your job, at home, at school?" "How clearly defined is your role at home? At work?" "What attitudes or ideas have you changed to function in your job, at home?" "What do you do when excessive demands are placed on you at home, at school, at work?" "Have you or a family member been arrested, tried, or convicted of a crime? If so, what was the crime?"

5. Cultural factors: to determine cultural influences on client's behavior
a. Traditions
 	
b. Customs
 	
c. Norms
	"What are some of your family traditions (for example, Christmas and birthday celebrations)?"
	Consider cultural influences of:
	  Age on dress and speech
	  Expressing emotions (anger, grief)
	  Eye contact
	  Background (urban or rural)
	  Child-rearing practices
	  Family makeup (nuclear or extended)
	  Life-style
	  Authority figures
	  Decision makers
	"What general things are done in your culture for persons with similar symptoms?"

DETAILED OUTLINE FOR A HOLISTIC ASSESSMENT—cont'd

ASSESSMENT	COMMENTS AND CONSIDERATIONS
6. Environmental factors: to elicit information regarding significant health hazards in the environment; to provide possible clues about the cause of the client's illness	

a. Stressors	Consider major situational stressors:
	  Change in residence
	  Hospitalization
	  Traffic violation
	  Marital separation, divorce, marriage
	  Job loss
	  Retirement
	  Jail sentence
	  Death of friend
	  Death in the family

b. Safety factors	Consider:
	  Job security
	  Financial security
	  Home environment
	  Recreational and leisure outlets
	  General health
	  Support systems

c. Resources	Consider:
	  Ability to ask for help
	  Client's strengths
	  Family strength
	  Available community services

Spiritual Dimension	
1. Philosophy of life: to elicit client's general attitude about life in terms of beliefs, values, morals, and ethics	"What are your thoughts and feelings about life in general?" "What kinds of things add meaning to your life?" "What do you see as your life's purpose?"

a. Life values: to elicit client's views concerning what is important in life and what influence these views have on the client's illness	Consider that client may demonstrate values more realistically than he or she articulates them. Observe client's behavior regarding:
	  Health
	  Sex
	  Spending money
	  Personal appearance
	  Family commitment
	  Education
	  Marriage
	  Religion
	  Community action
	  Recreation

b. Beliefs about illness: to assist in understanding client's health and illness behavior	"Tell me what you think caused your illness." "What did you do to treat your illness at home?" "From whom do you seek treatment?" "What are some home remedies you routinely use?" "Have you engaged in faith healing, folk remedies?"
2. Concept of deity: to plan spiritual experiences that promote health and healing	
a. Religion: to assess client's religion, beliefs, and practices; to determine whether these are a source of comfort to client	"What religion are you?" "How frequently do you attend religious services?" "How much satisfaction do you get from your religious life?" "Would you say you are a religious person? What do you do that demonstrates this?" "Do you pray, meditate?"

ASSESSMENT	COMMENTS AND CONSIDERATIONS
b. Spiritual beliefs: to elicit client's deeper meaning and purpose for life	Consider ways client demonstrates own purpose in life (through children, work, conservation of natural resources). "What kinds of things contribute meaning to your life?"
c. Perception of faith: to understand client's view of faith and its relationship to health and illness	"From where (whom) do you get strength?" Consider amount and quality of faith that client demonstrates about his life situation.
3. Sense of transcendence: to determine client's ability to accept illness (limitations and losses) and be a nurturing, productive person	
a. Hope or despair: to elicit client's sense of hope and confidence or sense of despair and futility about his illness	"Do you feel hopeless?" "Are you so depressed that you feel like giving up?" "Have you thought of killing yourself?"
b. Suicide: to assess client's potential for suicide	"How would you do it?" "What gives you the strength to go on?" Consider evidence that client has risen above the limitations of illness and committed self to a higher purpose (helping others).
4. Self-actualization: to determine client's ability to live a rewarding, enriched life	"As you look back, how satisfying has your life been?" "What does the future hold for you?" Consider client's ability to balance work, play, and love in a healthy manner.
a. Creativity: to elicit client's ability to feel self-satisfaction when expressing self creatively	"What are your artistic abilities?" "How much satisfaction do you derive from them?"
b. Aesthetic sense: to elicit client's ability to appreciate nature and beauty	"What do you enjoy about nature?" "What is your favorite season?" "What kind of beauty gives you a special sense of pleasure?"
c. Beliefs about life and death: to determine value client places on life and his ability to face death realistically and prepare for it	Consider client's past responses to separation and losses. Consider purpose of defenses when the client denies his illness. Initiate opportunities for the client to talk about his feelings concerning life and death. "What do you think will happen to you when you die?"

CLIENT BEHAVIORS

Part Two presents guidelines for behaviors commonly seen in mental health—psychiatric settings. The five steps of the nursing process—assessment, analysis, planning, implementation, and evaluation—provide the foundation for the organization of these guidelines.

First, the behavior is defined in a brief introduction and disorders related to the behavior and classified according to the *Diagnostic and Statistical Manual of Mental Disorders* (DSM-III-R) are listed in the principles section along with other conditions that may relate to the behavior. For each step of the nursing process, data are organized according to the five dimensions of the person. In the assessment section, which follows principles, data that apply specifically to the behavior are identified. It is important to note that only the predominant characteristics found in a specific behavior are identified. Appropriate principles are applied in the analysis of the data, and nursing diagnoses are developed. Nursing diagnoses approved by the Tenth North American Nursing Diagnosis Association (NANDA), and Psychiatric Mental Health Nursing Diagnoses (PMH) are used. An asterisk (*) indicates the PMH nursing diagnoses. All others are NANDA. Long-term and short-term goals and outcome criteria are described in the planning section, which is followed by discharge plans, an implementation section that lists nursing actions with rationale, and an evaluation section. Each behavior guideline concludes with a bibliography.

Amnesia

Amnesia is a complete or partial loss of memory. Amnesia usually occurs during highly stressful events from which the individual wishes to escape. Psychogenic amnesia and psychogenic fugue are two types of amnesia. The individual with psychogenic amnesia is unable to recall events that occurred during a certain period of time, usually the first few hours following a profoundly traumatic event. The stress often involves a threat of physical injury or death. The amnesic episode is characterized by perplexity, disorientation, and purposeless wandering. Termination of amnesia is typically abrupt and recovery is complete.

Individuals with psychogenic fugue may suddenly and unexpectedly travel away from home or their usual place of work following severe psychosocial stress. They are unable to recall their past and may establish a new identity for themselves. Travel and behavior appear more purposeful than the confused, wandering behavior seen in the person with psychogenic amnesia. Usually the fugue is of brief duration, from hours to days, and involves limited travel.

Related DSM-III-R disorders

Dissociative disorders
Organic mental disorders

Other related conditions

Shock
Military combat
Sleepwalking
Head injury

The original content for this section was contributed by Mary Flo Bruce, R.N., Ph.D.

PRINCIPLES

▶ Physical Dimension

1. Basic habit patterns remain intact; the person can talk, eat, write.
2. Amnesia may be associated with a head injury.

▶ Emotional Dimension

1. Amnesia is an unconscious response to anxiety.
2. Amnesia prevents the instinctual urges of the id from getting out of control.
3. A situation that is threatening to self may contribute to amnesia.
4. When a person becomes aware of an unacceptable, intolerable drive, anxiety is produced with possible amnesia.

▶ Intellectual Dimension

1. Amnesia is a learned behavior.
2. The behavior is impelled by anxiety and reinforced when the amnesia reduces anxiety.
3. Amnesia is an approach-avoidance situation in which an individual goes toward a stressful goal; as the goal gets closer, anxiety increases and the individual avoids the situation by becoming amnesic.
4. Forgetting is a way of avoiding stress while gratifying needs.
5. The individual denies personal responsibility for unacceptable behaviors.

▶ Social Dimension

1. Amnesia evolves from experiences in infancy that are poorly understood.
2. These experiences become a personification of the "not me" self system.

3. The self learns to avoid situations that cause intense anxiety.
4. Amnesia is a self-defense tactic called *dissociation*.
5. Psychogenic amnesia involves thoughts or feelings that are basically intolerable or threatening to the self.

▶ **Spiritual Dimension**

1. Loss of authentic self causes existential anxiety.
2. The individual is unable to face not being true to self.
3. When an individual is not true to self, he or she has no authentic goal; anxiety is aroused and may result in amnesia.

ASSESSMENT

▶ **Physical Dimension**

I. History

A. Habits
  1. Excessive use of alcohol
  2. Excessive use of medications and drugs
B. Health history
  1. Recent or past cranial trauma
  2. Toxic metabolic factors

II. Diagnostic tests

A. Arteriogram
B. Brain scan
C. Cerebral angiogram
D. Computed tomography scan (CT scan)
E. Electroencephalogram (EEG)
F. Test for orientation, memory, abstract thought
G. Questioning under hypnosis or amobarbital (Amytal)

▶ **Emotional Dimension**

CLIENT DATA	ANALYSIS	NURSING DIAGNOSIS
Has severe anxiety	May contribute to amnesia. Attempts to relieve stress by escape, that is, by loss of memory with or without flight. Leads to an inability to deal with stressful situations.	Ineffective individual coping: loss of memory related to severe anxiety

▶ **Intellectual Dimension**

CLIENT DATA	ANALYSIS	NURSING DIAGNOSIS
Has distorted perceptions	Inability to recall certain periods may lead to distortion of present environment. Impairment of perception because of organically caused amnesia.	Altered thought processes: distorted perceptions related to loss of memory. Altered thought processes: related to organically caused loss of recall
Has loss or partial loss of memory	Unable to recall all or certain events because of severe stress, physical injury, or organic deterioration.	Altered thought processes: inability to remember related to stress
Is disoriented	Disoriented about certain events or time, person, or place. Response to severe stress or to organic problem.	Altered thought processes: disorientation related to severe stress; disorientation related to organic problem
Lacks sufficient information	Because of inability to recall recent or past events, client has insufficient information.	Altered thought processes: insufficient information related to loss of memory
Lacks insight	Aware that there is loss of memory but is unable to relieve stress in any other manner.	Altered thought processes: lack of insight related to severe stress
Uses concrete thinking	Focuses on escaping and does not consider consequences. Is not able to search for other methods of resolving conflict.	Altered thought processes: impaired abstract thinking related to loss of memory

▶ **Intellectual Dimension—cont'd**

CLIENT DATA	ANALYSIS	NURSING DIAGNOSIS
Uses repression	Present conflict arises from conflict in early childhood. Individual has repressed earlier conflict and is attempting to resolve present conflict by escape. Ego defends itself against anxiety.	Ineffective individual coping: loss of memory related to inappropriate use of repression
Uses denial	To avoid conflict.	Ineffective individual coping: denial related to conflict
Thinks rigidly	Coping pattern is rigid and self-defeating. Unable or unwilling to look at other methods.	Ineffective individual coping: related to rigid thinking and an inability to consider other options

▶ **Social Dimension**

CLIENT DATA	ANALYSIS	NURSING DIAGNOSIS
Is confused about self-identity	Individual's concept of self forced back into unconsciousness. Does not know certain factors of own life. May not know own identity.	Personal identity disturbance: related to loss of memory
Has low self-esteem	Unable to resolve conflict in positive manner. Feels ineffective.	*Altered self-concept: related to feeling ineffective
Is dependent	Maladaptive dependence. Inability to recall all or certain events places the individual in a dependent position.	Ineffective individual coping: dependence related to loss of memory.
Lacks support system	Deficit in support system. Degree of deficit depends on amount of loss of recall. Total loss of memory with fugue may constitute total loss of support system.	Social isolation: lack of support system related to loss of recall
Has reduced ability to function in social role	Unable to function in usual social role. Degree of impaired functioning depends on degree of amnesia.	Altered role performance: related to loss of memory.
Has a loss of familiar setting	In severe cases, unable to recognize usual environment. In some cases, flees from own environment.	Altered thought processes: inability to recognize environment related to loss of memory
Is lonely	Inability to remember significant others.	Social isolation: related to inability to remember significant others
	With flight, caused by being in an unknown place with unknown people.	Social isolation: related to loss of memory
Has a loss of significant roles	Inability to remember disrupts significant roles.	Altered role performance: related to loss of memory

▶ **Spiritual Dimension**

CLIENT DATA	ANALYSIS	NURSING DIAGNOSIS
Has conflicts in personal values	Unable to resolve deep-seated conflict, which is reawakened under certain stress situations.	Spiritual distress: conflict in personal values related to anxiety
Lacks hope and faith	Unable to believe that stress can be relieved and conflict worked out. Uses escape to reduce anxiety.	Spiritual distress: lack of faith related to inability to resolve conflict
Sees sin as a basis for distress	Underlying anxiety based on client's conception of something client did that was "sinful." Unacceptable thoughts and impulses.	Spiritual distress: related to belief that underlying anxiety is due to "sinful" deeds or thoughts

PLANNING

Long-Term Goal

To develop an effective method of dealing with conflict and the resulting anxiety
without a loss of memory (amnesia)

SHORT-TERM GOALS	OUTCOME CRITERIA
Physical Dimension To identify stressors leading to amnesia	1. Verbalizes life story 2. Lists events causing anxiety in past 3. Explores feelings concerning these events 4. Verbalizes maladaptive methods used to handle stress 5. Lists events precipitating present problem 6. Relates feelings involved in dealing with problem 7. Identifies other methods of working through problem besides escape 8. Verbalizes thoughts and feelings concerning use of these other methods
Emotional Dimension To identify anxiety as source of memory loss To manage anxiety contributing to memory loss	1. Verbalizes present feelings 2. Relates specific instances of anxiety 3. States ways used to cope with present anxiety 4. Identifies other methods of reducing anxiety 5. Discusses consequences of each action 6. Chooses method to deal with present 7. Tests options 8. Evaluates results
Intellectual Dimension To improve or regain memory	1. Identifies areas of recall 2. Establishes method to use to improve ability to recall (for example, use of desensitization, hypnosis, or biofeedback) 3. Uses identified method to further memory recall
Social Dimension To develop a relationship of trust with caregivers	1. Verbalizes feelings concerning relationship with caregivers 2. Uses time with caregiver to work through feelings and fears 3. Ceases to attempt to manipulate caregiver 4. Demonstrates trust in caregiver by complying with treatment regimen
To develop positive interpersonal relationships	1. Establishes relationships with others 2. Verbalizes feelings about previous relationships with significant others 3. Verbalizes feelings about present relationships 4. Explores degree of autonomy 5. Lists methods that a person can use to become more autonomous 6. Verbalizes methods that can establish positive relationships with others
Spiritual Dimension To resolve value conflicts that contribute to amnesia and life distress	1. Explores conflicts 2. Clarifies values contributing to conflict 3. Identifies conflict and its relationship to amnesia
To use energy to live a productive, satisfying life rather than to flee from life	1. Identifies problems and present methods of resolving them 2. Uses healthy problem solving to resolve problem and promote satisfying life-style

Discharge Planning

The following client behaviors demonstrate readiness for discharge:
1. Identifies stress situations that result in using escape as a method of coping
2. Verbally confronts the underlying feelings that result in amnesia
3. Explores personal values, spiritual beliefs, moral code
4. Identifies support system
5. Increases self-esteem and self-awareness
6. Demonstrates methods to handle anxiety
7. Verbalizes a willingness to continue treatment regimen, if necessary

IMPLEMENTATION

NURSING ACTIONS	RATIONALE
Physical Dimension	
1. Do not allow client to manipulate caregiver into doing things that client can do for self.	To avoid being "used" by the client and to promote awareness of behavior.
2. Explore with client how the body responds physically to underlying feelings of anxiety.	To identify the body's physical responses to anxiety and increase awareness of the onset of anxiety.
3. Provide safe, protected environment.	To reduce stress and allow for reflection on events that led to the amnesic episode.
Emotional Dimension	
1. Explore with client the feelings that led to the acute amnesic phase.	To promote awareness and self-understanding.
2. Assist client in verbalizing feelings associated with amnesia: guilt, anger, powerlessness, loneliness, anxiety	To relieve tension, to indicate acceptance of feelings, to foster self-worth through acceptance, and to establish trust.
3. Help client relieve or reduce anxiety with stress-reduction techniques.	To provide socially acceptable alternatives for the expression of anxiety.
Intellectual Dimension	
1. Explore manner in which client's perception is distorted.	To reinforce reality and separate the real from the unreal. To promote an opportunity to question the distortion.
2. Assist client with orientation to time, place, and who he or she is.	To present reality and prevent distortions. To affirm self-identity.
3. Explore with client stressors that led to choosing loss of memory as method of dealing with stress.	To identify causative factors and to establish a basis for planning care.
4. Reinforce client's memory as client becomes willing to recover memory.	To support progress with positive reinforcement. To allow client to progress at own pace.
5. Assist client with decision-making until memory returns.	To alleviate the stress of decision-making while recovering memory.
6. Assist client in assuming responsibility for method chosen to deal with stress by offering options and allowing client to select preferred option.	To help client see consequences of behavior on self and others. To create in client a sense of self-responsibility for own behavior and to show that client has a choice in choosing ways to behave.
7. Arrange for psychotherapy.	To increase insight and self-awareness.
8. Explore with client methods of dealing with feelings that do not involve escape.	To help client explore other ways to express troubled thoughts and feelings and to promote mental health.
9. Encourage client to develop methods of dealing with unacceptable thoughts and impulses by talking about them with a supportive person.	To grant permission for the client to have unacceptable thoughts and impulses and to help client find acceptable ways to express them.
10. Offer feedback about appropriateness of methods client develops to deal with unacceptable thoughts and impulses.	To reinforce progress.
11. Assist client in identifying defense mechanisms used when anxious or under stress.	To increase awareness and insight and to encourage use of alternative methods for relieving anxiety.
12. Teach client problem-solving methods (see Appendix C).	To help client deal with problems rationally rather than emotionally. To increase self-esteem and feelings of competence.
13. Teach client positive methods of dealing with underlying stress and anxiety, such as relaxation, stress reduction, deep breathing.	To give client several options from which to choose for relief of anxiety.

IMPLEMENTATION—cont'd

NURSING ACTIONS	RATIONALE
Social Dimension	
1. Give client accurate positive feedback	To create feelings of competence and strengthen the ego to increase self-esteem and reduce anxiety.
2. Teach client methods of increasing own self-esteem when interacting with others.	To help client have positive feelings from interactions with others and avoid those who promote negative feelings.
3. If client does not remember significant others, work with client and significant others to establish a relationship.	To experience success and pleasure in relationships.
4. Assist client in identifying support system.	To develop a sense of success in social communication by sharing experiences and intimacy with others.
5. Work with client to build a new support system, if necessary.	To reinforce the importance of having someone with whom to talk.
6. If client is in a strange environment, assist in identifying location.	To present reality and trigger recovery of memory.
7. Assist client in identifying unknown objects in the environment.	To present reality and prevent feelings of ineffectiveness.
8. Include the family in treatment planning if secondary gains from amnesia are part of the problem.	To help the family understand their contribution to the client's problem and to plan ways to intervene.
Spiritual Dimension	
1. Explore with client the meaning of escape for client.	To determine what escape means to client and what client is avoiding or fears confronting.
2. Assist client in identifying values and moral code that may have been violated.	To help client see relationship between behavior and moral code that was violated and led to overwhelming anxiety.
3. When appropriate, refer client to clergy or other spiritual leaders to clarify belief system.	To sustain client's religious beliefs, to collect additional data about memory loss, and to offer encouragement, support, and hope.
4. Refrain from making judgments concerning client's values or belief system.	To demonstrate empathy and unconditional acceptance.
5. Encourage client to confront violation of underlying values or moral code through values clarification exercises.	To prevent denying or avoiding the issue.
6. Assist client in using creative energy in a positive manner.	To develop a sense of success and achievement in positive, growth-producing ways.
7. Promote self-awareness and self-actualization within the client's capabilities by observation, and giving feedback, and helping client meet basic needs.	To increase understanding of amnesic episodes and prevent future episodes.
8. Allow client the right to choose escape as a method of handling stress and anxiety.	To promote a sense of autonomy.
9. Avoid placing own values and mores on client.	To demonstrate unconditional acceptance of client values even though different from those of the nurse.

EVALUATION

Measurable goals and outcome criteria provide the basis for evaluating the client's recovery from an amnesic episode. In addition, the client's self-reports, nurse observations, and family reports supply information about the client's progress. The following behaviors indicate a positive evaluation:

1. Identifies stressful situations
2. Expresses feelings verbally about the stressful situation
3. Clarifies personal values and moral code
4. Has a support system
5. Relates escape to the stressful situation
6. Uses adaptive coping skills to handle stress

BIBLIOGRAPHY

Boss B: Memory impairments: forgetfulness versus amnesia, *J Neurosci Nurs* 20(3):151, 1988.

Corston R et al: Transient global amnesia in four brothers, *J Neurol Neurosurg Psychiatry* 114:734, 1982.

Foote A: Transient global amnesia, *J Neurosci Nurs* 21(1):14, 1989.

Garrett A, Jones G: Maybe the patient has pta . . . post traumatic amnesia, *Nurses J* 19(11):10, 1990.

Godwin-Austin R: Where am I? *Br Med J* 10:285, 1982.

Gudjansson G et al: Case report—hysterical amnesia as an alternative to suicide, *Med Sci Law* 22(1):68, 1982.

Hirst W: The amnesic syndrome: descriptions and explanations, *Psychol Bull* 91(3):435, 1982.

Jackson R, Mysiw W, Corrigan J: Orientation group monitoring system: an indicator for reversible impairments in cognition during posttraumatic amnesia, *Arch Phys Med Rehabil* 70(1):33, 1989.

Kiklstrom I: Spontaneous recovery of memory during post-hypnotic amnesia, *Int J Clin Exp Hypn* 31(4):309, 1983.

MacHovec F: Hypnosis to facilitate recall in psychogenic amnesia and fugue states: treatment variables, *Am J Clin Hypn* 24(1):7, 1981.

Mysiw W et al: Prospective assessment of posttraumatic amnesia: a comparison of the GOAT and the OGMS, *J Head Trauma Rehab* 5(1):65, 1990.

Parker V: Amnesia towards a cure? *Nurs* 2(24):695, 1984.

Scharter D: Amnesia observed: remembering and forgetting in a natural environment, *J Abnorm Psychol* 92:236, 1983.

Spanos N et al: Disorganized recall, hypnotic amnesia and subjective faking: more disconfirmatory evidence, *Psychol Rep* 50(2):383, 1984.

Warkham A, Barre T: Escaping from the past . . . hysterical amnesia, *Nurs Times* 84(46):52, 1988.

Anger

Anger is a feeling of extreme displeasure, annoyance, indignation, exasperation, or hostility. The feeling is both physical and emotional and may be directed toward self or others. When the attainment of a goal is frustrated and a person feels inadequate, anger is one of the emotions that surfaces. Aggression is related to anger. In aggression hateful ideas manifest themselves in destructive behavior. Aggression may take the form of verbal attacks (for example, manipulation or undermining) or violent acts resulting in personal injury or destruction of property. Other characteristics include hostility, threats, abuse of self or others, agitation, and rigid body language (clenched fists and tight jaws).

Anger can be described on a continuum from mild annoyance to rage. The feeling occurs in response to anxiety when a person feels threatened and may be expressed directly, indirectly, or through physical symptoms. Anger is both positive and negative. Positive aspects include its energizing effects, the sense of control over situations, and motivation for change. Negative aspects include inappropriate expression as in depression, physical illness, passive-aggressive behavior, or violence. Anger is frequently seen during adolescence, when it is expressed as profanity, hostile interactions, and destruction.

Effective handling of anger implies that people accept their right to be angry and the rights of others to be angry. Nurses need to be aware of their own methods of coping with anger to demonstrate an appropriate expression of anger to an angry client.

Related DSM-III-R disorders

Anxiety disorders
Schizophrenia
Delusional (paranoid) disorder
Somatoform disorders

Dissociative disorders
Personality disorders
Psychological factors affecting physical condition
Psychoactive substance use disorders
Sexual disorders

Other related conditions

Crisis situations
Rape, abuse, or assault
Phobias
Compulsions
Obesity
Tension headache
Migraine headache
Angina pectoris
Neurodermatitis
Gastric ulcer
Nausea and vomiting
Colitis
Enteritis
Rheumatoid arthritis
Asthma
Painful menstruation
Masturbation
Sexual dysfunction

PRINCIPLES

▶ Physical Dimension

1. The limbic system is the regulator of aggression.
2. A lesion in the hypothalamus and amygdala may increase or decrease aggressive behavior.
3. Neurophysiology has identified specific areas of the brain that are responsible for particular emotional responses, both aggressive and inhibitory.
4. The release of norepinephrine is directly related to aggressive behavior. Modification of aggressive behavior is accomplished by adjusting the rate of metabolism of dopamine, norepinephrine, and serotonin.

The original content for this section was contributed by Judith Seidenschnur, R.N., M.S.N.

5. Chemical and endocrine disorders such as hypoglycemia or allergies may produce aggressive behavior.
6. Increased blood levels of male sex hormones, particularly testosterone, correlate with an increase in aggressive action.
7. Premenstrual decrease in progesterone blood levels correlates with irritability and increased hostility in women.
8. Genetic factors may determine an individual's capacity for aggressive or violent behavior.

▶ **Emotional Dimension**

1. Aggression evolves from two instinctual drives: eros, the life drive expressed through sexuality, and thanatos, the death drive expressed through aggression (Freud).
2. Life is a struggle to maintain a balance between the two drives.
3. Aggression is seen as an innate trait not under willful control and as an expression of the death instinct.
4. The aggressive drive is extremely strong, and individuals are prone to destructive behavior.
5. Aggressive energy is diminished when directly expressed.
6. Self-destructive behavior occurs when the death drive predominates.
7. Anger is a response to anxiety.
8. Lack of self-esteem increases feelings of frustration and anger.

▶ **Intellectual Dimension**

1. A conflict may exist between verbal messages and behavior demonstrated; for example, violence is unacceptable, but spanking children is tolerated.
2. Violence-prone individuals view frustration as provocation and do not have the cognitive or verbal ability to respond differently. These individuals demonstrate inadequate problem-solving and social relationship skills, and violence is their only known alternative.
3. Anger is an emotional response to provocation and is determined by three response modalities: cognitive, somatic-affective, and behavioral.
   a. Cognitively, anger is a function of appraisals, attributions, self-statements, and images.
   b. Somatic-affective anger is exacerbated by tension and agitation; physiological tension potentiates the anger response.
   c. Behavioral responses include withdrawal, which contributes to anger by leaving the situation unchanged, and antagonism, which escalates the provocation sequence by providing cues from which the person infers anger.

▶ **Social Dimension**

1. People use anger to avoid feeling anxiety. Anger is an attempt to destroy the object or situation that produced the anxiety.
2. Threats to self-esteem produce anxiety.
3. Anger wards off anxiety. When anger does not drive the threat away, the individual becomes frustrated and rage results.
4. If anger is not expressed, three outcomes are probable: (1) conforming, (2) rebelling, (3) behaving malevolently.
5. The impulse to behave aggressively is subject to the influence of learning, socialization, and experience.
6. Aggression is learned behavior under voluntary control.
7. Learning takes place as a result of observation of a significant other's method of venting anger.
8. Learning aggressive behavior is accomplished through direct experience. An individual feels angry, behaves aggressively, and feels relief. The behavior brings reward and is strengthened.
9. Aggression or anger may contribute to child or spouse abuse.
10. Environmental factors determine an individual's capacity for violent and aggressive behavior.
11. The aggressor selects the situation in which the aggression occurs.
12. Aggressive acts may serve to maintain an individual's reputation, social status, and self-image.
13. Violence-prone individuals generally have interpersonal orientations in which they perceive, process, and respond to social situations in a way that produces violent interactions.
14. Aggression may result from an experience of frustration.
15. Thwarted goal achievement results in frustration.
16. The more valued the goal, the greater the frustration.
17. The greater the frustration, the greater the degree of aggression.
18. Aggressive behavior may be learned by imitation and may be related to the family, the subculture, or symbolic models.
19. Inability to satisfy needs with positive constructive behavior may result in need satisfaction through negative destructive behavior.

▶ **Spiritual Dimension**

1. Anger is a component of a person's total being.
2. Gratification of a person's spiritual needs provides the individual with meaningful identity, purpose, hope, and confidence without undue frustration and anger.

3. The experience of a trusting relationship with God or a higher power enables the individual to formulate a positive existence without undue anger.
4. Lack of meaning in a person's life frequently leads to a frustration-anger cycle.
5. Spirituality influences thoughts, determines which new ideas a person is willing to consider, and serves as a framework within which the individual integrates anger into his or her life.

ASSESSMENT

▶ Physical Dimension

I. History
  A. Activities of daily living
    1. Nutrition
      a. Loss of appetite
      b. Weight loss
    2. Sleep
      a. Inability to sleep (insomnia)
      b. Excessive sleep (withdrawal)
    3. No special recreation, hobbies, or interests
    4. Physical activities
      a. Excessive energy
      b. Lack of energy
    5. Sexual activity
      a. Hypersexual when agitated
      b. Impotent when enraged
  B. Habits
    1. Excessive alcohol intake
    2. Misuses both legal and illegal medications and drugs
  C. Destructive behavior
    1. Impulsive
    2. Homicidal
    3. Suicidal
  D. Health history
    1. Ineffective coping
  E. Family health history
    1. Substance abuse
    2. Depression
    3. Schizophrenia
  F. Physical abuse
    1. Abuse as a child
  G. Review of systems
    1. General
      a. Inability to sleep
      b. Generalized fatigue
      c. Weight loss
    2. Skin
      a. Excessive perspiration
    3. Ears
      a. Ringing
      b. Pounding
    4. Eyes
      a. Blurring of vision
    5. Cardiovascular
      a. Tachycardia
    6. Respiratory
      a. Shortness of breath
    7. Gastrointestinal
      a. Indigestion
      b. Nausea
      c. Vomiting
      d. Diarrhea
    8. Genitourinary
      a. Frequency
      b. Urgency
    9. Reproductive
      a. Impotent after explosive episodes
    10. Musculoskeletal
      a. Tenseness
      b. Rigidity
      c. Backaches
      d. Tense posture
    11. Neurological
      a. Nervousness
      b. Mood changes
      c. Headaches

▶ **Physical Examination**

CLIENT DATA	ANALYSIS	NURSING DIAGNOSIS
Tachycardia Blood pressure increase	Physiological response to anger from action of autonomic nervous system (secretion of epinephrine).	Anxiety: related to feelings of unresolved anger
Flushed or blanched face, piercing glares, tightened jaws, flared nostrils, protruding neck veins, clenched fists	Neurohumeral, neurovascular, and neuromuscular responses to stress.	Ineffective individual coping: related to anger

▶ **Emotional Dimension**

CLIENT DATA	ANALYSIS	NURSING DIAGNOSIS
Irritable, volatile rage, fury	Hypersensitive to disappointment. Inept social relationship skills because of low self-esteem and frustration tolerance.	Ineffective individual coping: related to excessive anger
Frustration or exasperation	Needs for attachment, concern, affection not met; blocked goals.	Ineffective individual coping: anger related to frustration or exasperation
Annoyed, aggravated, or belligerent	Inadequate problem-solving skills.	Ineffective individual coping: anger related to inadequate problem-solving skills
Feels inadequate, insecure, or intimidated	Needs for recognition and acceptance not fulfilled.	*Altered self-concept: feelings of inadequacy related to anger
Depression, hopelessness	Unable to express anger. Viable alternatives for coping with anger unknown.	*Anger: related to depression and hopelessness
Powerlessness	Unwilling to take responsibility for self; dependence. Frustration with feelings of powerlessness influences aggression.	Ineffective individual coping: anger related to reluctance to accept responsibility for self

▶ **Intellectual Dimension**

CLIENT DATA	ANALYSIS	NURSING DIAGNOSIS
Sarcastic, ridiculing, verbally abusive, argumentative	Projection of negative feelings regarding self onto others; dependency conflicts.	Ineffective individual coping: anger related to dissatisfaction with self
Blaming, rejecting, scolding, screaming, shouting	Acting out resentment toward others. Frustration over blocked goals. Attempts to produce guilt in others to get own needs met.	Impaired verbal communication: related to frustration-anger cycle
Demanding, arguing, belligerent, quarrelsome	Insecurity, dissatisfaction with self; protection from discovery of self by others.	High risk for violence: related to anger
Rumination	Preoccupation with anger. Inadequate problem-solving skills; unclear thoughts and feelings caused by frustration and anger when needs not fulfilled.	Altered thought processes: ruminations related to preoccupation with anger
Fixed, rigid beliefs	Preoccupied with anger-producing event or situation. Unable to see alternative actions.	Altered thought processes: fixed rigid beliefs related to anger
Fault finding	Feels cornered and not able to get what is desired.	Altered thought processes: fault finding related to anger
Overconfident, grandiose	Overcompensates for inadequate feelings.	Self-esteem disturbance: overconfident, grandiose related to anger

▶ **Social Dimension**

CLIENT DATA	ANALYSIS	NURSING DIAGNOSIS
Avoiding, withdrawing, isolating self from others	Negative self-concept; condemning others to avoid risk of closeness.	Social isolation: avoidance or withdrawal from others related to anger
Domineering, revengeful, vindictive	Fear of close relationships; projecting previous hurt; lack of trust.	Impaired social interactions: domineering, revengeful, vindictive related to anger
Teasing, harassing, threatening, intimidating	Fear of rejection; air of superiority to avoid intimate relationship; inadequate problem-solving skills.	Impaired social interactions: teasing, harassing, threatening, intimidating related to anger
Agitated	Agitation related to anxiety and anger buildup.	High risk for violence: related to agitation
Overly compliant (passive-aggressive)	Excessive compliance, politeness, and sweetness in attempt to produce guilt or manipulate others.	Ineffective individual coping: overly compliant related to inability to achieve satisfying social relationships

▶ **Spiritual Dimension**

CLIENT DATA	ANALYSIS	NURSING DIAGNOSIS
Demoralized, cheated, hurt	Inability to experience love and appreciation and to value self.	Spiritual distress: lack of self-love related to anger
Self-doubt	Insecurity, inability to accept self.	Spiritual distress: self-doubt related to anger, frustration
Bitterness	Generalized frustration, hostility, and resentment toward society.	Spiritual distress: bitterness over inequities in life related to anger
Dissatisfied	Inability to be where one wants to be in life.	Spiritual distress: anger related to inability to succeed and accomplish life goals
Disillusioned	Void of a sense of purpose or direction in life.	*Altered meaningfulness: anger related to lack of personal meaning and hope

PLANNING

Long-Term Goals

To express anger in ways that are not injurious to self or others
To develop ability to deal with tension without becoming combative

SHORT-TERM GOALS	OUTCOME CRITERIA
Physical Dimension	
To prevent injury to self, others, and property	1. Does not inflict injury on self and others 2. Acknowledges and accepts feelings of anger 3. Increases insight into causes and ramifications of aggressive behavior 4. Develops impulse control and does not physically act out feelings of aggression 5. Avoids or manages threatening situations
To decrease agitation and restlessness	1. Increases involvement in therapeutic milieu 2. Feels safe and secure in environment and decreases fears, anxiety, and agitation 3. Requests help when unable to control agitation and restlessness 4. Uses the energy of anger in physical activity

SHORT-TERM GOALS	OUTCOME CRITERIA
Emotional Dimension To develop socially acceptable ways of expressing feelings of anxiety, anger, fear	1. Expresses feelings of self-worth and self-esteem 2. Describes angry feelings verbally 3. Directs hostility, anger into socially acceptable channels 4. Uses outlets for verbal and nonverbal expression of aggression 5. Decreases manipulation of authority figures 6. Develops adequate skills to deal with life, adapt to change, cope during crisis 7. Identifies escalating anger and seeks time-out 8. Accepts need for medication (if appropriate) 9. Increases physical and competitive activities
Intellectual Dimension To decrease verbal abuse	1. Decreases outburts of hostility and aggression 2. Decreases sarcasm, teasing, intimidation 3. Recognizes feelings of stress, anger, and anxiety 4. Develops effective coping strategies 5. Decreases suspicion and establishes a trust relationship
Social Dimension To tell others when angry	1. Identifies when angry 2. States angry feelings to others 3. Knows the difference between angry feelings and actions 4. Talks about anger without threatening, belittling, intimidating, blaming, arguing 5. Uses "I" statements when expressing anger
Spiritual Dimension To decrease bitterness, disappointments about life situation	1. Expresses feelings of bitterness, disappointment 2. Forms a relationship with a caring person 3. Establishes support systems 4. Initiates activities and interactions that result in success and pleasure 5. Moves from pessimism to optimism 6. Is confident that life situation can improve as responsibility is taken for improving it

Discharge Planning

The following client behaviors demonstrate readiness for discharge:
1. Identifies angry feelings in self
2. Verbalizes angry feelings appropriately to others
3. Uses methods to reduce anger
4. Seeks help when beginning to feel out of control

IMPLEMENTATION

NURSING ACTIONS	RATIONALE
Physical Dimension 1. Observe for indicators of agitation, for example, increased motor activity, verbal aggression.	To indicate anger may be escalating and intervene.
2. Decrease environmental stimulation such as noise, activity.	To prevent overstimulation that may contribute to client's anger.
3. Remove to a quiet environment.	To promote calming effect.
4. Be aware of client's personal space and be careful not to invade.	To support client's need for space, to convey respect, and to prevent client from feeling overpowered or dominated by persons in authority.

IMPLEMENTATION—cont'd

NURSING ACTIONS	RATIONALE
5. Plan a physical exercise program, for example, swimming, walking, running, punching bag, volleyball, as an alternative to cope with aggressive feelings and increased level of energy.	To reduce the energy that accompanies anger.
6. Remain with client at all times if restrained unless staff presence increases agitation level of client.	To provide protection and control until client can maintain self-control.
7. Medicate as presented.	To lessen danger or destructiveness to client, others, or property.
8. Clear immediate environment of potential items that can be used as weapons or can obstruct in transporting client to the seclusion room. Provide clear instructions for staff members. Enlist assistance of additional staff as necessary. Remove any visitors or clients from the environment; do not request their assistance.	To protect client and others from injury.
9. If decision is made to physically restrain client, respond as a team, coordinating actions in a rapid, smooth, and consistent fashion with one person as designated leader.	To remove client quickly with a minimum of confusion among staff members.
10. Observe client's eyes when he is agitated; he will look at body part that will be attacked.	To prepare self or others for an impending attack and plan for distracting client or removal to a safe area.

Emotional Dimension

1. Communicate warmth, empathy, respect, and genuineness to encourage verbalization of angry feelings.	To help client feel safe expressing anger.
2. Give client encouragement for choosing acceptable methods of managing angry, hostile, or aggressive feelings, for example, verbalizing angry feelings versus physically acting out angry feelings.	To reinforce positive behaviors.
3. Inform client of responsibility for controlling own behavior, recognizing feelings, and choosing the method of dealing with them.	To create in the client a sense of responsibility for own angry feelings and help client learn that choices exist in ways to respond.
4. Encourage client to practice verbalizing angry feelings in a safe situation such as group therapy.	To gain skill and confidence in handling anger with help from a skilled therapist and a supportive group.
5. Help client identify consequences of anger.	To develop awareness of effects of anger on self and others.
6. Help client reduce anxiety (see Anxiety, p. 48).	To prevent anger resulting from anxiety.
7. Provide outlets for expression of feelings, such as punching bags, sports, and music.	To provide acceptable outlets for expressing anger when client is unable to express it verbally.
8. Provide feedback on nonverbal behavior to help client identify anger.	To assist client to recognize own behavior when angry.
9. Refrain from conveying fear of client by demonstrating confidence and self-assurance.	To prevent client from losing control. If the nurse appears fearful, the client lacks the security of knowing nurse will set limits on client's behavior when client cannot do this for self.

Intellectual Dimension

1. Encourage positive self-statements.	To increase client's self-worth. Often angry clients have a low opinion of themselves.
2. Help client identify alternative coping strategies for anger and tension, such as expressing feelings and releasing physical energy.	To increase client's repertoire of coping skills.
3. Encourage client to request the assistance of staff when sensing a buildup of anger.	To prevent anger from escalating and help client to learn to talk about anger rather than acting on it.
4. Ask client to discuss feelings when anger has subsided.	To give client time for emotional reaction to lessen and think more rationally.
5. Communicate that you accept the client as a person but that certain behaviors are unacceptable.	To give recognition to client. To increase client's feelings of worth while letting client know his or her behavior is not acceptable.

NURSING ACTIONS	RATIONALE
6. Give information in a low, calm voice; address client's affect and communicate that you are here to help.	To help client hear clearly what is said with as few words as possible. Client's anger may be reduced with a calm voice and deliberate words.
7. Inform client that you will help him or her control behavior. Provide seclusion and physical restraints if client is unable to control behavior.	To promote feelings of security and safety. Angry clients fear losing control and knowing that the nurse will not let that happen is reassuring.
8. Assist client in identifying sources of anger or frustration.	To help client learn to handle the situation causing anger, avoid it, or accept it.
9. Confront client with behavior after a relationship is established.	To maintain a therapeutic relationship. Confrontation early in the relationship may interfere with establishing a trusting relationship.
10. Set limits on inappropriate angry behavior by communicating expectations.	To prevent injury to self others, or property. To communicate in a positive way that behavior is not acceptable. To clarify expectations of client.
11. Help client discuss conflicts objectively.	To clarify conflicts. Talking about the anger generated from conflicts lessens the intensity of the emotion.
12. Develop goals with client for appropriate expression of anger.	To increase client's self-concept by requesting client's participation in decisions about own care.
13. Explore client's past experiences with anger and any rewards anger achieves for client.	To determine if client is receiving secondary gains from angry behavior.
14. Avoid accusatory approach.	To prevent client from feeling threatened.
15. Avoid increasing guilt by use of matter-of-fact statements.	To prevent further burdening with guilt. It is likely that client has guilt feelings about angry behavior and any additional guilt may overburden client.
16. Take threats of physical aggression seriously.	To prevent injury to self, others, or property and to let client know he or she has been heard.
17. Teach relaxation for underlying anxiety manifested in aggressive behavior.	To reduce intensity of the emotion and promote a relaxed body and mind.
18. Teach stress inoculation to help client substitute positive coping statements for statements that bring about anxiety.	To increase self-esteem with the use of positive self-statements.
19. Discuss situations in which expressing anger is appropriate or inappropriate.	To increase client's awareness of appropriate and inappropriate expressions of anger so that appropriate expressions can be reinforced.
20. Discuss relationship between anger and anxiety.	To give information that may help client to understand own behavior.
21. Discuss with client thoughts that occur in conjunction with feelings of anger.	To help client link thoughts to behavior and to consider alternatives for behaving.
22. Discuss options for expressing anger.	To let client know he or she has choices concerning responses to anger.
23. Refrain from responding to client's threatening behavior in an angry manner.	To model a rational response to another's anger and to avoid a power struggle.
24. Be aware that own anxiety may stimulate an angry response.	To increase insight about the relationship of anger to anxiety and promote a therapeutic response to client.
25. Assist client in rehearsing situations that result in anger and in using effective methods to cope with anger.	To build confidence in client's methods of expressing anger and to experiment with different approaches to determine which ones work best for client.
26. Teach client self-reinforcement for getting through an anger-producing situation.	To help client boost self-esteem with appropriate behavior, to become more autonomous, and to lessen need to rely on others for reinforcement.

Social Dimension

1. Use role playing to facilitate expression of feelings of anger.	To practice expressing anger in a safe setting.
2. Involve client in planning goals for treatment.	To increase esteem by requesting client's participation in making decisions about own care.
3. Expect client to take responsibility for self; clearly define expectations.	To increase autonomy, self-responsibility.

IMPLEMENTATION—cont'd

SHORT-TERM GOALS	OUTCOME CRITERIA
4. Withdraw attention if client is verbally abusive.	To avoid attention-seeking behaviors, providing there is no imminent danger to client or others.
5. Set and enforce limits of what is acceptable behavior.	To prevent inappropriate expressions of anger. All staff needs to be aware of limits and expectations and enforce them consistently.
6. Interact early with a physically aggressive client.	To prevent anger from escalating and the need for more severe interventions such as medications or isolation.
7. Discuss effects of anger and aggression on others.	To help client see consequences of own behavior on others and the trouble it creates for self.
8. Develop behavior and modification approaches for selected angry behaviors.	To use external controls until client is able to develop self-controls.
9. Reward acceptable behavior.	To reinforce appropriate behavior helps client continue to use appropriate behavior.
10. Involve family in therapy.	To help family understand client's angry behavior and reinforce client's new learnings.
11. Provide group therapy.	To offer a safe setting for client to learn new ways to cope with anger, his or her own and others'.

Spiritual Dimension

1. Communicate acceptance of client through caring actions.	To give recognition to client as a unique individual with a problem with anger.
2. Help client identify personal beliefs or values that produce angry feelings.	To separate beliefs about anger that are rational or irrational, for example, it is wrong to get angry (irrational belief).
3. Assist client in clarifying meaning and purpose underlying anger.	To help client understand reasons or causes of own anger and gain insight about anger.
4. Assist client in developing confidence that anger can be controlled by increasing self-esteem.	To promote internal security in client so that in time and with help client can learn to control anger.
5. Recognize the positive worth and value of client.	To help client value self and emphasize positive attributes.
6. Reinforce client's previous accomplishments and potential for achievement.	To help client focus on positive experiences in life while working on limitation—anger.

EVALUATION

Measurable goals and outcome criteria provide the basis for evaluating a client's inappropriate expression of anger. The client's self-reports, nurse observations, and family reports supply additional information about the client's progress. The following behaviors indicate a positive evaluation:

1. Identifies angry feelings in self
2. Verbalizes angry feelings appropriately
3. Uses appropriate methods to reduce anger
4. Seeks help when beginning to feel out of control
5. Demonstrates congruency between the feeling of anger and behavior

BIBLIOGRAPHY

Bandura A: *Aggression: a social learning analysis,* Englewood Cliffs, NJ, 1973, Prentice-Hall, Inc.

Biaggio M: Clinical dimensions of anger management, *Am J Psychother* 41:417, 1987.

Clunn P: Nurses' assessment of violence potential. In Babich K, editor: *Assessing patient violence in the health care setting,* Boulder, Colo., 1981, Western Interstate Commission for Higher Education.

Comstock G, Strasburger V: Deceptive appearances: television violence and aggressive behavior, *J Adolesc Health Care* 11:31, 1990.

Dollard J, Miller N: *Frustration and aggression,* New Haven, Conn., 1939, Yale University Press.

Eichelman B: Neurochemical basis of aggressive behavior, *Psychiatr Ann* 17(6):371, 1987.

Grainger R: Anger within ourselves. *Am J Nurs* 90(7):12, 1990.

Kalogjera I: Impact of therapeutic management on use of seclusion and restraint with disruptive adolescent patients, *Hosp Community Psychiatry* 40(3):280, 1989.

Lanza M: Origins of aggression, *J Psychosoc Nurs Ment Health Serv* 21(6):11, 1983.

Maynard C, Chitty K: Dealing with anger: guidelines for nursing interventions, *J Psychiatr Nurs* 17:37, 1979.

Meddaugh D: Reactance: understanding aggressive behavior in long term care, *J Psychosoc Nurs Ment Health Serv* 28(4):28, 1990.

Turnbull J et al: Turn it around: short-term management for aggression and management, *J Psychosoc Nurs Ment Health Serv* 28(6):7, 1990.

Williams R: The trusting heart: type a's, take note: ambition won't kill you; it's hostility that can be fatal. *New Age J* 6(May—June):26, 1989.

Anorexia and Bulimia Nervosa

Anorexia nervosa is an eating disorder characterized by self-imposed restrictions of food intake. It usually begins with the adolescent's desire to lose weight and occurs predominantly in females 12 to 18 years of age because more females than males diet during adolescence. The condition results in a failure to maintain normal body weight, sometimes to the point of self-starvation and death. Although the person restricts food intake, she is intensely interested in and obsessed with food. To control the appetite, the person engages in elaborate rituals with occasional binging (bulimia nervosa) followed by vomiting. Some persons with anorexia nervosa have bulimia nervosa, but most persons with bulimia are not anorexic. Those with anorexia nervosa deny their problem and typically do not volunteer for treatment. It is the weight loss that usually causes the client to be hospitalized, and most are hospitalized more than once. Anorexia nervosa may be the result of delayed or fixated psychosexual development; no known physical disease causes this life-threatening disorder. The illness may be an attempt to control the person's life or body and a way to achieve a sense of identity. Restoring nutritional intake, enhancing the person's self-concept, and improving family relations offer challenges for nursing care.

Related DSM-III-R disorders

Depressive disorders
Anxiety disorders
Bulimia nervosa
Obsessive-compulsive personality disorder
Sexual disorders
Dependent personality disorder
Parent-child problem
Psychoactive substance—use disorders

The original content for this section was contributed by Paul Deyoub, PhD.

PRINCIPLES

▶ Physical Dimension

1. Adolescent girls with changing bodies are threatened with a status change at home, at school, and with boys and other girls. Suddenly they are concerned solely with their appearance and less invested in achievement and competence. Avoidance of foods is a way to establish control and hold on to power that would be lost with sexual development. In the effort to gain power, the client is self-defeating as she becomes physically weak and dependent on others.

2. The anorectic client tries to hide her female body in a self-defeating attempt to deal with sex, power, mothering, and assertion.

3. Both obese, compulsive eaters and anorectic clients seek to escape the status of sex object. The obese person gains power through largeness, whereas the anorectic person tries to disappear.

4. Treatment focuses on consciousness raising, preferably in groups of women who are anorexics and compulsive eaters.

5. Inadequate nutritional intake with less than minimum daily requirements impairs physiological functioning.

6. Anorexia and bulimia nervosa occur almost exclusively in girls and young women (90% to 95%).

7. Male obligatory running and the eating disorders in females are parallel conditions.

8. Anorexia nervosa is closely related to compulsive eating, bulimia, and obesity. The anorexic is as obsessed as the compulsive eater and the obese person.

9. Biochemical or hormonal imbalances may perpetuate anorexia/bulimia once it has begun.

10. Estimates of mortality range between 1% and 15%; cases of mortality are equally divided between suicide and medical complications.

▶ **Emotional Dimension**

1. Anorexia nervosa symbolically expresses an internalized sexual conflict.
2. Anorexia and bulimia nervosa represent regression to the infantile stage of development.
3. Anorexia nervosa is an effort to repress drives. Oral satisfaction is unconsciously connected to hostile and aggressive impulses.
4. The ego is impaired and fails to differentiate between biological experiences and emotional interpersonal experiences.

▶ **Intellectual Dimension**

1. Anorexia nervosa is ambivalence and rebellion against femininity. There is both a denial of femininity and an exaggeration of it by becoming petite.
2. The anorectic client is perfectionistic. She believes that if she is not perfect, others will not love her or approve of her.
3. If the anorectic client loses weight, she thinks this will make her more attractive and liked by others. She irrationally thinks her weight is how other people judge her.
4. The anorectic or bulimic client has a cognitive disturbance and cannot correctly evaluate body size and what constitutes a normal amount of food.

▶ **Social Dimension**

1. Anorexia nervosa is learned behavior that has been rewarding for the client.
2. It is an eating phobia in which failing to eat helps avoid anxiety that has been associated with eating.
3. Behavioral control works well in the hospital where contingencies can be controlled. However, on discharge the uncontrollable environment often leads to further self-starvation if the learning has not been generalized.
4. Family organization is often related to development and maintenance of anorexia nervosa during adolescence.
5. The illness plays an important role in maintaining the family system, and all members of the family are involved in the illness.
6. In the anorexic's family the client gains power through starvation, remains the child that mother and father want, and achieves other neurotic goals for the sake of family members.
7. When family dynamics change for better or worse, then the symptoms of the anorectic client change for better or worse.
8. The anorectic client's family is enmeshed, overprotective, rigid, and incapable of conflict resolution.
9. The thinness of the client reflects society's worship of the thin, frail woman. Anorexia nervosa is dieting out of control in response to notions about femininity that the client and society share.
10. Families of anorectic and bulimic clients tend to emphasize achievement.

Spiritual Dimension

1. The anorexic's general philosophy of life reflects little meaning and purpose.
2. The self is seen as being without worth or value.
3. The client despairs over the futility of the illness.
4. The client alienates and isolates herself from significant relationships.
5. The client allows self few pleasures from life.
6. The client believes death may be a solution to problems.

ASSESSMENT

▶ **Physical Dimension**

I. History
  A. Activities of daily living
    1. Nutrition
      a. Appetite
        (1) Intense interest in food
        (2) Sustained appetite
        (3) Drastic reduction in food intake
      b. Weight
        (1) Loss of 20% to 40% of original body weight
    2. Sleep
      a. Ranges from normal to severe insomnia
    3. Physical activities
      a. Excessive and nonstop
    4. Sexual activity
      a. Little or none
  B. Destructive behavior
    1. Self-starvation
    2. Use of large amounts of laxatives
    3. Use of frequent enemas
    4. Self-induced vomiting
  C. Body image
    1. Sees self as overweight or normal when, in fact, emaciated
  D. Review of systems
    1. Gastrointestinal
      a. Vomiting following binges
      b. Constipation
      c. Uses laxatives, enemas excessively

2. Reproductive
  a. Amenorrhea
II. Diagnostic tests
  A. Hemoglobin
  B. Serum albumin
  C. Serum transferrin or iron-building capacity
  D. Lymphocytes
  E. Thyroid function
  F. Electrolytes
  G. Urinalysis and renal function
  H. ECG
  I. Luteinizing hormone secretion test

▶ Physical Examination

CLIENT DATA	ANALYSIS	NURSING DIAGNOSIS
Emaciated appearance	Results from self-starvation and excessive exercise.	Altered in nutrition: less than body requirements related to fear of obesity and excessive exercise
Deterioration in physical condition	Inadequate nutritional intake with less than minimum daily requirements impairs physiological functioning.	Altered in nutrition: less than body requirements related to inadequate nutritional intake as evidenced by
Brittle nails		Brittle nails
Lanugo (neonatal-like hair)		Lanugo
Bluish color to hands and feet		Bluish color to feet and hands
Dental lesions		Dental lesions
Lack of fatty layers		Lack of fatty layers
Atrophied skeletal muscles		Atrophied skeletal muscles
Edematous feet and calves		Edematous feet and calves
Changes in electrolyte balance		Changes in electrolyte balance
Drop in basal metabolic rate		Drop in basal metabolic rate
Reduced elimination of estrogen		Reduced elimination of estrogen
Hypotension		Hypotension
Bradycardia		Bradycardia
Electrolyte imbalance		Fatigue related to electrolyte imbalance
Edematous feet and calves		High risk for fluid volume deficit: related to inadequate fluid intake, food intake, or both
Dry skin		Impaired skin integrity: related to edema
Poor skin turgor		High risk for impaired skin integrity: related to dehydration

▶ Emotional Dimension

CLIENT DATA	ANALYSIS	NURSING DIAGNOSIS
Cold, indifferent, angry, depressed, anxious	Rigid defense against loss of control results in hostile overcontrolled affect.	Fear of losing control: related to eating disorder
Unconcerned about weight loss	Reports everything under control, which is not congruent with client's affect or appearance. Has virtually no insight and is unable to appreciate the seriousness of the disorder.	Altered thought processes: related to malnutrition
Reports feeling good	Obvious that client is not well. Anger is expressed when not justified. Out of touch with own feelings and moods.	*Unpredictable behaviors: related to being out of touch with own emotions
Fears sexual maturity	Emotional development has not kept up with physical development.	Impaired adjustment: related to sexual role development
Feels helpless, incompetent	New social and emotional requirements are overwhelming.	Impaired adjustment: related to adult role development

▶ **Intellectual Dimension**

CLIENT DATA	DATA ANALYSIS	NURSING DIAGNOSIS
Distorted perception of body	Thinks she is unattractive when she may not be, that she is overweight when emaciated, or that she will become overweight when she will not. Thinks she looks good when she is a walking skeleton.	Altered thought processes: inaccurate perception of self related to body image distortion
Does not admit seriousness of the problem	Denies life-threatening nature of the disorder. Rationalizes that she eats normally. Others perceive disorder to be matter of life and death. Excuse is she does not like most foods, especially high-calorie foods, feels too bloated to eat, likes salads and tuna, rather than realizing she will not eat anything that will make her gain weight.	Ineffective denial: related to psychological conflicts, malnutrition, or both
Phobia of food	Fear of losing control means she closely supervises all she eats and never eats what she has an impulse to eat. Will go to any length to avoid foods not on her list of approved foods. At the same time, she is obsessed with food and devotes much time to planning and eating. Prefers to eat alone and dreads eating in public.	Self-care deficit, feeding: fear of losing control of food intake related to morbid fear of obesity
Delusional thinking about body size, threat of becoming overweight, importance of thinness, and need to be loved	Irrational perception; cannot evaluate size of body, attempts perfection to gain love.	Body image disturbance: related to delusions regarding body size
Believes she is judged by her weight	Thinks weight loss will make her more attractive.	Altered thought processes: related to belief that she is judged by weight
Selective memory	Is on the defensive and avoids unpleasant thoughts. Poor historian of family background.	Altered thought processes: related to selective memory
Self-centered, immature, concrete in thinking	Does not worry about the effects on family members. Anorexia nervosa affects all aspects of cognition, including judgment and insight. Thinks she is an expert on food and nutrition and uses selective information to justify behavior. Has narrow range of interests. Has impaired judgment particularly when it comes to food. Cannot see how her disease includes family dynamics and how food is a weapon of self-control.	Altered thought processes: impaired judgment and insight
Refuses to talk about food, is sarcastic, irritable, and critical	Becomes defensive and stubborn. Main symptom, refusal to eat, is not a topic for discussion.	Impaired verbal communication: related to refusal to talk about food
Uses defense mechanisms (repression, regression)	To allay anxiety, retreats to a more infantile state; resists mature forms of anxiety.	Ineffective individual coping: use of defense mechanisms (repression or regression) related to eating disorder
Ambivalence	Both denies and exaggerates femininity by becoming excessively thin.	Anxiety: related to ambivalence about sexual role

▶ **Social Dimension**

CLIENT DATA	DATA ANALYSIS	NURSING DIAGNOSIS
Discrepancy between ideal and real self	Disturbed self-concept bears little resemblance to the actual self. Strives to be perfect and suffers because she cannot obtain perfection. Ideal self is someone who is perfect, always in control, beautiful, and very thin. She has lots of friends, a boyfriend who adores her, and a life where everything is under control. Actual self is someone who is not perfect as is and who is actually out of control physically, emotionally, intellectually, and socially.	Self-esteem disturbance: related to inaccurate perception of self
Strained family relations	Psychopathological functions of entire family are required to produce an anorectic client. Parents have neurotic conflicts. Mother is usually the dominant figure in family and the person most likely to be in conflict with client.	Ineffective family coping: related to dysfunctional family patterns
Rejects input of family members	Tendency to reject input from family members. With therapist she becomes sullen.	Ineffective individual coping: related to rejection of family input
Superficial communication	Likes to move from one subject to another as long as no one penetrates her defenses.	Impaired verbal communication: related to lack of meaningful communications as a defensive maneuver
Domineering, aggressive, critical mother, passive father	Anorectic client may be victim of intense mother-daughter conflict. Mother transmits her own conflicts to the daughter. Mother prevents daughter from having her own opinions and attitudes. Emotional development is impaired, and anorectic client feels self-conscious about herself emotionally, socially, and intellectually. Mother often has conflict about food and ambivalence regarding the nourishing of her daughter.	Altered parenting: related to mother-daughter conflict
Dependent on mother for opinions	Client alternates between extreme dependence and independence. Conflict over own boundaries and sphere of influence. Anorectic client is involved in intense conflict over dependence, independence, and interdependence.	Ineffective individual coping: related to conflict over dependence and independence
Seeks constant approval from others and cannot tolerate criticism	Low self-esteem. Poor insight and judgment. Self-critical and preoccupied with self.	Self-esteem disturbance: related to self-criticism
Disturbed emotions exist as long as family continues to reinforce client's behavior	Whole family is disturbed, even though they insist they are normal.	Ineffective family coping: related to dysfunctional patterns of behavior
Gains power through starvation	Client's behavior distracts from family issues as a way to avoid problems by focusing on client.	Ineffective family coping: related to family members acting as enablers

▶ **Spiritual Dimension**

CLIENT DATA	DATA ANALYSIS	NURSING DIAGNOSIS
Lacks meaning and purpose to life	Poor physiological condition limits individual's motivation for emotional growth with a sense of purpose to life.	Spiritual distress: related to poor physiological condition
Feels decreased self-worth and value	Self-concept is poor; client is struggling to achieve own identity.	Spiritual distress: related to decreased self-worth and value
Unable to accept self with strengths and weaknesses	Lacks a healthy self-love. Sees mostly weaknesses in self.	Spiritual distress: related to inability to accept self
Believes extreme thinness is normal and healthy	Beliefs about health and illness are erroneous and based on distorted perceptions.	Spiritual distress: related to irrational beliefs about health and illness
Has few pleasures in life	Isolates and alienates self from significant relationships and lacks ability to receive pleasure from activities.	Spiritual distress: related to denial of pleasure in life
Values thinness	Assumes values of society, which places much emphasis on thinness.	Ineffective individual coping: related to overidentification with social values of thinness

PLANNING

Long-Term Goals

To eat normally, gain weight, and mature in all areas of self
To maintain at least 90% of expected body weight

SHORT-TERM GOALS	OUTCOME CRITERIA
Physical Dimension	
To experiment with new foods and increase amounts of food eaten	1. Understands that past food preferences ("I like salads") have been defensive and self-serving to maintain anorexia 2. If bulimic, begins eating with others instead of alone and secretly 3. Tries small amounts of new foods; discovers there is nothing to fear in food 4. Keeps a diary of when hunger is felt, writes time and what would satisfy that hunger, then acts on the feeling 5. Learns there is no "good" or "bad" food, only food that satisfies hunger; different foods satisfy hunger at different times 6. Sets a reasonable ideal weight and when the ideal weight is reached, decides how to stay within the desired range
To decrease malnutrition	1. Increases caloric intake 2. Stays within agreed planned caloric intake 3. Gains weight consistently 4. Exercises in moderation
To correct electrolyte and fluid imbalances	1. Normal lab reports 2. Normal vital signs 3. Adequate intake and output 4. Moist mucous membranes 5. Energetic
To maintain skin integrity	1. Increased skin turgor 2. Maintains skin integrity

PLANNING—cont'd

SHORT-TERM GOALS	OUTCOME CRITERIA
Emotional Dimension To develop and mature emotionally	1. Verbalizes fears of sexual development and of responsibilities of adulthood 2. Becomes confident that others will not and cannot dominate her emotionally or sexually 3. Verbalizes the fear that physical development will result in separation from parents 4. Demonstrates emotional intimacy with one other person 5. Examines religious beliefs to determine if they are being used to hide behind, justifying sexual inactivity 6. Sees that sexual behavior is under self-control 7. Recognizes difference between sexuality and being a sex object
Intellectual Dimension To admit that a problem exists over which she has control	1. Admits she is underweight 2. Admits everything is not perfect at home with the family 3. Admits she has a fear of weight gain 4. Admits her choice of foods is not a preference, but a compulsion
Social Dimension To change perfectionist behavior and attitudes	1. Becomes more emotionally mature so that thinness is not the most important part of life 2. Decides that everyone cannot like or love her all of the time 3. Expects less from other people, since they also cannot be perfect 4. Learns that others cannot read her mind and that communication is necessary 5. Decides that eating cannot be a perfect experience every time she sits down for a meal
To examine family relations so contributions to the disorder can be discovered	1. Explores relationship with mother, father, and siblings; discusses problems she has with each person 2. Understands that social values regarding food were learned 3. Explores how family dynamics influence client's use of food 4. Learns how anorexia nervosa is an expression of dysfunctional family patterns 5. Gains legitimate power in family so that power through starvation can be abandoned
Spiritual Dimension To find meaning in own existence in spite of eating difficulties	1. Examines own life, stating reasons for existing 2. Verbalizes no suicide ideas 3. Expresses confidence or hope that life has been more pleasant in the past and can be again with time and help 4. Moves from working all the time, obsessively concerned with details, to a more balanced life where fun and leisure are important
To accept self as a person of value	1. Makes statements indicating acceptance of self 2. Makes statements indicating a valuing of self

Discharge Planning

The following client behaviors demonstrate readiness for discharge:
1. Eats adequate amounts of nutritious food to sustain health
2. Continues therapy on outpatient basis
3. Has stopped vomiting, if this was a problem
4. Is more independent from parents
5. Has a realistic self-image

IMPLEMENTATION

NURSING ACTIONS	RATIONALE
Physical Dimension	
1. Have the bulimic client eat with others in the dining room. Tray is filled with amount of food prescribed by hospital nutritionist. Client is not allowed to be alone for at least 30–45 minutes after each meal. If there is evidence of vomiting, then client cannot be alone anytime except when sleeping.	To promote social interactions at mealtimes, to provide nutritional restitution necessary for life, and to prevent her from being alone and possibly inducing vomiting.
2. Allow a choice of foods.	To help client gain a sense of control in her life.
3. Have client in clothes one size larger than current size.	To provide motivation to gain weight and be attractive.
4. Promote discussion of sexuality.	To help client understand her maturing body, accept the changes, and appreciate her sexuality.
5. Agree upon a contract for a weight goal and renegotiate as needed.	A mutually agreed-upon contract will reduce resistance to treatment and promote client's control and responsibility.
6. Monitor for signs and symptoms of infection if on hyperalimentation.	To prevent infection since susceptibility to infection is greater if malnourished.
7. Administer hyperalimentation or tube feedings.	Malnutrition may be life threatening if caloric intake is insufficient to sustain metabolic needs.
8. Provide tube feedings in nonpunitive manner.	A nonjudgmental attitude encourages cooperative behavior.
9. Stay with client following tube feeding for 30–45 minutes.	To prevent vomiting or siphoning feeding in an effort to prevent weight gain.
10. Present and remove food without comment. Do not coax or use bribes to get client to eat.	To avoid power struggles in the area in which she has exercised control.
11. Provide liquids and foods with fiber.	To avoid the use of laxatives. Client may have used them for weight control.
12. Observe and record physical activity.	To insure that the client is not secretly exercising in the bathroom.
13. Develop an individualized exercise program.	To help client limit excessive exercising.
14. Observe intake and output.	To insure that client is receiving adequate amounts of fluid.
15. Weigh every other day before breakfast in the same clothing and after voiding. Do not approve or disapprove of weight gain or loss.	To assure consistency since client may attempt to increase weight by wearing heavier clothing or by retaining urine. To maintain a nonjudgmental attitude. Approval or disapproval of the client is not food related.
16. Monitor lab reports.	To assure electrolyte balance and renal function.
17. Provide skin care.	To prevent skin breakdown resulting from poor nutrition.
Emotional Dimension	
1. Assist client in expressing feelings about herself and sexuality.	To help her become aware of feelings about herself and her sexuality and be comfortable expressing them to trusted persons.
2. Involve client in individual therapy.	To help her understand herself, her illness, to receive feedback about her behavior from a supportive person.

IMPLEMENTATION—cont'd

NURSING ACTIONS	RATIONALE
3. Help client understand relationship between self-starvation and a desperate attempt to control own life.	To promote awareness of factors contributing to the eating problem and help client consider areas in her life that she can control in a healthy manner.
4. Confront client with her self-destructive behavior and point out how she is driving others away, how she avoids intimacy.	To help her see the effects of her behavior on herself and on others.
5. Discuss fears associated with physical development of body.	To decrease anxiety associated with physical growth and provide information.
Intellectual Dimension	
1. Have client look in a full-size mirror with little or no clothing. Ask her to describe what she sees and how she would like to be.	To assist client to realistically appraise her body.
2. Discuss irrational and unrealistic perceptions of her body.	To cast some doubt on the way she perceives her body.
3. Discuss expectations of herself functioning in an adult role.	To promote positive expectations of adult functioning.
4. Discuss irrational beliefs of needing to be perfect.	To find out possible sources of irrational beliefs, to give permission to be less than perfect and still be a worthwhile person.
5. Discuss vocational and career plans.	To encourage realistic, attainable career goals.
6. Assist client in developing realistic beliefs about food, weight, and beauty.	To break the cycle of anorexia nervosa, to lessen preoccupation with food and weight, and to promote a more healthy, productive life-style.
7. Provide assertiveness training.	To help the client learn to ask for what she wants directly, thus gaining control in her life.
8. Involve client in sex education.	To provide client with accurate information about sexuality, sexual behavior, and sexual issues.
Social Dimension	
1. Enhance client's self-concept.	To increase self-esteem and help her see self as a person with abilities and value.
2. Provide family therapy to teach family new ways of relating, changing dominance of mother and rebellion of daughter.	To promote comfort and intimacy in relationships.
3. Teach client to see herself as worthwhile in context of heterosexual relationships.	To encourage independence and separation from parental conflicts.
4. If she is over 18, encourage client to move out of family home if appropriate.	To prevent family from continuing efforts to control client and to limit discussion of food.
5. Encourage family to visit client in hospital on a limited basis and to avoid discussions of food. Food should not be an issue in the family since client needs to become solely responsible for food management.	To increase interactions with others, gain insight into her behavior, and receive support from members of the group.
6. Discuss irrational aspects of societal value of thinness.	To encourage client to think independently.
Spiritual Dimension	
1. Help client learn to see self as worthwhile and of value.	To decrease self-destructive behavior and increase feelings of importance.
2. Help client to like self as she is.	To help client treat herself kindly and lovingly, be less critical of herself, and accept imperfections in herself.
3. Facilitate client's acceptance of self as a female human being.	To assist client in enjoying the pleasures of being female.
4. Help client lessen alienation from others by establishing meaningful relationships.	To prevent isolation and loneliness.
5. Help client enjoy life.	To enhance the quality of client's life.

EVALUATION

Measurable goals and outcome criteria provide the basis for evaluating the client's recovery from anorexia nervosa. In addition, nurse observations and family reports supply information about the client's progress. Self-reports from the client that all is well are unreliable; anorexics typically have poor insight. The following behaviors indicate a positive evaluation:

1. Eats adequate amounts of nutritional food regularly
2. Does not vomit
3. Has a positive and realistic self-concept
4. Has laboratory values that are normal
5. Has increased weight to near normal limits
6. Interacts with others
7. Is becoming independent from parents
8. Continues in therapy on an outpatient basis

BIBLIOGRAPHY

Agras WS: *Eating disorders: management of obesity, bulimia, and anorexia nervosa,* New York, 1987, Pergamon Press, Inc.

Amizo SA, Oda EA: Anorexia nervosa: psychological consideration for nutrition counseling, *J Am Diet Assoc* 88(1):49, 1988.

Biley F: Mirror images of anorexia . . . behavior therapy is not necessarily the most appropriate form of treatment, *Nurs* 3(43):20, 1989.

Brockdopp D: Eating disorders: a teenage epidemic, *Nurs Pract* 9(4):32, 1984.

Bruch H: *Eating disorders, obesity, anorexia nervosa and the person within,* New York, 1973, Basic Books, Inc.

Canaday M: Anorexia nervosa: distorted body image, *Issues Health Care Women* 3(5):281, 1981.

Carino C: Disorders in eating in adolescence: anorexia nervosa and bulimia, *Nurs Clin North Am* 18(2):343, 1983.

Covey M et al: Cardiovascular consequences of anorexia nervosa, *Prog Cardiovasc Nurs* 3(4):137, 1988.

Dardis PO, Hofland SL: Anorexia nervosa: fluid-electrolyte and acid-base c, *J Child Adolesc Psychiatr Ment Health Nurs* 3(3):85, 1990.

Edelstein OK, Haskew P, Kramer JP: Early clues to anorexia and bulimia, *Patient Care* 23(13):155, 1989.

Flood M: Addictive eating disorders, *Nurs Clin North Am* 24(1):45, 1989.

Geary MC: A review of treatment models for eating disorders: toward a holistic nursing model, *Holistic Nurs Pract* 3(1):39, 1988.

Gross M: Hypnosis in the therapy of anorexia nervosa, *Am J Clin Hypn* 26:175, 1984.

Grossniklaus D: Nursing interventions in anorexia nervosa, *Perspect Psychiatr Care* 18:11, 1980.

Johnson M: Anorexia nervosa: a framework for early identification and intervention, *Issues Ment Health Nurs* 4(2):87, 1982.

Keltner N: Bulimia: controlling compulsive eating, *J Psychosoc Nurs Ment Health Serv* 22(8):24, 1984.

Kiecolt-Graser J: Post adolescent onset male anorexia, *J Psychosoc Nurs Ment Health Serv* 22(1):10, 1984.

Maloney M: Eating attitudes and behaviors of anorexia nervosa patients and their sisters, *Gen Hosp Psychiatry* 5(4):285, 1983.

Marcus RN: Inpatient care of the substance-abusing patient with a concomitant eating disorder, *Hosp Community Psychiatry* 41(1):59, 1990.

Marks R: Anorexia and bulimia: eating habits that can kill, *RN* 84(1):30, 1984.

Miner DC: The physiology of eating and starvation, *Holistic Nurs Pract* 3(1):67, 1988.

Minuchin S, Rosman B, Baker L: *Psychosomatic families: anorexia nervosa in context,* Cambridge, Mass., 1978, Harvard University Press.

Muscari ME: Impaired coping and the eating disordered client, *Adv Clin Care* 5(2):22, 1990.

Muscari ME, Lobisser M: Teaching the eating disordered client, *Adv Clin Care* 5(1):20, 1990.

Nusbaum JG, Drever E: Inpatient survey of nursing care measures for treatment of patients with anorexia nervosa, *Issues Ment Health Nurs* 11(2):175, 1990.

Palmer TA: Anorexia nervosa, bulimia nervosa: causal theories and treatment, *Nurs Pract* 15(4):12, 1990.

Plehn KW: Anorexia nervosa and bulimia: incidence and diagnosis, *Nurse Pract* 15(4):22, 1990.

Sanger E: Eating disorders: avoiding the power struggle, *Am J Nurs* 84(1):30, 1984.

Seligman J: A deadly feast and famine, *Newsweek* 101(10):59, 1983.

Werry JS: Behavior therapy with children and adolescents: a twenty-year overview, *J Am Acad Child Adolesc Psychiatry* 28(1):1, 1989.

White M: Anorexia nervosa: a transgenerational system perspective, *Fam Process* 22(3):225, 1983.

Williamson DA: *Assessment of eating disorders: obesity, anorexia, and bulimia nervosa,* New York, 1990, Pergamon Press, Inc.

Yates A: Current perspective on the eating disorders: II. Treatment, outcome, and research directions, *J Am Acad Child Adolesc Psychiatry* 29(1):1, 1990.

Yates A: *Compulsive exercise and the eating disorders: toward an integrated theory of activity,* New York, 1991, Brunner/Mazel, Inc.

Anxiety

Anxiety is a state in which the individual feels uneasy and apprehensive and the autonomic nervous system activates in response to a nonspecific threat. The source is generally unknown or unrecognized. Anxiety is differentiated from fear, which arises from the threat of danger to a person's existence from a known cause. Anxiety ranges in intensity from mild to severe. It accompanies the developing personality and is felt whenever the individual is exposed to new situations. The formation of defense mechanisms, personality traits, and interpersonal behaviors results from anxiety. When anxiety is severe and defense mechanisms fail, serious problems—such as acting-out behavior, physical illness, and schizophrenia—may result.

Anxiety may be directly felt or may not be felt at all because of the relief measures instituted by the individual. Over time, relief behaviors occur automatically, and patterns are established that provide comfort and protection from anxiety. These relief measures may use the energy of anxiety in a constructive or destructive manner.

Anxiety is expressed in multiple ways, and nurses can become skillful in recognizing and dealing with the anxious client and family. Nurses themselves become anxious, and it is helpful for them to recognize and deal with their own anxieties so they can respond effectively to their clients and families.

Related DSM-III-R disorders

Anxiety disorders
Schizophrenia
Delusional (paranoid) disorder
Somatoform disorders
Dissociative disorders
Psychological factors affecting physical condition
Psychoactive substance-use disorders
Sexual disorders
Sleep disorders

Other related conditions

Crisis situations
Rape, abuse, or assault
Phobias
Compulsions
Obesity
Tension headache
Migraine headache
Angina pectoris
Neurodermatitis
Gastric ulcer
Nausea and vomiting
Colitis
Enteritis
Rheumatoid arthritis
Asthma
Painful menstruation
Masturbation
Sexual dysfunction

PRINCIPLES

▶ **Physical Dimension**

1. General health has an effect on person's predisposition to anxiety.
2. Fatigue increases irritability and feelings of anxiety.
3. Anxiety is manifested through physical changes in all body systems via the autonomic nervous system.
4. The process of birth is the person's first experience with anxiety.
5. Feelings of anxiety continue as the infant develops; the possibility exists that the physical needs of hunger, thirst, and comfort may not be met.

▶ **Emotional Dimension**

1. Anxiety is a subjective warning of an unknown danger.
2. Anxiety is first communicated through the emotional bonding by mother to the infant.
3. Anxiety is increased by fear that id impulses, or instincts, will get out of control and cause the person to do something for which he or she will be punished.
4. The individual guards against anxiety by disregarding certain undesirable aspects of the personality.
5. Mild or moderate anxiety is frequently expressed as anger.
6. Anxiety arises from feelings of inferiority.
7. A person with a high predisposition for anxiety is one who is easily threatened and has a low self-esteem.
8. A discrepancy between the perceived self and the ideal self exists in persons with high anxiety.
9. Individuals exposed to intense fears in early life are more likely to demonstrate a high disposition to anxiety in later life.

▶ **Intellectual Dimension**

1. Defense mechanisms protect the ego from the threat to the self system and prevent awareness of anxiety.
2. Defense mechanisms are primarily unconscious and involve a degree of self-deception and reality distortion.
3. Anxiety serves to motivate a person's behavior.
4. Anxiety arises through conflicts in which the individual has two opposing interests and must choose between them.

▶ **Social Dimension**

1. Anxiety is a product of interpersonal relationships and is communicated interpersonally.
2. Anxiety arises from interpersonal situations in which the individual perceives he or she will be viewed unfavorably by another whose opinion is valued.
3. Anxiety is felt because of a threat to the individual's autonomy.
4. Whatever interferes with an individual's ability to achieve a desired goal causes frustration and anxiety.
5. Blocks to achieving goals, which result in anxiety, can be external (loss of job) or internal (unreal self-expectations).
6. The ability to tolerate anxiety is important for the individual's mastery of the environment.
7. Anxiety is a learned drive based on an innate desire to avoid pain.
8. Parental influences are instrumental in developing feelings of security in a child.

▶ **Spiritual Dimension**

1. Anxiety arises from being in a world as a finite being who is faced with fear of the unknown and eventual death, the ultimate destiny of self.
2. Situations such as confronting freedom, authority, opposing values, and death cause anxiety.
3. Anxiety is apprehension caused by the threat to some value the individual considers essential to existence.
4. Anxiety is a phenomenon of human existence that every individual experiences when confronting a situation that threatens his being.
5. Anxiety serves as an incentive to further growth.

ASSESSMENT

▶ **Physical Dimension**

I. History
  A. Activities of daily living
    1. Nutrition
      a. Inadequate or more than adequate diet
      b. Weight loss or weight gain
    2. Sleep
      a. Difficulty sleeping
      b. Fatigue
    3. Physical activities or limitations
      a. Overly active
      b. Pacing
      c. Restlessness
      d. Immobilized
    4. Sexual activity
      a. Sexual dysfunction (impotence)
  B. Habits
    1. Alcohol
      a. Increased or excessive intake
    2. Smoking
      a. Chain smoking
    3. Medications and drugs
      a. Over-the-counter drugs

b. Increased use or abuse of prescription drugs, especially the antianxiety agents diazepam (Valium) and chlordiazepoxide hydrochloride (Librium)

c. Illegal drugs

4. Caffeine

a. Increased intake

5. Destructive behavior

a. Impulsive acts

C. Health history

1. Illnesses

a. Any illness or disease, acute or long-term, related to any body part or the loss of a body part

2. Injuries

a. Fractures

b. Wounds

c. Lacerations

d. Assault, abuse, rape, molestation

3. Allergies

a. May result in anxiety or be a response to anxiety

4. Hospitalizations

a. Unknown diagnosis

b. Tests and laboratory procedures

c. Invasive procedures

d. Dying

5. Surgeries

a. Any operation

D. Review of systems

1. General

a. Change in weight

b. Change in sleep habits

2. Skin

a. Rash, hives, "goose bumps"

b. Excessive perspiration

c. Flushed face

d. Cold hands

3. Ears

a. Deafness

4. Eyes

a. Dilated pupils

5. Nose and throat

a. Dry mouth

6. Cardiovascular

a. Tachycardia

b. Palpitations

c. Chest pain

d. Syncope

7. Respiratory

a. Cough

b. Shortness of breath

c. Increased respiratory rate

d. Shallow breathing

8. Gastrointestinal

a. Nausea

b. Diarrhea

c. Indigestion

d. Loss of appetite or increased appetite

9. Genitourinary

a. Frequency

b. Urgency

10. Reproductive

a. Male—impotence

b. Female—irregular menses

11. Musculoskeletal

a. Muscle rigidity

b. Muscle tenseness

c. Backache

d. Arthritis

e. Paralysis

12. Neurological

a. Fainting spells

b. Dizziness

c. Forgetfulness or memory loss

d. Nervousness

e. Tremors

f. Headaches

II. Diagnostic tests

A. Blood studies

B. Urinary studies

► **Physical Examination**

CLIENT DATA	ANALYSIS	NURSING DIAGNOSIS
Mild Anxiety		
Physiological responses	Mild physiological responses to stress	Altered health maintenance:
Increased heart rate		Increased heart rate related to mild anxiety
Increased blood pressure		Increased blood pressure related to mild anxiety
Rapid breathing		Rapid breathing related to mild anxiety
Slowed digestive process		Slowed digestive process related to mild anxiety
Inhibited salivation		Inhibited salivation related to mild anxiety
Tightened muscle tone		Tightened muscle tone related to mild anxiety
Dilated pupils		Dilated pupils related to mild anxiety
Increased blood sugar		Increased blood sugar related to mild anxiety
Cold skin and extremities		Cold skin and extremities related to mild anxiety
Increased alertness		Increased alertness related to mild anxiety
Moderate Anxiety		
Increased physiological responses	Moderately severe physiological responses to stress.	Altered health maintenance: increased physiological responses related to moderate anxiety
Decreased response to stimuli (seeing, hearing)	Responses to stimuli are diminished with moderate anxiety (e.g., tunnel vision).	Altered health maintenance: decreased vision, hearing, grasping stimuli related to moderate anxiety
Severe Anxiety		
Survival response (fight or flight)	Instinctual responses to severe anxiety: to flee or to fight	*Social isolation/withdrawal: behavior related to severe anxiety; assaultive behavior related to severe anxiety
Sympathetic nervous system activation: Increased epinephrine Increased blood pressure, pulse, respiration Skin vasoconstriction Increased body temperature Diaphoresis Dry mouth Urinary urgency Loss of appetite Decreased blood to digestive system Increased glucose production by liver	Severe physiological responses to stress.	Altered health maintenance: increased physiological responses related to severe anxiety
Sensory changes: Decreased hearing Dilated pupils Fixed vision Decreased pain perception		Altered health maintenance: Decreased hearing, vision related to severe anxiety Decreased pain perception related to severe anxiety
Tense, rigid muscles		Tense, rigid muscles related to severe anxiety

▶ **Physical Examination—cont'd**

CLIENT DATA	ANALYSIS	NURSING DIAGNOSIS

Panic Anxiety
Continued, increased physiological responses:
 	
   Blood returns to major organs (individual is pale)
   Lowered blood pressure
 	
   Minimum response to pain, noise, stimuli
   Poor motor coordination
	Severe physiological responses to stress with disorganization.	Altered health maintenance:
		   Increased physiological responses to panic level of anxiety
		   Pallor related to panic level of anxiety
		   Lowered blood pressure related to panic level of anxiety
		   Minimum response to pain related to panic level of anxiety
		   Poor motor coordination related to panic level of anxiety

▶ **Emotional Dimension**

CLIENT DATA	ANALYSIS	NURSING DIAGNOSIS
Anxiety	Fear of the unknown (such as a diagnosis), fear of success or failure, fear of punishment, aging, or death results in anxiety.	Anxiety: related to unknown origin
Apprehension, helplessness, nervousness, irritability, anger, discomfort, fear, frustration, resentment, crying	Expressions of anxiety: anxiety is expressed in multiple ways.	Anxiety: related to feelings of helplessness, nervousness, irritability, anger, discomfort, fear, frustration, resentment, crying

▶ **Intellectual Dimension**

CLIENT DATA	ANALYSIS	NURSING DIAGNOSIS
Perceptions *Severe anxiety* Perceptual field greatly reduced	Feelings of increasing threat, reduced ability to handle threat.	Ineffective individual coping: increased feelings of threat related to severe anxiety
Hypervigilant	Response to stress, increased alertness.	Ineffective individual coping: hypervigilance related to severe anxiety
Panic Perceptual field closed or distorted	Disorganization and inability to handle situation.	Ineffective individual coping: related to panic level of anxiety
Memory *Severe anxiety* Impaired memory, increased forgetfulness	Increased feelings of threat cause lapses in recall of thoughts and an inability to learn.	Altered thought processes: memory impairment related to severe anxiety
Panic Unable to remember simple instructions, directions (The following characteristics are impaired in both severe and panic levels of anxiety with the most dysfunctional symptoms occurring in the panic levels of anxiety.)	Increased feelings of threat result in disorganization and inability to retain information.	Altered thought processes: severe memory impairment related to panic level of anxiety

▶ **Intellectual Dimension—cont'd**

CLIENT DATA	ANALYSIS	NURSING DIAGNOSIS
Orientation Distorted sense of time, place	Response to severe stress.	Altered thought processes: disorientation to time and place related to severe or panic anxiety
Judgment and Insight Lack of awareness Inability to make decisions	Reponses to severe stress.	Altered thought processes: lack of insight, inability to make decisions related to severe or panic anxiety
Abstract Thinking Inability to think in abstract terms	Responses to severe stress are concrete.	Altered thought processes: concrete thinking related to severe or panic anxiety
Thought Content Selective inattention in severe anxiety	Severe anxiety impairs ability to listen, comprehend.	Altered thought processes: selective inattention related to severe anxiety
Focuses on scattered details	Response to severe threat.	Altered thought processes: scattering related to severe anxiety
Unable to problem solve	Anxiety impairs ability to think logically and reasonably.	Altered thought processes: inability to problem solve related to severe or panic anxiety
Highly distractible	Severe anxiety interferes with attention span.	Altered thought processes: distractibility related to severe or panic anxiety
Unable to concentrate	Severe anxiety impairs concentration and learning.	Altered thought processes: inability to concentrate related to severe or panic anxiety
Unable to understand directions	Responses to stress, disorganization, scattering.	Altered thought processes: inability to understand directions related to severe or panic anxiety
Questions repetitiously	Responses to stress, disorganization, scattering.	Altered thought processes: repetitious questioning related to severe or panic anxiety
Defense Mechanisms Projection Denial Rationalization	Unconscious mechanisms used to reduce anxiety.	Defensive coping: pathological use of defense mechanisms related to severe or panic anxiety
Communication Pressured speech	Response to stress.	Impaired verbal communication: pressured speech related to severe or panic anxiety
Habitual responses	Sameness reduces anxiety: speech is automatic.	Impaired verbal communication: habitual responses related to severe or panic anxiety
Blocking	Thinking stops; thoughts create too much anxiety, are too threatening.	Impaired verbal communication: blocking related to severe or panic anxiety.
Overtalkative	Response to stress indicating anxiety.	Impaired verbal communication: overtalkative related to severe or panic anxiety
Flood of talk	Response to stress indicating anxiety.	Impaired verbal communication: flood of talk related to severe or panic anxiety
Stammering	Response to stress indicating anxiety.	Impaired verbal communication: stammering related to severe or panic anxiety

▶ **Intellectual Dimension—cont'd**

CLIENT DATA	ANALYSIS	NURSING DIAGNOSIS
Slips of speech	Response to stress indicating anxiety.	Impaired verbal communication: slips of speech related to severe or panic anxiety
Arguing	Response to stress indicating anxiety.	Impaired verbal communication: arguing related to severe or panic anxiety
Complaining	Response to stress indicating anxiety	Impaired verbal communication: complaining related to severe or panic anxiety
Blaming	Response to stress indicating anxiety.	Impaired verbal communication: blaming related to severe or panic anxiety
Demanding	Response to stress indicating anxiety.	Impaired verbal communication: demanding related to severe or panic anxiety
Scattered thoughts	Increased anxiety may result in client focusing on many unrelated thoughts.	Impaired verbal communication: scattered thoughts related to severe or panic anxiety
Ruminations	Increased anxiety leads to client focusing on one particular thought over and over.	Impaired verbal communication: ruminations related to severe or panic anxiety
Communication difficult to understand	Response to stress indicating panic level of anxiety.	Impaired verbal communication: related to panic level of anxiety

▶ **Social Dimension**

CLIENT DATA	ANALYSIS	NURSING DIAGNOSIS
Lowered self-esteem	Events are more threatening than to those with high self-esteem.	Self-esteem disturbance: related to severe anxiety
Seeks out others to talk to without discretion or withdraws from others	Those with high levels of anxiety will stop and talk to anyone who will listen or they may withdraw from others.	Self-esteem disturbance: seeking of attention from others or withdraws from others related to severe anxiety
Little or no family support	Clients with high anxiety levels associated with excessive verbalization and cognitive dysfunctions tend to alienate families.	Impaired social interaction: lack of support systems related to severe anxiety
Impaired functioning in social roles	High anxiety interferes with social role functioning.	Altered role performance: related to severe anxiety
Environmental stressors: for example, loss of valued possessions, hospitalization, moving, retirement, new job	High level of anxiety may result when factors in environment are stressful or crisis producing.	Anxiety: related to environmental factors, for example, loss of valued possessions, hospitalization, moving, retirement, new job

▶ **Spiritual Dimension**

CLIENT DATA	ANALYSIS	NURSING DIAGNOSIS
Indifference to life values	Anxiety interferes with client's ability to think clearly and formulate decisions, hence the indifference.	Spiritual distress: indifferences to previously held values related to anxiety
Feels that life lacks meaning	The need to handle immediate anxiety-producing situation prevents client from experiencing deeper meaning to life.	*Altered meaningfulness: lack of meaning to life related to anxiety

▶ **Spiritual Dimension—cont'd**

CLIENT DATA	ANALYSIS	NURSING DIAGNOSIS
Questions previously held ethical beliefs	Immediacy of situation and need to handle it quickly may cause client to question previously held beliefs.	Anxiety: related to questioning previously held ethical beliefs related to anxiety
Despairs	Sense of hopelessness and loss of control contribute to despair.	Spiritual distress: hopelessness and loss of control related to anxiety
Is unable to move beyond self	Preoccupied with self and anxiety-producing situation.	Spiritual distress: preoccupied with self and situation related to anxiety
Seeks sameness, is unable to reach out	Sameness creates security and freedom from threatening situations.	Spiritual distress: inability to take risks related to anxiety
Moans and wails for God's or other supreme power's help or rejects faith	Anxiety inhibits problem solving. Client ruminates over help from God (or a religious leader) or may completely reject faith.	Spiritual distress: lack of comfort from religious belief related to anxiety
Withdraws from usual religious practices	A response to anxiety-producing situation (flees)	Spiritual distress: withdrawal from usual religious practices related to anxiety
Has reduced creativity	Decreased cognitive abilities and functioning	Spiritual distress: impaired creativity related to anxiety
Is unable to enjoy beauty	Too preoccupied with self.	Spiritual distress: inability to enjoy beauty related to anxiety
Alienated from relationships with others	Anxiety interferes with establishing, accepting, and nurturing relationships.	Spiritual distress: alienation from others related to anxiety
Afraid of future, death	Threatened by fears of unknown; focuses on past rather than present or future.	Spiritual distress: fear of future or death related to anxiety

PLANNING

Long-Term Goals

To identify, accept, and learn to live with anxiety
To cope with anxiety effectively

SHORT-TERM GOALS	OUTCOME CRITERIA
Physical Dimension To identify the symptoms of anxiety	1. States times when feelings of anxiety occur 2. Identifies body responses and behavior related to anxiety 3. States he or she is feeling anxious (nervous, uptight) 4. Is able to stay with and experience the feelings of anxiety 5. Discusses similarities of the immediate situation and past experiences in which anxiety was felt
Emotional Dimension To reduce the level of anxiety	1. Is less restless 2. Listens to information given 3. Is able to follow instructions 4. Sleeps restfully without interruption 5. Makes decisions 6. Reduces alcohol intake 7. Makes fewer (or no) derogatory statements about self 8. Discusses fears 9. Is able to remember events

PLANNING—cont'd

SHORT-TERM GOALS	OUTCOME CRITERIA
	10. Is able to problem solve 11. Makes eye contact 12. Is able to talk about death 13. Verbalizes feelings; is relaxed, comfortable
Intellectual Dimension To identify sources of anxiety	1. Identifies events and situations that precipitate anxiety 2. Verbalizes anxiety when client thinks he or she will be viewed unfavorably 3. Verbalizes threats that arouse anxiety 4. States bad feelings about self that arouse anxiety 5. States conflicts in values that arouse anxiety 6. Verbalizes anxiety when feeling fatigued
To identify coping mechanisms used	1. Identifies ways of coping with anxiety in past and at present 2. Identifies effective coping mechanisms 3. Identifies ineffective coping mechanisms 4. Identifies other ways to deal with anxiety
To develop effective coping mechanisms	1. Uses effective coping mechanisms 2. Gives self positive feedback when effective coping mechanisms are used
Social Dimension To relate to another person without undue anxiety	1. Is comfortable interacting with others 2. Feels safe expressing feelings and concerns to another 3. Listens to another's feelings and concerns 4. Establishes a support system for self 5. Contacts supportive person when feeling anxious
Spiritual Dimension To live with some anxiety	1. Identifies own anxiety 2. Knows ways to reduce anxiety 3. Accepts anxiety as a challenge, an opportunity, and a part of life

Discharge Planning

The following client behaviors demonstrate readiness for discharge:

1. Identifies feelings of anxiety and identifies responses to anxiety
2. Copes effectively with anxiety
3. Knows and uses several techniques for managing anxiety
4. Gains insight by identifying precipitating factors and linking them to anxious feelings
5. Seeks help when anxiety begins to escalate

IMPLEMENTATION

NURSING ACTIONS	RATIONALE
Physical Dimension	
1. Provide recreational and diversional activities such as swimming, jogging, walking, running errands, simple tasks, repetitive activities.	To use the energy activated by anxiety to reduce anxiety, to decrease amount of time available for introspection and preoccupation.
2. Promote sleep with comfort measures (warm bath, music, back rub, quiet presence of a significant person).	To assist client to relax and obtain a restful sleep.
3. Provide medication as prescribed for sleep when indicated.	To assist client in relaxing when anxiety is severe and sleep is disturbed.
4. Assist client in relaxing with relaxation exercises and deep breathing and in reducing hyperventilation.	To help client assume responsibility for decreasing anxiety and to increase feelings of control.
5. Help client limit smoking and caffeine intake and substitute raw vegetables or popcorn.	To inhibit the stimulating action of nicotine and caffeine and substitute nutritious foods.
6. Help client refrain from attempts to quit smoking during periods of high anxiety.	To prevent additional stress generated by attempts to quit smoking.
7. If client is a victim of rape, assault, abuse, or molestation, refer to appropriate professional person if you are unable to help client deal with the anxiety.	To provide client with the most competent, qualified person with specialized training in rape or assault.
8. Walk with client who is pacing or restless.	To provide support while using the energy of anxiety effectively.
9. Treat physical complaints matter-of-factly.	To prevent undue focus on physical complaints, to help client identify relationship of physical symptoms to anxiety.
10. Help client refrain from dwelling on physical complaints through distractions such as music or physical activity.	To prevent incapacitation from and preoccupation with complaints.
11. Give positive feedback when client is symptom-free.	To reinforce client's ability to cope with anxiety.
12. Provide nutritious, regular meals.	To encourage healthy eating patterns and to prevent increased anxiety associated with irregular meal times.
13. Protect from impulsive acts with one-to-one supervision or hospitalization.	To prevent client from harm to self or others.
14. Maintain appropriate eye contact even when client avoids it.	To convey genuine interest, concern, and that the nurse is listening.
15. Use touch on hand, back, or shoulder as appropriate and comfortable for client and nurse.	To convey warmth, understanding, and support to client.
16. Provide client with telephone number for emergency or crisis situations (hotline clinics, emergency rooms, mental health centers).	To facilitate client's ability to contact help when anxious.
Emotional Dimension	
1. Facilitate expression of feelings of anxiety by listening actively, showing respect, and expressing empathy.	To help client identify anxiety and possible causes, to assess the level of anxiety, and to set priorities for care. To talk about anxious feelings with another person diminishes the intensity of the anxiety.
2. Identify level of anxiety	To provide a base for intervention.
3. Help client identify threat causing anxiety.	To provide clues to the anxiety-producing situation.
4. Identify duration of stress.	To gain an understanding of the severity of the anxiety.
5. Explore meaning of threat to client by discussing effects of threat on self and health.	To gain an understanding of the client's perception of the situation that triggered the anxiety.
6. Help client acknowledge and accept feelings of anxiety.	To promote self-awareness and help client understand that some anxiety is normal and appropriate.
7. Accept client's feeling of anxiety.	To promote client's ability to acknowledge and express feelings and that to do so appropriately is healthy and normal.
8. Sit quietly with client who cries.	To convey acceptance of crying as an expression of a normal feeling.
9. Increase client's feelings of security and control.	To reduce unknowns, thus reducing anxiety. Structuring the environment, giving information, and allowing client to participate in decisions provide client with security and sense of control.

IMPLEMENTATION—cont'd

NURSING ACTIONS	RATIONALE
10. Ask client if he or she is fearful or anxious when nonverbal behavior indicates that is the case.	To assist client in identifying anxious feelings.
11. Provide feedback on behavior that indicates anxiety.	To promote client's awareness of own anxiety.
12. Help client find other ways to express anxious feelings, for example, by physical activity or talking with a supportive person.	To promote adaptive coping with anxiety. The more skills client has for coping with anxiety, the less likely client is to be overwhelmed by it.
13. Identify behaviors that indicate that anxiety is mounting such as restlessness, pacing, tenseness, or irritability.	To intervene before anxiety is severe or out of control.
14. Discuss with client fears and worries.	To gain insight about events and situations that cause fears or worries and help client find ways to avoid or accept them without undue anxiety.
15. Allow specified "worry time" (e.g., 15 minutes each day at 10 AM).	To set limits on worrying.
16. Accept client's anxiety without being provoked into reciprocal anxiety.	To prevent feelings of anxiety from being communicated to nurse.
17. Avoid transferring own anxiety to client.	To prevent feelings of anxiety from being communicated to client.
18. Provide feelings of security to client by presence and confidence of nurse.	To decrease anxiety through the therapeutic use of self.
19. Refrain from false reassurance.	To promote a trusting relationship.
20. Allow denial of anxiety when appropriate and continue to facilitate communication of feelings.	To prevent taking away client's defenses before client is ready or before the defenses are replaced with other adaptive coping skills.
21. Be aware of responses to client's anxiety; helplessness, anger, demands, repetitive questions.	To prevent feelings from being communicated and interfering with the therapeutic relationship. To be aware of the many faces of anxiety.
22. Help client make connections between feelings of anxiety and subsequent behavior.	To help the client gain insight about behavior by linking anxious feelings to client's responses to them.
Intellectual Dimension	
1. Speak slowly and calmly.	To convey a relaxed attitude by using self therapeutically.
2. Use simple, short sentences.	To help the client understand the message. Anxious clients have difficulty concentrating and processing information.
3. Give brief, concise directions.	To facilitate understanding.
4. Refrain from making demands on or requiring decisions from client.	To lessen stress and tension associated with making decisions.
5. Enforce rules consistently.	To promote security; uncertainty and inconsistency create anxiety.
6. Respond to requests promptly.	To promote security and help client learn to trust.
7. Use reflection and empathy.	To let client know he or she is understood. To use self therapeutically.
8. Discuss what relieves client's anxiety.	To help client become aware of relief measures, those that help and those that do not.
9. Initiate problem solving when anxiety is lessened (Appendix C).	To help client learn problem-solving skills at a time when readiness is indicated.
10. Focus on present situation that is producing anxiety.	To emphasize what is happening and deal with it rather than the past.
11. Assist client in identifying sources of frustration, unmet needs, and conflicts that cause anxiety.	To help client recognize situations producing anxiety and learn to handle them.
12. Help client identify consequences of maladaptive coping with anxiety.	To promote understanding of client's methods of handling anxiety and introduce alternative methods.
13. Set limits on demands by stating clearly and simply what is expected.	To help client know what is expected and decrease anxiety.
14. Give positive reinforcement for not exceeding limits.	To reinforce positive behavioral change.
15. Help client assess threats as realistic or distorted.	To help client question his or her own conclusions about reality of threat.
16. Give specific information on all tests, procedures, and expectations.	To reduce anxiety by giving specific information.

NURSING ACTIONS	RATIONALE
17. Help client participate in decisions.	To enhance feelings of control, autonomy, trust, and security.
18. Provide desensitization.	To reduce the intense anxiety of phobias that interfere with functioning in life.
19. Help client learn to control behavior by setting limits and rewarding positive behavioral changes.	To promote feelings of self-responsibility and increasing self-esteem.
20. Motivate client to assume responsibility for lessening anxiety by involving client in decisions about care and treatment.	To promote self-responsibility for controlling behavior and the confidence that client can control own anxiety.

Social Dimension

1. Stay with client.	To indicate that help is available.
2. Remove client from excessive stimulation.	To calm or relax client.
3. Provide a safe environment with prompt attention to requests.	To increase trust and safety, both physical and emotional.
4. Limit contact with others (for example, other clients or family members who are anxious).	To prevent feelings of anxiety from being transferred to client.
5. Explore secondary gains clients may be receiving from others through their anxious behavior.	To prevent client from receiving benefits and satisfaction from anxious behavior.
6. If client is unemployed or relocated because of anxiety problems, refer to a social worker for services.	To initiate rehabilitation and prevent incapacitation.
7. Identify client's support system.	To help client recognize need for supportive persons.
8. Enhance client's self-esteem so that life is less threatening by focusing on client's positive attributes, skills, and talents.	To promote confidence in self and an ability to deal with life situations.
9. Help client discuss concerns with one consistent person initially.	To avoid rejection or alienation from others that further deflate self-esteem.
10. Change environment, hospitalize, or have client stay with another family member.	To reduce stressors.
11. Provide group and family therapy.	To discuss the problems associated with anxiety, to change behavior, to receive support, and to increase self-esteem.
12. Provide counseling for retirement, widowhood, or widowerhood, if source of anxiety.	To provide information; information reduces anxiety.
13. Provide privacy to ensure confidentiality and build trust.	To avoid situations that may increase client's anxiety level.
14. Refer to self-help groups, such as worry clinics, if appropriate and available in the community.	To promote responsibility for own mental health and to share feelings with others.

Spiritual Dimension

1. Refrain from discussion of beliefs, values that require decisions, until anxiety decreases.	To prevent escalation of anxiety when issues are emotionally charged.
2. Help client add peace and contentment to life by increasing confidence in self and abilities.	To add quality to client's life without excessive anxiety.
3. Help client see anxiety as a challenge and an opportunity to add meaning to life by changing from focusing on problems to emphasizing opportunities for growth.	To promote sense of mastery of anxiety, to learn problem-solving skills, to increase self-esteem and autonomy.
4. Provide opportunities for client to help others to gain self-satisfaction, increase self-esteem, and enrich life.	To receive satisfaction from helping others promotes a sense of satisfaction with self, increases self-esteem, and adds an enriching quality to life, one's own and others'.
5. Provide pleasures that client enjoys (painting, books, gardening).	To enhance self-concept, to promote success and achievement.
6. Promote relationships with others in similar religious groups to lessen alienation and reduce anxiety.	To promote interactions with people of similar religious backgrounds may lessen anxiety.
7. Assist client in being creative (writing, drawing, dancing) as a way to reduce anxiety when expressing it verbally is difficult.	To help client express anxious feelings in mediums other than verbalization.

IMPLEMENTATION—cont'd

NURSING ACTIONS	RATIONALE
8. Help client accept dying and death without undue anxiety by helping client verbalize feelings about death, dying.	To reduce the anxiety associated with death and dying.
9. Refer client to clergy or religious leader for assistance with anxiety about dying and death.	To offer the help of a religious, comforting person.
10. Help client learn from the experience of anxiety so that pain and anguish are replaced with something more useful and appropriate.	To prevent client from denying or avoiding anxiety, to assist client in growing emotionally, and to promote mental health.
11. Discuss cultural and religious influences and implications for anxiety-producing situations (divorce, abortion, out-of-wedlock pregnancy, rape, incest, mental illness, mercy killing).	To help client understand cultural and religious influences on situations that may contribute to anxiety.

EVALUATION

Measurable goals and outcomes provide the basis for evaluating the client with anxiety. Client self-reports, nurse observations, and family reports provide information about the client's progress. The following behaviors indicate a positive evaluation:

1. Is relaxed
2. Identifies feelings of anxiety
3. Verbalizes feelings of anxiety
4. Identifies effects of anxiety on self and others
5. Uses appropriate methods to handle anxiety, such as relaxation, exercise, or other stress reduction techniques
6. Seeks help from others when unable to reduce the anxiety

BIBLIOGRAPHY

Goodwyn J: Post-traumatic symptoms in abused children, *J Traum Stress* 1(4):475, 1988.

Grainger R: Anxiety interrupters, *Am J Nurs* 90(2):14, 1990.

Haack M: Collaborative investigation of adult children of alcoholics, *Arch Psychiatr Nurs* 4(1):62, 1990.

Katon W, Sheehan D, Whole T: Panic disorder: a treatable problem, *Patient Care* 2(6):148, 1988.

Koenig H: Religious behaviors and death anxiety in later life. *Hospice J* 4(1):3, 1988.

Kreitler S, Kreitler H: Trauma and anxiety: the cognitive approach, *J Traum Stress* 1(1):35, 1988.

Long C, Bluteau P: Group coping skills training for anxiety and depression: its application with chronic patients, *J Adv Nurs* 13(3):358, 1988.

Lyons J, Keane T: Implosive therapy for the treatment of combat-related PTSD, *J Traum Stress* 2(2):137, 1989.

Martin P: A feeling that needs expressing: helping patients manage their anxiety, *Prof Nurse* 5(7):374, 1990.

May R: *The meaning of anxiety,* New York, 1977, W.W. Norton & Co.

May R: Value conflicts and anxiety. In Kutash I, editor: *Handbook on stress and anxiety,* San Francisco, 1980, Jossey-Bass Inc., Publishers.

McNally R: Preparedness and phobias: a review, *Psych Bull* 101(2):283, 1987.

Sluckin A: Psychotherapy with an acutely anxious six year old, *Health Visit* 61(6):184, 1988.

Titlebaum H: Relaxation, *Holistic Nurse Pract* 2(3):17, 1988.

Trimpey M: Self-esteem and anxiety: key issues in an abused women's support group, *Issues Ment Health Nurs* 10:297, 1989.

Trygstad L: Simple new ways to help anxious patients, *RN* 80(12):28, 1980.

Valente S: Children, adolescents, and nuclear war anxiety, *J Child Adolesc Psychiatr Ment Health Nurs* 1(1):36, 1988.

Weeks C: *Peace from nervous suffering,* New York, 1983, Bantam Books, Inc.

Chronic Pain

Pain is generally defined as a state in which the individual has an uncomfortable sensation accompanied by physical and emotional reactions. Pain may be acute, as in response to a noxious stimuli with a definable causative organism. Pain may be chronic, lasting over a period of years as with certain types of back pain or with chronic disease. In chronic pain the complaint of pain may be in excess of what is expected from the physical findings. Psychogenic pain may occur in the absence of any physical finding. In this situation the pain is inconsistent with the anatomical distribution of the nervous system and cannot be accounted for by organic pathological findings after extensive diagnostic evaluation. The focus of this chapter is on pain of a chronic nature, regardless of the cause.

Physical and emotional factors have potential for producing pain. Contributing factors may be physiological, such as dysfunctions in any body system. Situations and events may also contribute to an individual's pain; these include trauma, diagnostic tests, invasive procedures, immobility, chronic illness, and pregnancy. Responses to pain are highly individual and depend on the person's pain threshold, personality, stressors, the meaning of the illness or disability, benefits received, and cultural norms.

The person in pain may report the pain verbally. Other defining characteristics include an increase in blood pressure, pulse, and respirations; diaphoresis; and dilated pupils. The person may also remain in a guarded position, have a pained facial expression, and cry or moan. Whatever the cause, the pain is real to the client. The challenge is to provide comfort measures to assist the client in relieving the pain or in learning to live with it.

The experience of pain is unique to each individual and varies depending on the disease process, emotional state, personality, relationships, interpretation, religion, cultural factors, and values. It becomes important, then, for the nurse to fully recognize that the client, not the nurse, is the expert on the client's pain. Thus the nurse's approach of empathic, personal warmth is essential when working with the client in pain.

Related DSM-III-R disorders

Somatoform pain disorder
Somatization disorder

Other related conditions

Injury
Pregnancy
Diagnostic tests
Invasive procedures
Chronic or terminal illness
Depression
Malingering

PRINCIPLES

▶ Physical Dimension

1. Pain accompanies nearly all chronic and terminal illnesses.
2. Pain stimuli are allowed in or closed out from the cerebral cortex (gate control theory) depending on the meaning the individual attaches to the stimuli.
3. Pain may be a secondary symptom, as in peptic ulcer or other psychophysiological disorders, when the discomfort originates with the organ damage.
4. Pain may be a conversion symptom originating in the mind but felt as though it were in the body.
5. Pain is a signal of actual or potential danger to body tissues and to the person.
6. Intense stimulation from other sources (for example, music) can reduce or abolish pain.
7. Activities that narrow attention, such as yoga and self-hypnosis, may diminish painful sensations.

▶ Emotional Dimension

1. Pain is a subjective experience; there is no way to measure it.

2. Common responses to pain are crying and moaning.
3. At times of severe stress, emotions associated with conflict may be converted to a symptom, pain.
4. An individual's feeling state influences the attention paid to pain. Individuals tend not to notice events that have little personal meaning and to pay great attention to those events that interest them deeply.
5. Anxiety is an important factor that influences the perception of pain.

▶ Intellectual Dimension

1. Meaning and symbolism are important components of pain.
2. Unconscious conflicts resulting from traumatic experiences in childhood that are reawakened in adult life by a similar trauma may cause psychological pain.
3. The individual who is unable to express the feeling aroused by a conflict because of guilt, fear of retribution, fear of loss of love, or fear of loss of control feels pain.
4. Consciousness, attention, and self-concern are necessary for a person to have pain.
5. Pain is influenced by psychological factors such as emotional state, personality, past experiences, and defense mechanisms.

▶ Social Dimension

1. Psychological pain occurs in a social setting; therefore the treatment needs to occur within the person's social and cultural belief system.
2. Conversion pain provides a different way of relating, a sick role, that is socially acceptable and removes the person from the disturbing life situation.

3. Conflicts resulting in pain involve clashes between dependence and independence, hostile and sexual impulses and opposing inhibitions, and ideals or cultural mores.
4. Children who receive love and attention only when suffering from a painful injury or disease learn to exaggerate a symptom to regain sympathy and concern; thus pain is a bridge that enables them to have a relationship with another person.
5. Behavior exhibited by others in pain influences an individual's pain behavior.
6. Children associate pain with punishment and see it as a way to control behavior.
7. The degree of environmental support influences an individual's feeling of pain and pain tolerance.
8. Positive and negative reinforcers can modify or eliminate pain behaviors.
9. Specific painful experiences in childhood influence how a person perceives and feels pain in later life.
10. Ethnic groups vary in their behavior toward and emotional response to pain; some may be stoic, others expressive.
11. Chronic pain may be a learned behavior.
12. The family's attitude toward pain influences the expression of pain.

▶ Spiritual Dimension

1. Western beliefs associate pain with concepts of suffering, punishment, and repentence.
2. A dominant image of the Western world is that of the crucifixion, indicating the importance of pain and suffering in western culture.
3. Pain may disrupt the quality of a person's life.

ASSESSMENT

▶ Physical Dimension

I. History
  A. Activities of daily living
     1. Nutrition
        a. Impaired food intake if nausea and vomiting accompany pain
     2. Sleep
        a. Disturbed sleep if pain is severe
     3. Recreation, hobbies, and interests
        a. Limited or none when pain is severe
     4. Physical activities
        a. Limited
        b. Invalidism
  B. Habits
     1. Alcohol
        a. Excessive use
        b. Misuse or abuse
     2. Medication or drugs
        a. Excessive use, misuse, or abuse of over-the-counter drugs and pain medications (legal or illegal)
  C. Destructive behavior
     1. Suicide attempts with prolonged pain
  D. Health history
     1. Injuries

a. Childhood trauma (physical or emotional)
2. Injuries
    a. Fractures
    b. Strains/sprains
    c. Falls
3. Surgery
    a. Major surgery
E. Review of systems
1. Mark on drawings the location of pain—*E,* external; *I,* internal; *E* and *I,* both external and internal (see Assessment, p. 9)

II. Physical examination
A. Examine specific areas associated with pain

III. Diagnostic tests—any diagnostic test to rule out pathological condition related to pain
  A. Blood chemistry profile
  B. Hematology
  C. Urinalysis
  D. Pap smear
  E. Stool specimen
  F. Serology
  G. Chest x-ray examination
  H. Cytological examination
  I. Hormone elevation
  J. Proctoscopy
  K. ECG
  L. EEG

▶ Emotional Dimension

CLIENT DATA	ANALYSIS	NURSING DIAGNOSIS
Anguish and suffering	Pain is real to client; responds with anguish and suffering.	Pain: related to . . . ; evidenced by anguish and suffering
Anger or rage	May be directed toward world in general or toward those around him who are healthy and free of pain.	Pain: related to . . . , evidenced by anger (rage)
Depression	Unable to express feelings of anger appropriately.	Pain: related to misery and depression
Worried, frowning appearance	Physical responses to pain.	Pain: related to . . . , evidenced by worried look and frowning
Fears dreaded disease associated with pain (for example, brain tumor with headache, heart attack with chest pain)	Irrational fears continue even when diagnostic tests have been performed to rule out organicity; personality, emotional state, past experiences influence pain.	Ineffective individual coping: irrational fears related to pain
Emotional conflict	Expressed as pain.	Pain: related to emotional conflict
Suicidal feelings	Result of severe, continuous, chronic pain.	High risk for self-directed violence related to severe, persistent pain

▶ Intellectual Dimension

CLIENT DATA	ANALYSIS	NURSING DIAGNOSIS
Distorted perception of pain	Pain is excessive, out of proportion to what is expected from the physical findings.	Pain: related to distorted perception
Complaining	May be excessive for what is expected from the physical findings.	Pain: related to . . . , evidenced by excessive complaints
Preoccupied with pain	Life is dominated by presence of pain.	Pain: related to . . . , evidenced by preoccupation with pain
Conflicts	Expressed as pain (for example, headache).	Pain: related to conflicts
Conveys message "pay attention to me"	Pain is symbolic expression of need for more attention.	Ineffective individual coping: attention-seeking behavior related to pain
Communicates with physical symptoms (pain)	Unable to express wants and needs directly, focuses on symptoms.	Impaired verbal communication: related to pain

▶ **Social Dimension**

CLIENT DATA	ANALYSIS	NURSING DIAGNOSIS
Sees self as an invalid	Assumes sick role, receives secondary gains from symptoms.	Self-esteem disturbance: invalidism related to pain
Lowered self-esteem	Actions and activities are designed to confirm identity as a suffering person, a way to receive secondary gains.	Self-esteem disturbance: related to pain
Uses pain games	Attempts to manipulate and control others with pain, to receive secondary gains.	Ineffective individual coping: manipulation and receiving secondary gains related to pain
Avoids intimacy	Alienates self from others with pain behavior.	Impaired social interactions: related to pain
Avoids responsibility for own life	Relies on others.	Ineffective individual coping: dependence with failure to accept responsibilities related to pain
Satisfies needs for care by remaining sick, receiving medications and sustenance through disability compensations	Ways to meet dependence needs.	Ineffective individual coping: dependence related to pain
Manipulates others	To meet own comfort needs, to reinforce life-style.	Ineffective individual coping: manipulation related to pain
Demanding of others	To meet own comfort needs and to promote a life-style of invalidism.	Ineffective individual coping: demanding behavior related to pain
Disturbed social role and occupational functioning or totally incapacitated and hospitalized	Unable to perform social roles and occupational roles.	Altered role performance: related to pain
Disabled	Leads to time-out from aversive situations.	Altered role performance: disability related to pain
Helplessness	Unable to meet own comfort needs.	Ineffective individual coping: helplessness related to pain
Dependence	Relies on others to meet comfort needs.	Ineffective individual coping: dependence related to pain
Feels inadequate	Lacks confidence in self to meet comfort needs.	Self-esteem disturbance: feelings of inadequacy related to pain
Cultural factors Meaning of pain differs depending on individual's culture	Ethnic groups may vary in their responses to pain.	Pain: related to . . . , evidenced by cultural factors

Environmental factors contributing to pain:
  Separation
  Divorce
  Death
  Illness
  Move
  Jail
  Loss of job
  Promotion in job
  Injury
  Marriage
  Pregnancy
  Business readjustment
  Change in financial status
  Vacation
  Christmas or other holidays
	Any situation that requires a social readjustment may cause pain.	Pain: related to environmental stressors

Iatrogenic factors (e.g., prescribed medications) contributing to pain	Physicians who prescribe medications may reinforce the pain behavior.	Pain: related to iatrogenic factors

▶ **Spiritual Dimension**

CLIENT DATA	ANALYSIS	NURSING DIAGNOSIS
Believes having no control over pain	Lacks insight and fails to accept any responsibility for pain, feels no control over own life and destiny.	Spiritual distress: lack of control over own life and destiny related to pain
Believes pain is associated with suffering, punishment, and lack of repentance	Religious background influences beliefs about pain.	Spiritual distress: related to religious beliefs about pain
Despairing	Robbed of sleep and energy, client is irritable and is prevented from doing enjoyable activities: so preoccupied with pain that client excludes all pleasures, fights pain in self-defeating ways.	Spiritual distress: despair related to pain
Lacks an enriched personal life	Unable to participate in social, occupational, and recreational functions that add quality to life.	Spiritual distress: impaired quality of life related to pain

PLANNING

Long-Term Goals

To be free of pain that interferes with daily functioning and achievement of life goals

To decrease focus on pain through pain management

SHORT-TERM GOALS	OUTCOME CRITERIA
Physical Dimension To accept some pain	1. Discontinues doctor shopping for a cure for pain 2. States that he thinks he has taken reasonable steps to reduce pain and nothing further can be done 3. Says, "I'll learn to live with it" with conviction 4. Identifies stressors that trigger pain and takes measures to avoid or prevent their occurrence
Emotional Dimension To express feelings of pain	1. Verbalizes feelings of pain 2. Describes duration, severity, intensity of pain 3. Verbalizes feelings about pain 4. States ways pain interferes with life-style 5. Identifies other feelings associated with pain: anger, helplessness
Intellectual Dimension To identify sources of pain	1. Names situations or events that precipitate pain 2. Links situations or events to pain
To identify relationship of stress and conflicts to pain	1. Names stressful events and conflicts that contribute to pain
To state relief measures for pain	1. Identifies ways for relieving pain: (a) recreationally, (b) diversionally, (c) noninvasively
To state openly and directly what is wanted	1. Does not manipulate, using pain, to meet needs
To cope with pain effectively	1. Identifies work-related goals 2. Changes area of work if no longer able to perform job 3. Builds a positive identity for self with new work or new skills 4. Does not feel sorry for self or elicit sympathy from others 5. Participates in fun activities 6. Looks forward to pleasurable activities as a time-out from pain

PLANNING—cont'd

SHORT-TERM GOALS	OUTCOME CRITERIA
	7. Improves social relationships
	8. Listens to others' problems
	9. Allows self limited time to experience pain when severe
	10. Uses self-hypnosis and relaxation techniques to deal with pain
Social Dimension	
To relate to others without pain complaints	1. Forms relationships with others
	2. Decreases focus on pain in relating to others
Identifies impact of culture on pain	1. Verbalizes ways culture influences pain responses
To increase confidence in own ability to control or manage pain	1. Demonstrates confidence in managing or controlling own pain
To use multiple methods of pain management: music, relaxation, imagery, social interactions	1. Uses multiple methods for pain management
	2. Used community resources for pain management
Spiritual Dimension	
To use religious faith for comfort	1. Goes to church, temple, or other religious setting for comfort
To seek relationships and activities that provide pleasure and diminish focus on pain	1. Participates in relationships and activities that promote pleasure and enrich client's life

Discharge Planning

The following client behaviors demonstrate readiness for discharge:
1. Verbalizes situations that influence the occurrence and severity of pain
2. Uses diversional and recreational activities to reduce pain
3. Uses noninvasive pain relief measures (relaxation, imagery)
4. Verbalizes the role of stress in pain behavior
5. Knows community resources available for receiving treatment and counseling for pain

IMPLEMENTATION

NURSING ACTIONS	RATIONALE
Physical Dimension	
1. Promote adequate nutrition by relieving nausea and vomiting associated with pain.	To maintain adequate nutritional status and show interest and concern for client's well being.
2. Provide comfort measures that promote sleep: hygienic measures, position, room temperature, decaffeinated drinks, reduced noise level, nonconstricting bedding.	To promote a relaxed state and provide a respite from pain.
3. Encourage client to pursue hobbies, interests, and recreational activities.	To refocus attention away from self and pain with activities that are pleasurable.
4. Monitor factors that increase or decrease pain, for example, activities, persons, noise, inattention.	To provide a base for interventions.
5. Encourage physical exercise.	To increase level of pain tolerance.
6. Establish a baseline pain tolerance level, then set exercise quotas below tolerance level and systematically increase until exercise quota is attained.	To decrease client's perception of pain and increase level of tolerance for pain.

NURSING ACTIONS	RATIONALE
7. Observe closely for medication abuse, suspected addiction, or severe habituation.	To prevent drug addiction.
8. Monitor closely for alcohol abuse for pain relief.	To prevent alcohol addiction.
9. Give pain medication on fixed time schedules around the clock and independent of client needs for medication to lessen the individual's systemic association with the occurrences of pain.	To decrease actual pain perception and promote comfort.
10. Prepare and assist client with any diagnostic tests for pain.	To prevent increasing anxiety that may trigger pain.
11. Reinforce results of diagnostic tests after physician discusses results with client.	To decrease anxiety and reinforce reality of the facts.
12. Prevent suicidal acts when client despairs over severity of pain and lack of cure for it.	To prevent client from impulsive acts of self-destruction.
13. Observe client at different times to determine intensity of pain and relief measures.	To obtain a baseline for interventions by noting site, frequency, type, duration, possible causes, contributing factors and feelings prior to onset of pain.
14. Use of pain flow sheet to monitor pain and medications used to relieve it (see below).	To provide a daily record of pain, the time, severity, medications, vital signs, and client response.
15. Use a daily diary to monitor pain and medications with relation to activities (see p. 68).	To provide a daily record of pain and assist client to become aware of relief measures.
16. Provide distractions (games, television, rubs, massages, conversation).	To help client focus on other activities.
17. Refer to specialist to provide transcutaneous electrical nerve stimulation (TENS).	To alleviate pain.
18. Refer to pain clinic.	To help client understand own pain, discuss it with others, receive support, and learn to live with it.

Emotional Dimension

1. Listen to client's expressions of anguish, suffering, anger, depression, fears, feelings of inadequacy, and helplessness.	To show concern and interest and obtain a baseline for interventions.
2. Empathize with client ("You are hurting," "Nothing seems to help") to convey understanding.	To demonstrate understanding of client's pain.
3. Promote client's expression of anger at what is happening, rather than at persons involved with client, as a motivator to do something for self.	To promote self-awareness, to help client assume responsibility for initiating relief measures, to preserve interpersonal relationships.
4. Assist client in finding other ways to express feelings when stressed: for example, physical activity, tearing up telephone books, pounding pillows.	To provide outlets for expression of feelings that are appropriate for the client.
5. Provide information to reduce anxiety and fears related to pain: fear of addiction to medications, fear of losing control, fear that medication will not be effective, fear that family doubts client's pain.	To reduce client's fears about pain and lessen preoccupation with pain.
6. Remain with client and give emotional support when client is angry or despairing.	To set limits if angry and to provide hope if despairing by using the therapeutic use of self.

PAIN FLOW SHEET

Time	Pain Rating	Medication	R	P	BP	Response

Pain rating: A number of different scales may be used. Indicate which scale is used and use the same one each time. Two common examples: 0 to 10 with 0 being no pain and 10 being the most severe. Scale 0 = no pain, 1 = mild; 2 = discomforting; 3 = distressing; 4 = horrible; 5 = excruciating.

DAILY DIARY

Date: _____   Name: _____

Time	Major Activity	Pain Medication Taken	Other Pain Relief Method	Pain Estimate*
Midnight 12				
1				
2				
3				
4				
5				
6				
7				
8				
9				
10				
11				
Noon 12				
1				
2				
3				
4				
5				
6				
7				
8				
9				
10				
11				

*Scale: 0 to 10 with 0 being no pain and 10 being the most severe. Comments.

NURSING ACTIONS	RATIONALE
Intellectual Dimension	
1. Involve the client in establishing goals for pain management.	To increase feelings of control and autonomy by participating in making decisions about care.
2. Explore conflict situations with client.	To shed insight on possible causes or contribution factors of pain.
3. Be honest with client: explain that nothing more can be done to relieve the pain.	To help client face reality.
4. Listen to complaints.	To gather data about severity of pain.
5. Distract client from preoccupation with pain by listening to music, engaging in activities, or interacting with supportive persons.	To promote interest in other activities and lessen the concern with pain.
6. Teach client ways to manage pain: relaxation, biofeedback, yoga, medication, skin stimulation (heat and cold application), massage, imagery, music, activities.	To promote responsibility for relief of pain and become less dependent on others or medications.
7. Use behavior modification techniques.	To reinforce healthy responses to pain.
8. Explore with client effective ways to cope with pain by asking client what helps and what does not.	To give client several alternatives to cope with pain, to increase feeling of power and control.
9. Be aware of your response to client with pain. Disbelief, annoyance, or lack of concern may be communicated to client.	To prevent personal feelings about pain from interfering with your care of client.
10. Explore with client the nonverbal message of the statement, "I want out of these responsibilities."	To gain an understanding of client's reasons for pain; for some, secondary gains are beneficial.
11. Enhance client's verbal communication to the point where client feels ready to face conflicts.	To promote clear, direct communication of wants and needs without using pain.
12. Promote client's participation in decisions.	To increase feelings of having control of self and ability to manage pain.
13. Administer pain questionnaire (see below).	To gather data about client's pain.
14. Avoid judgmental statements.	To remain objective and establish a therapeutic relationship.
15. Explain relationship of pain to physical findings.	To present reality and help client accept the findings as accurate.
16. Foster client's motivation and willingness to participate in new treatments.	To stimulate client to consider several different options for dealing with pain.
Social Dimension	
1. Increase self-esteem by emphasizing client's positive attributes, skills, talents.	To bolster client's self-concept and help client feel more "in charge" in order to prevent invalidism.
2. Assist client in designing actions and activities that promote a healthy identity rather than one that confirms an identity as a suffering person.	To promote positive self-concept.

PAIN QUESTIONNAIRE

1. Describe in your own words your discomfort.
2. What are you doing that adds to your discomfort?
3. What can you do to lessen your discomfort?
4. What activities or habits does your discomfort prohibit you from doing?
5. What is the frequency of your discomfort?
6. What is the nature of your discomfort? Throbbing, sharp, dull, or what?
7. What is the duration of your discomfort?
8. What other feelings do you have that accompany this discomfort?
9. How often do you have pain-free periods? What is the length?
10. Approximately how old were you when you first felt any similar discomfort?
11. What do others do when you have discomfort?
12. How do others know that you have discomfort?
13. Has anyone in your family had similar discomfort? If so, describe.
14. Were you considered a healthy child?
15. What are your most enjoyable hobbies? When did you last participate in these?
16. What happens to your discomfort if you relax?
17. Does tension add to your discomfort?
18. If your pain were magically removed, how would your life be different?

IMPLEMENTATION—cont'd

NURSING ACTIONS	RATIONALE
3. Provide activities and tasks that client can do with others.	To feel useful, to experience pleasure with others, to distract from pain.
4. Recognize client's perception of self as unable to cope.	To demonstrate empathy.
5. Help client be aware that irritable, pain-filled behavior toward others promotes isolation and alienation.	To help client gain insight about own behavior and its effect on others.
6. Assist client in enlarging support systems.	To prevent a sense of aloneness.
7. Encourage client to take responsibility for own life, with or without pain by communicating confidence in client.	To prevent incapacity from pain and to increase autonomy.
8. Prevent manipulation to obtain medications.	To avoid possibility of addiction, to confront client with own manipulative behavior.
9. Be aware of pain games client plays with family and health care providers.	To prevent manipulation.
10. Prevent client from obtaining secondary gains with pain.	To prevent dependency and invalidism.
11. Enlist support of family in treatment of client's pain.	To broaden support system and help family understand client's pain behavior. To prevent family from contributing to it.
12. Teach family ways to prevent reinforcing pain behavior and providing secondary gains by including them in the treatment plans.	To support client in efforts to deal with pain at home and in functioning in usual roles.
13. Teach those in working environment ways to prevent reinforcing pain behavior.	To support client in efforts to deal with pain at work and function at optimum level.
14. Explore with client ways in which pain leads to freedom from responsibilities.	To promote awareness of secondary gains.
15. Be sensitive to cultural meanings associated with pain (for example, it is acceptable for men to cry in some cultures).	To demonstrate sensitivity to cultural influences that affect the expression of pain.
16. Promote acceptable responses to pain.	To help client respond to pain in ways that do not alienate others.
17. Be aware of iatrogenic factors that reinforce pain behavior.	To prevent the treatment from creating other serious problems, for example, addiction to a medication.
18. Have client talk with others who have successfully managed their pain.	To receive support and maintain hope.
19. Explore with client environmental factors that precipitate pain.	To gather data for interventions.
20. Promote control over daily activities by allowing client to make own decisions.	To motivate client toward autonomy and independence in spite of pain.

Spiritual Dimension

NURSING ACTIONS	RATIONALE
1. Explore with client the meaning of pain and suffering (for example, punishment for sins).	To support client's endeavors to find meaning in pain and suffering.
2. Be aware that each client has own unique responses to pain.	To individualize care.
3. Avoid imposing judgments of client's pain from your point of reference.	To promote the idea that client is the expert on own pain and to avoid alienating client.
4. Encourage client to participate in life, to endure some pain, and to realize ways to move beyond pain.	To add quality to client's life, to prevent despair.
5. Assist client in participating in activities and events that provide a feeling of significance to life, in spite of pain.	To promote a sense of worthwhileness and importance.
6. Provide reassurance to client and family while client is learning to cope and find meaning in pain.	To support both client and family in their endeavors to cope.
7. When client is alone or alienated from others refer client to clergy or other religious leader to explore meaning of pain. When client is alone or alienated from others.	To provide spiritual comfort.
8. Instill attitude that pain has meaning, that no individual is without merit, usefulness, and significance.	To enhance client's self-concept.

NURSING ACTIONS	RATIONALE
9. Help client accept self with limitations (pain) and continue with life.	To be accepting of self with limitations helps client to accept others with their limitations and may strengthen relationships, thus enhancing the quality of life.
10. Use analogies and parables to help client find meaning and purpose in pain, for example, the biblical story of Job.	To increase self-awareness and expand client's thinking.
11. Share personal experiences with client when time and occasion are appropriate.	To self-disclose demonstrates you are human with limitations also, as well as strengths.
12. Listen to client's discussion of religious beliefs about pain without arguing or belittling ideas.	To gather data about client's beliefs about pain.
13. If client is suicidal, explore reasons to continue living in spite of pain (see suicide behavior).	To provide positives in the client's life that may motivate client toward life.

EVALUATION

Measurable goals and outcomes provide the basis for evaluating the amount of pain in the client's life and the amount of relief client feels with pain reduction measures. Both verbal and nonverbal responses from the client provide clues about the effectiveness of the client's management of pain. Nurse observations and reports from the family add additional data for evaluation. The following behaviors indicate a positive evaluation:

1. Shows awareness of situations or events that trigger pain
2. Manages pain with appropriate reduction techniques such as recreation, diversional activities, music, or imagery
3. Accepts the fact that some pain is inevitable
4. Knows community resources available for treatment and counseling

BIBLIOGRAPHY

Broome A: A psychological approach to chronic pain, *Nurs Times* 80(6):136, 1984.

Covino N: The pain clinic: hypnosis and the management of pain, *Hosp Practitioner* 20(2):486, 1985.

Cowan P, Lovasik D: American chronic pain association: strategies for surviving chronic pain, *Orthop Nurs* 9(4):47, 1990.

Escobar P: Management of chronic pain, *Nurs Pract* 10(1):24, 1985.

Geach G: Pain and coping, *Image* 19(1):12, 1987.

Graber R: Stopping pain before it's chronic, *Patient Care* 18(2):51, 1984.

Graffam S, Johnson A: A comparison of two relaxation strategies for the relief of pain and its distress, *Pain Sympt Manage* 2:292, 1987.

Grainger S: No cause, no cure . . . but he's still in pain, *RN* 50:43, 1987.

Gruber M, Beavers F, Amodeo D: Trying to care for the great pretender, *Nurs Grand Rounds* 17:76, 1987.

Jamison R, Sbrocco R, Parris W: The influence of physical and psychosocial factors on accuracy of memory for pain in chronic pain patients, *Pain* 37:289, 1989.

Jenkins P: Psychogenic abdominal pain, *Gen Hosp Psychiatry* 13:27, 1991.

Koeze T, Williams A, Reiman S: Spinal cord stimulation and the relief of chronic pain, *J Neurol Neurosurg Psychiatry* 50:1424, 1987.

Kores R: Predicting outcome of chronic pain treatment via a modified self-efficacy scale, *Behav Res Ther* 28:165, 1990.

McCaffery M, Beebe A: *Pain: clinical manual for nursing practice,* Philadelphia, 1989, Mosby—Year Book.

Miller T, Kraus R: An overview of chronic pain, *Hosp Community Psychiatry* 41:433, 1990.

Murphy K: Prediction of chronicity in low back pain, *Arch Phys Med Rehabil* 65(6):334, 1984.

Pilowski I, Barrow C: A controlled study of psychotherapy and amitriptyline used individually and in combination in the treatment of chronic intractable psychogenic pain, *Pain* 40:3, 1990.

Roy R: Pain clinics: reassessment of objectives and outcomes, *Arch Phys Med Rehabil* 65(8):448, 1984.

Sherman R: Phantom pain: a lesson in the necessity for careful clinical research on chronic pain problems, *J Rehabil Res Dev* 25:vii, 1988.

Weh-Hsein W: *Pain management, assessment, and treatment of chronic and acute syndromes,* New York, 1987, Human Sciences Press.

Wood D, Weisner M, Reiter R: Psychogenic chronic pelvic pain: diagnosis and management, *Clin Obstet Gynecol* 33:179, 1990.

Compulsions

Compulsions are repetitive and seemingly purposeful behaviors that are performed according to certain rules or in a stereotyped fashion and are contrary to a person's wishes and standards. The behavior is designed to produce or prevent some future event or situation. However, either the activity is not connected in a realistic way with what it is designed to produce or prevent, or it may be clearly excessive. The activity is performed with a driving force. The individual generally recognizes the senselessness of the behavior and does not derive pleasure from carrying out the activity although it provides release from tension. The most common compulsions are hand washing, counting, checking (for example, to see if doors are locked or if stove is turned off), and touching.

Compulsions differ from obsessions. Obsessions are recurring or persistent ideas or thoughts that invade the consciousness and are experienced as repugnant or senseless. Compulsions are the acts that may follow the obsessions. Obsessions and compulsions are generally grouped together as obsessive-compulsive behavior. The two are discussed separately in these guidelines to provide an understanding of each.

Compulsive (ritualistic) behaviors can range from mild forms, which are viewed as normal and healthy and permit the person to function well in a situation that requires orderliness, frugality, and neatness, to forms that are severe and cause almost total incapacitation of a person's ability to function.

Related DSM-III-R disorders

Obsessive-compulsive disorder
Schizophrenia
Organic mental disorders
Anxiety disorders
Paraphilias

Other related conditions

Drinking
Gambling
Overeating
Undereating
Excessive use of antianxiety medications
Stealing
Setting fires

PRINCIPLES

▶ Physical Dimension

1. Compulsive behaviors can cause serious physical problems when the behaviors are exhausting or excessive.

▶ Emotional Dimension

1. Anxiety is discharged through compulsive behavior.
2. Relief of the anxiety is only transient.
3. Although transient, the relief brought about by performance of the compulsive act reinforces the act.
4. The psychogenesis of compulsive behavior lies in a disturbance in normal growth and development during the period of 1 to 3 years of age.
5. A specific ritualistic act reduces the anxiety attached to the compulsion.
6. Rituals and compulsive acts prevent, control, and undo the effects of forbidden thoughts and impulses.
7. Fears and tensions are often disguised in ritualistic acts.
8. Preventing the compulsive act may result in terror for the client.

▶ Intellectual Dimension

1. Conflict plays an integral part in the development of compulsive behavior.
2. Conflicts arise from an individual's conscience and unacceptable desires.
3. An underdeveloped conscience may be a cause.
4. Compulsive behavior is a substitute for the verbal expression of anxiety.
5. Defense mechanisms of isolation and reaction formation determine the quality and characteristics of compulsions.
6. The person recognizes the compulsion as irrational and as a threat.
7. A relationship exists between compulsive behavior and magical thinking.
8. Compulsive acts are attempts to control or modify a primary obsession.
9. The more chronic and fixed the symptom pattern, the less amenable the disorder is to modification.
10. The usefulness of psychotherapy for the compulsive client depends on:
    a. Prominence of situational precipitating events
    b. Ability to relate to others
    c. Stable work patterns
    d. Ability to tolerate stress
    e. Ability to express emotions
    f. Intelligence
    g. Ability to be introspective
    h. Flexibility in thinking and behaving
    i. Supportive social network

▶ Social Dimension

1. Compulsions, since they reduce anxiety, are self-perpetuating.
2. The learned pattern of behavior (ritualistic act) blocks the learning of new and adaptive behavior.
3. Compulsions are ego alien (foreign to a person's perception).
4. Compulsive behavior occurs as a drive to do a procedure in the same way.
5. Compulsive acts may be reinforced by keeping the person from certain uncomfortable situations.
6. Because of its usefulness in reducing anxiety, the act becomes a learned behavior pattern.

▶ Spiritual Behavior

1. The compulsive person has little personal freedom for change or growth.
2. Security and relief from anxiety are primary goals, which prevent risk taking and involvement in new experiences.
3. The obsessive-compulsive individual has a strong sense of justice, honesty, property, and rights.

ASSESSMENT

▶ Physical Dimension

I. History
  A. Activities of daily living
     1. Nutrition
        a. Compulsion to eat
        b. Compulsion to vomit
     2. Sleep
        a. Rituals on getting up or at bedtime
     3. Physical activities and limitations
        a. Excessive handwashing
        b. Excessive touching
        c. Excessive exercising
           (1) Running
           (2) Jogging
           (3) Working out with weights
     4. Sexual activity
        a. Paraphilias
  B. Habits
     1. Alcohol
        a. Compulsion to drink
     2. Medications
        a. Misuse of antianxiety medications
  C. Destructive behavior
     1. Impulsive acts
     2. Aggressive acts
     3. Violent acts
     4. Self-mutilation
     5. Stealing
     6. Gambling
     7. Setting fires
     8. Overeating
     9. Vomiting

▶ **Physical Examination**

CLIENT DATA	ANALYSIS	NURSING DIAGNOSIS
Excessive cleanliness	Overemphasis on tidiness and neatness based on disturbances in the period of development from 1 to 3 years: may pose a threat to health.	Ineffective individual coping: compulsion related to need for excessive cleanliness
Grooming rituals	Relief from anxiety is felt through performance of ritual, which becomes fixed as a pattern of behavior; anxiety is discharged through compulsive behavior.	Ineffective individual coping: compulsions related to grooming rituals

▶ **Emotional Dimension**

CLIENT DATA	ANALYSIS	NURSING DIAGNOSIS
Disguises anxiety	High level of anxiety is disguised in symbolic acts.	Ineffective individual coping: compulsions related to high level of anxiety
Feels guilty	Feels he or she has done something wrong and compulsive act will atone for the sin and reassure that things are all right; rituals prevent, control, undo effects of forbidden thoughts and impulses.	Ineffective individual coping: compulsions related to guilt
Is emotionally distant, formal, sober	Refrains from expression of emotions. Control enhances sense of security and protects from feelings of helplessness in a world full of unpredictables and unpleasant surprises.	Ineffective individual coping: compulsions related to overcontrol of emotional expression
Lacks spontaneity in emotional expression	Has restricted ability to express warm and tender emotions.	Ineffective individual coping: lack of spontaneity in emotional expression related to compulsiveness
Is obstinate, stubborn when challenged or contradicted	Insists that others submit to his or her way. Lacks awareness of feelings elicited by own behavior.	Ineffective individual coping: obstinacy and stubbornness related to compulsiveness
Fears he or she will harm someone or something	Often expresses unconscious fears in a disguised form through symbolism.	Ineffective individual coping: disguised fears related to compulsive acts

▶ **Intellectual Dimension**

CLIENT DATA	ANALYSIS	NURSING DIAGNOSIS
Denies feelings	Has limited ability to express feelings; compulsion is substitute for verbal expression of anxiety.	Ineffective individual coping: compulsive behavior related to denial of feelings
Uses isolation, undoing, reaction formation, regression, and magical thinking	Person protected from anxiety by use of defense mechanisms.	Ineffective individual coping: compulsive behavior related to excessive use of defense mechanisms
Has doubts	Is indecisive, wards off feared consequences of ideas and forbidden urges.	Ineffective individual coping: compulsive behavior related to doubts
Is cautious, deliberate, thoughtful in approach to life and problems	Has valued characteristics, which may become a liability when carried to an extreme that leads to dysfunction.	High risk for ineffective individual coping: excessively cautious related to compulsions

▶ Intellectual Dimension—cont'd

CLIENT DATA	ANALYSIS	NURSING DIAGNOSIS
Emphasizes reason and logic at expense of feelings and intuition	Has limited ability to express emotions, is overly controlled.	Altered thought processes: excessive reason and logic related to compulsive behavior
Is objective, avoids being carried away with enthusiasm	Has limited ability to express emotions.	High risk for altered thought processes: rigidly objective and lacks spontaneity related to compulsive behavior
Shows steadiness of purpose and reliability, is conscientious	Has valued characteristics, which become liabilities when excessive.	High risk for altered health maintenance: excessive reliability, conscientiousness related to compulsive behavior
Shows cautiousness, likes predictability	Has valued characteristics, which relieve anxiety. Client inflexible and not open to new ideas when behavior is excessive.	High risk for altered health maintenance: excessive cautiousness related to compulsive behavior
Needs to control self and others	Fears consequences of urges and impulses or fears making a mistake; rituals prevent anxiety, control and undo effects of forbidden urges and desires.	Ineffective individual coping: need to control related to compulsive behavior
Uses seemingly nonsensical words	Wards off underlying impulses.	Impaired verbal communication: use of nonsensical words related to compulsiveness
Uses long, involved sentences with many stereotyped expressions	Is preoccupied with trivial details, rules, order, organization, schedules, and lists.	Impaired verbal communication: use of long, involved sentences related to compulsive behavior
Ends conversation with difficulty, will come back and add information	Strives for perfection. To be sure message is understood, goes on and on with it; is driven to complete message.	Impaired verbal communication: difficulty ending a conversation related to compulsive behavior
Relies on rational argument	Has limited ability to express feelings.	High risk for impaired verbal communication: rational argument related to compulsive behavior
Talks in intellectual terms	Uses isolation as a defense mechanism to protect from underlying feelings.	High risk for impaired verbal communication: use of intellectualization related to compulsive behavior
Recalls events in detail with painful attention to accuracy and completeness	Strives for perfection.	Impaired verbal communication: excessive attention to detail related to compulsive behavior
Resists hurrying, cutting time short	Change threatens security; preventing completion of compulsion may result in terror.	Ineffective individual coping: resistiveness related to compulsive behavior
Adheres rigidly to preconceived plan of action.	Change threatens comfort and security.	Ineffective individual coping: rigid adherence to preconceived plans related to compulsive behavior

▶ Social Dimension

CLIENT DATA	ANALYSIS	NURSING DIAGNOSIS
Has low self-esteem	Alleviates feelings of inadequacy and insecurity with compulsive acts and rituals.	*Altered self-concept: related to compulsive behavior
Has strong dependency needs	Wants reassurance that impulses and urges are not out of control.	Ineffective individual coping: dependence related to compulsive behavior
Lacks ability to develop warm, meaningful relationships	Has limited ability to express emotions.	Impaired social interaction: inability to form warm, meaningful relationships related to compulsive behavior

▶ **Social Dimension—cont'd**

CLIENT DATA	ANALYSIS	NURSING DIAGNOSIS
Has impaired social role functioning	Insists that others submit to his or her way; lacks awareness of the feelings elicited by this behavior, which interferes with social and occupational functioning.	Altered role performance: related to compulsive behavior
Shows excessive devotion to work and productivity	Excludes pleasure and meaningful relationships; avoids anxiety of interpersonal relationships. Is driven to complete tasks.	Ineffective individual coping: excessive devotion to work related to compulsive behavior
Is bothered by changes in environment (e.g., rearranged furniture)	Becomes anxious with any deviation from usual.	Ineffective individual coping: anxiety with changes in the environment related to compulsive behavior
Needs to control environment	Gets comfort and security from "a place for everything and everything in its place."	Ineffective individual coping: need to control related to compulsive behavior
Manages own resources frugally, is stingy	Is stingy and miserly, does not part with possessions.	Ineffective individual coping: frugality, stinginess related to compulsive behavior.

▶ **Spiritual Dimension**

CLIENT DATA	ANALYSIS	NURSING DIAGNOSIS
Has strong sense of justice, honesty, property, and rights	Shows rigid thinking. Alienates others with rigid, fixed conclusions.	High risk for spiritual distress: excessive sense of justice, honesty, property, and rights related to compulsive behavior
Has impaired creativity and spontaneity	Prevents spontaneity and creativity with ritualistic acts. Gets comfort and security from sameness. Lacks personal freedom to change and grow.	Spiritual distress: impaired creativity and spontaneity related to compulsive behavior

PLANNING

Long-Term Goal

To cope with anxiety adaptively without compulsive behavior

SHORT-TERM GOALS	OUTCOME CRITERIA
Physical Dimension	
To maintain physical health	1. Maintains physical health 2. Wears gloves if handwashing is excessive 3. Reduces need for antianxiety medications
To decrease compulsive behavior	1. Demonstrates fewer episodes of compulsive actions 2. Shows awareness of need for compulsions by discussing anxiety with nurse 3. Controls compulsive actions 4. Gives self decreasing amounts of time to perform rituals if unable to control them 5. Recalls events with less detail
Emotional Dimension	
To identify anxiety underlying compulsive acts	1. Recognizes own anxiety 2. Identifies behaviors related to anxiety 3. Links anxiety to compulsive acts

SHORT-TERM GOALS	OUTCOME CRITERIA
To express genuine feelings	1. Expresses feelings of anxiety 2. Decreases intellectual responses 3. Shows enthusiasm 4. Shows warmth in relationships 5. Demonstrates affection
Intellectual Dimension To gain insight about fears and anxieties that cause compulsive acts	1. Verbalizes events and conflicts that precede an increase in anxiety and result in compulsive behavior 2. Discusses possible causes of anxiety 3. Develops awareness of conflicts 4. States what is being threatened and subsequent conflict 5. Relates present experience to past experiences with anxiety and compulsive behavior 6. States ways anxiety was reduced in the past 7. Identifies effective relief measures
Social Dimension To improve relationships with others	1. Expects less than perfection from self and others 2. Shows concern for others and less for self 3. Decreases workaholic behavior 4. Has less need to control others 5. Shows trust in others and has fewer doubts
Spiritual Dimension To experience a more spontaneous, creative way of life	1. Becomes less controlling of self and others 2. Enjoys the unpredictable and surprises 3. Shows more flexibility in thinking

Discharge Planning

The following client behaviors demonstrate readiness for discharge:
1. Deals with anxiety without compulsions
2. Increases quality of relationships
3. Uses relaxation techniques to reduce anxiety
4. Monitors self for increasing anxiety

IMPLEMENTATION

NURSING ACTIONS	RATIONALE
Physical Dimension	
1. Prevent potential self-imposed injuries (wears gloves for excessive handwashing).	To promote and maintain health status.
2. Treat self-imposed injuries (skin lotion on reddened hands).	To prevent further injury.
3. Allow adequate time to perform rituals or compulsive actions.	To interrupt or stop the ritual may result in increased anxiety or terror.
4. Refrain from interfering with compulsive actions.	To avoid increasing client's anxiety.
5. Prevent aggressive, violent, and self-destructive anxiety and removing client to a less stimulating environment.	To prevent harm to client or others.
6. Be aware of compulsions that result in illegal acts, for example, gambling, setting fires, stealing.	To understand legal implications of behavior.
7. Provide a structured environment to minimize anxiety and compulsive acts.	To promote security that comes with knowing schedule of daily activities.
8. Focus on the person, not the compulsion.	To acknowledge the person.
9. Watch for events that increase anxiety and rituals.	To gather data on possible factors that contribute to increased anxiety and ritualistic behavior.

IMPLEMENTATION—cont'd

NURSING ACTIONS	RATIONALE
10. Watch for activities that relieve rituals.	To gather data on possible factors that may relieve anxiety and ritualistic behavior.
11. Assign tasks that can be completed with a degree of perfection (folding towels, blankets).	To use client's perfectionistic qualities constructively.
12. Encourage client to assume responsibility for own health care (e.g., wear gloves).	To promote independence and autonomy.

Emotional Dimension

NURSING ACTIONS	RATIONALE
1. Observe client for mounting anxiety, and when possible intervene before the compulsive behavior begins.	To prevent need for compulsive behavior and increase client's awareness of anxiety.
2. Be aware that anxiety is disguised and may not be observable.	To understand that anxiety is outside of the client's conscious awareness.
3. Help client decrease anxiety or fears underlying the compulsive behavior by using stress reduction techniques.	To reduce the anxiety lessens the need for compulsions.
4. Assist client in feeling safe expressing feelings by using empathy statements.	To facilitate client's expression of feelings and decrease the need for the compulsive act.
5. Promote spontaneity in expressing feelings through jokes and funny stories.	To increase effectiveness and help client be a more feeling person.
6. Give positive feedback when feelings are expressed.	To reinforce positive behaviors.
7. Refrain from challenging stubbornness and obstinacy.	To prevent threatening client and increasing anxiety.
8. Weigh value of intervening in behavior that protects client from mental anguish against need to prevent physical harm caused by behavior.	To consider the implications of interventions, whether it is more essential to prevent physical damage or emotional pain.
9. Encourage client to ventilate feelings in ways that are appropriate for client.	To individualize care. It may be counterproductive to expect client to express feelings in a way that is inappropriate (culturally) for him or her.
10. Avoid pressure and prying.	To prevent threatening the client and increasing his or her anxiety.
11. Help client laugh and use humor.	To help client learn to have fun, to decrease client's serious, unemotional nature.

Intellectual Dimension

NURSING ACTIONS	RATIONALE
1. Avoid calling attention to compulsive acts.	To minimize the act. Client knows he or she is engaging in a compulsive act; reminders increase client's anxiety about them.
2. Assist client in identifying concerns and stressors.	To gather data about possible factors that contribute to anxiety.
3. Allow specific periods of time (for example, 10 minutes) for client to focus on concerns. Then encourage client to attend to other ideas. Gradually reduce time (e.g., to 5 minutes every 2 hours).	To help client set limits on own behavior.
4. Help client identify alternative methods for dealing with anxiety underlying the compulsion, e.g., physical activity or talking with a supportive person.	To increase client's repertoire of effective coping skills.
5. Verbally support client's efforts to decrease compulsions.	To reinforce positive behavior.
6. Avoid focusing of nonsensical use of words.	To minimize attention to compulsions.
7. Acknowledge nonverbal behavior.	To promote client's awareness of behavior.
8. Set reasonable limits	To allow client to meet expectations with minimum anxiety.
9. Listen attentively to client to understand difficulty client has in ending a conversation.	To let client know you are listening yet will need to set limits on the conversation.
10. Deal with the communication problem (client is a stickler for details, for example).	To set limits on client's striving for perfection with message.
11. Help client say directly what he or she wants.	To help client eliminate nonessential details and clarify communication.

NURSING ACTIONS	RATIONALE
12. Discuss original anxiety; what is the conflict?	To increase self-awareness; to plan interventions.
13. Develop alternatives to deal with original conflict.	To offer other options for dealing with the compulsions that are socially acceptable and contribute to emotional health.
14. Be time-conscious and consistent when making contacts.	To set limits on behavior.
15. Offer information about rituals and compulsions in everyday life.	To relieve client of anxiety about those that are useful and nonpathological.
16. Assist client in identifying ways of dealing with compulsions.	To help client consider other options for dealing with compulsions.
17. Discuss the compulsion following an episode since comfort level is increased at this time.	To increase learning. Learning takes place best when anxiety is low.
18. Help client decrease need to be perfect.	To let client know it is OK to make mistakes.
19. Teach relaxation techniques.	To reduce anxiety and need for compulsions.
20. Explore with client the purpose that the behavior fulfills in client's life.	To promote self-awareness in client.
21. Reinforce short, to-the-point conversations.	To give positive feedback for appropriate behavior.
22. Use desensitization techniques.	To reduce anxiety.
23. Stimulate client's motivation and willingness to participate in treatment by allowing client to participate in decisions about treatment.	To promote responsibility for own mental health. To increase sense of control and autonomy.

Social Dimension

1. Assure client that impulses and urges will not get out of control.	To increase feelings of safety and trust. Fears may be out of client's conscious awareness; thus your attitude and behavior will be more assuring than your words.
2. Work with dependence problem (see Dependence, p. 122).	To promote a sense of control and decrease feelings of resentment often associated with dependence. With decreased dependence client may experience feelings of closeness with another person.
3. Increase self-esteem by decreasing anxiety and subsequent compulsive actions.	To reduce anxiety boosts client's confidence in self as a capable and competent person.
4. Encourage client to share more of self and possessions.	To experience the pleasure of giving, both of self and things.
5. Refrain from changing environment, e.g., rearranging furniture.	To prevent increased anxiety. Sameness contributes to security.
6. Provide neat, orderly environment.	To reduce anxiety about tidiness.
7. Protect from criticism or ridicule by others.	To prevent lowering of self-esteem.
8. Provide group therapy.	To help client express feelings, change behavior, and receive support.
9. Refer to Alcoholics Anonymous, Gamblers Anonymous, or Overeaters Anonymous if appropriate.	To receive group support and learn about client's illness.
10. Avoid lengthy discussions of stealing; quietly and calmly have client return items to owners.	To make restitution.
11. Include client's family in treatment.	To help family understand client's illness and learn ways to deal with it.

Spiritual Dimension

1. Identify realistic strengths in client, such as strong sense of honesty, justice, property, and rights.	To boost self-esteem.
2. Promote self-satisfactions and pleasures in life by stimulating creativity and newness.	To help be comfortable with new activities and relationships, to expand client's horizons.
3. Increase quality of relationships with capacity for intimacy by teaching listening and communication skills.	To help client enjoy the satisfactions of close and intimate relationships.

EVALUATION

Measurable goals and outcome criteria provide the basis for evaluating progress or lack of progress in working with persons demonstrating compulsive behavior. Client self-reports, nurse observations, and family reports provide additional data about the client. Flow charts are useful in obtaining a baseline indicating the number of times per day or hour a particular behavior has occurred, events preceding the behavior, and relief measures used.

The following behaviors indicate a positive evaluation:

1. Identifies conflict situations
2. States when he or she feels anxious
3. Copes with anxiety without compulsive behavior
4. Uses adaptive coping skills
5. Shares feelings with others
6. Forms satisfying relationships with others.

BIBLIOGRAPHY

Barron J: Compulsive disorders: how to help when your patient has lost control, *Nurs* 21(10):83, 1990.

Boyd M: Polydipsia in the chronically mentally ill: a review, Arch *Psychiatr Nurs* 4(3):166, 1990.

Bromley S: Washing the pain away . . . compulsive neurosis, *Nurs Mirror* 156(22):43, 1983.

Griest J: Spotting the obsessive-compulsive, *Patient Care* 24(9):47, 1990.

Guthrie P: The mystery illness that was making me bald: "trichotillomania," the irresistable impulse to pull out one's own hair, *Good Housekeeping* 210(3):68, 1990.

Information about obsessive-compulsive disorder, *Patient Care* 24(9):74, 1990.

Isoniazid-related obsessive-compulsive neurosis (case study), *Nurses Drug Alert* 15(1):7, 1991.

Manley G: Treatment and recovery for sexual addicts, *Nurs Pract* 15(6):34, 1990.

Runck B: Research is changing views on obsessive-compulsive disorders, *Hosp Community Psychiatry* 34(7):597, 1983.

Schaffer S: The sexual addict: a challenge for the primary care provider, *Nurse Pract* 15(6):25, 1990.

Simoni P: Obsessive-compulsive disorder: the effect of research on nursing care, *J Psychosoc Nurs Ment Health Serv* 29(4):19, 1991.

Confusion

Confusion is a condition characterized by inattention and memory deficits, inappropriate verbalizations, disruptive behavior, noncompliance, and failure to perform activities of daily living. The individual lacks awareness of own position in terms of time, space, or other people and is unable to concentrate on the here and now.

Confusion can be categorized by origin, type of onset (rapid or slow), duration of symptoms, degree of severity, prognosis for recovery, and age of client. Confusion may be acute, temporary, reversible, or irreversible, or it may be a hopeless and permanent dementia. It is a constellation of behaviors, which include disorientation, decreased attention span, restlessness, anxiety, fright, verbosity, confabulation, rambling speech, belligerence, combativeness, and loss of memory.

Causes of confusion are numerous. Nurses can plan treatment for the confused client after making a holistic assessment of the client and knowing the medical diagnosis.

Related DSM-III-R disorders

Organic mental disorders
Panic disorder
Posttraumatic stress disorder
Psychogenic amnesia
Psychoactive substance use disorders

Other related conditions

Crisis situations
Infectious diseases (fever)
Alcohol intoxication and withdrawal
Drug intoxication and withdrawal
Brain tumor, lesion, or disease (Alzheimer's disease)
Brain injury
Any systemic illness affecting the brain (meningitis)
Arteriosclerosis
Toxic substances (insecticides, heavy metals)
Postoperative psychosis
Nutritional deficiencies
Natural disaster
Relocation (to a nursing home)
Culturally related conflicts
Side effects of prescribed medication
Metabolic imbalances
Dehydration
Pain

PRINCIPLES

▶ Physical Dimension

1. Confusion may be related to aging process.
2. Confusion arises from pathological conditions involving circulation, oxygenation, and metabolism of brain tissues.
3. Confusion associated with senile dementia—Alzheimer's type (SDAT) is not reversible.
4. With perceptual changes, the individual undergoes reality distortion and confusion.
5. Normal decline in capacity for mental functioning and subsequent confusion can be accelerated by illness or physical impairment.
6. A narrow range of temperature, pressure, nutrients, fluid, chemicals, and minerals exists for the brain to maintain physiological equilibrium.
7. The capacity for confusion exists when there are systemic problems that interfere with cerebral support, mechanical problems (obstruction), and presenile irreversible dementias.
8. Choline, a vitamin of the B complex, may slow the mind-destroying disease process and the resulting confusion.
9. Confusion varies with time, as in the "sundown syndrome" in which elderly clients suddenly become confused at night.
10. Sensory deficits (visual, hearing, tactile) contribute to confusion.

11. Altered physiological states contribute to confusion.
12. Confusion may be a side effect or reaction to medications.
13. Sensory overload or sensory deprivation can result in confusion.

▶ Emotional Dimension

1. Confusion is common during crisis states.
2. Feelings of helplessness and loss of control contribute to confusion.
3. Grief and depression lead to confused thinking.
4. Confusion is a characteristic of panic states.
5. An adolescent may be confused about his or her identity.
6. Confused clients may be excessively suspicious.

▶ Intellectual Dimension

1. Cognitive functions such as memory, reason, abstract thinking, calculation, judgment, and ability to follow directions are affected when the client is confused.
2. Distortions in cognition are seen in delusions and hallucinations and contribute to confused thinking.
3. The client's perception of changes reflects an ability to evaluate reality or become confused.
4. Language differences promote confusion.
5. The confused person has a faulty memory and the capacity to learn is compromised.
6. Lack of information and absence of newspapers, clocks, radios, and family members or friends contribute to confusion.

▶ Social Dimension

1. Lack of success in interacting with the environment may lead to confusion.

2. How successful a client is in interacting according to the expectations of others determines if the client will be judged as confused, whether or not he or she is.
3. Confused behavior can be produced by reinforcement.
4. Judgments made about confused behavior need to take into account the influence of historical events, aging, life-style, words, language, and culture.
5. Confusion may be based less on specific disease than on combined effects of poor nutrition, loneliness, and social deprivation.
6. Environmental factors (relocation, cultural change, catastrophe, or loss of familiar objects) contribute to confusion.
7. Loss of support system, as in rejection or separation, may evoke confused states.
8. Affectional relationships (people or pets who give and receive love) may prevent confusion by presenting reality.
9. Feelings of incompetency may create confusion.
10. Confusion often occurs at times of sociocultural stress.
11. A sense of independence and autonomy is decreased in the confused client.

▶ Spiritual Dimension

1. Confusion is lessened when values are clarified.
2. Every person has a basic need for a relationship with another person to experience love, forgiveness, and hope. At times, because of confusion, this relationship seems unreachable.
3. Confusion impairs the individual's ability for self-actualization.
4. Confusion leads to a loss of a sense of intactness and worthiness.

ASSESSMENT

▶ Physical Dimension

I. History
A. Activities of daily living
  1. Nutrition
     a. Inadequate food and fluid intake
     b. Vitamin deficiency
     c. Anemia
     d. Dehydration
  2. Sleep
     a. Dozes frequently
     b. Wanders at night
     c. Is drowsy
  3. Physical activities and limitations
     a. Is easily fatigued
     b. Is unaware of limitations
     c. Has less physical energy
     d. Shows restless, aimless motions
B. Habits
  1. Medications and drugs
     a. Takes many medications
     b. Misuses or abuses prescribed medications
C. Destructive behavior
  1. Physical neglect of self
     a. Leg ulcers
     b. Cellulitis
     c. Ingrown toenails
     d. Bleeding gums
     e. Chronic diarrhea
  2. Impulsive, combative, assaultive
  3. Noncompliance with medications, treatment, diet

D. Health history
  1. Illnesses
     a. Infections
     b. Metabolic disturbances
     c. Neurological conditions
     d. Drug intoxication
     e. Cardiovascular and respiratory distur-
        bances
     f. Drug and alcohol withdrawal
     g. Seizures
  2. Injuries
     a. Trauma
     b. Accidents
  3. Surgery
     a. Postoperative psychosis

E. Genetic factors
  1. Family history of organic mental disorders
F. Review of systems
  1. Neurological
     a. Memory loss
     b. Disorientation
     c. Short attention span
     d. Decreased concentration

II. Diagnostic tests
A. Blood studies
B. Urinalysis
C. EEG
D. Brain scan
E. Computerized axial tomography (CAT)
F. Laboratory workup related to physical history
   and findings from physical examinations

▶ **Physical Examination**

CLIENT DATA	ANALYSIS	NURSING DIAGNOSIS
Malnourished	With drug or alcohol abuse, forgets to eat. Decline in mental functioning is accelerated with illness or physical impairment.	Altered nutrition: less than body requirements related to confusion
Neglected personal hygiene, untidy grooming, and disheveled clothes	Impaired cognitive functions interfere with ability to perform self-care.	*Altered self-care: related to confusion
Inappropriate verbalizations	Difficulty with comprehension, attention, relevancy, and orientation.	Impaired verbal communication: related to confusion
Loss of skin turgor	Lessened elasticity with dehydration.	Fluid volume deficit: related to confusion
Tooth decay, lack of oral hygiene	Self-neglect; forgets oral hygiene; cognitive functions such as memory are affected when client is confused.	*Altered self-care: related to confusion
Increased or decreased blood pressure Pulse changes	Cardiovascular and altered physiological states contribute to confusion	Altered thought processes: confusion related to cardiovascular disturbances
Increased or decreased body temperature	Physiological dysfunction contributes to confusion.	Altered thought processes: confusion related to increased or decreased body temperature
Bladder or bowel incontinence	Genitourinary functions affected with confused states.	Altered patterns of urinary elimination: bladder or bowel incontinence related to confusion

▶ **Emotional Dimension**

CLIENT DATA	ANALYSIS	NURSING DIAGNOSIS
Is dazed, irritable, cantankerous, frightened, apprehensive, belligerent, anxious, or depressed	Changes in usual methods of functioning are threatening and provoke many different kinds of feelings.	Anxiety: related to changes in ability to function normally
Is hostile, angry, and assaultive	Inability to handle situation; becomes angry, hostile, and assaultive.	Ineffective individual coping: anger, hostility, and assaultiveness related to confusion
Is fearful and suspicious	Attempts of others to redelegate individual's responsibilities lead to fear and suspiciousness.	Fear: related to confusion

▶ **Emotional Dimension—cont'd**

CLIENT DATA	ANALYSIS	NURSING DIAGNOSIS
Lacks spontaneity in expressing feelings	Possible effect of depression.	Ineffective individual coping: lack of spontaneous expression of feeling related to confusion
Overreacts	Loss of ability to control emotions.	Ineffective individual coping: overreaction related to confusion
Is labile	Loss of ability to control emotions; may go from irritation to uncontrollable laughter.	Ineffective individual coping: lability related to confusion
Has inappropriate moods	Loss of ability to control moods.	Ineffective individual coping: inappropriate mood related to confusion
Fears losing control	Decreased ability to function evokes fear of losing control.	Ineffective individual coping: fear of losing control related to confusion
Fears abandonment	Lonely and alienated; confusion results from combined effects of poor nutrition, loneliness, and social deprivation.	Ineffective individual coping: fear of abandonment related to confusion

▶ **Intellectual Dimension**

CLIENT DATA	ANALYSIS	NURSING DIAGNOSIS
Is confused at night	Loss of familiarity with surroundings and darkness increase confusion, "sundown syndrome"; changes in perceptual functioning distort reality.	Sensory/perceptual alteration: confusion related to darkness
Interprets stimuli inaccurately	Impaired cognitive functioning.	Sensory/perceptional alteration: inaccurate interpretation of stimuli related to confusion
Hallucinates	Overwhelming anxiety or impaired cognitive functioning.	Sensory/perceptual alteration: hallucinations related to overwhelming anxiety.
Impaired recent memory	Impaired cognitive functioning.	Altered thought processes: impaired recent memory related to confusion
Disturbed ability to learn	Impaired cognitive functioning.	Altered thought processes: impaired ability to learn related to confusion
Impaired orientation with time, place, person	Impaired cognitive functioning.	Altered thought processes: disorientation related to confusion
Impoverished fund of information	Impaired cognitive functioning.	Altered thought processes: impoverished fund of information related to confusion
Decreased judgment abilities	Impaired cognitive functioning.	Altered thought processes: decreased ability to make judgments related to confusion
Has fluctuating levels of awareness	Impaired cognitive functioning.	Altered thought processes: fluctuating levels of awareness related to confusion
Altered abstractions	Thinking tends to become concrete with brain damage or lesions (for example, OMD).	Altered thought processes: inability to abstract related to confusion
Has delusions	Severe anxiety or impaired cognitive functioning.	Altered thought processes: delusions related to severe anxiety
Has limited comprehension	Impaired cognitive functioning.	Altered thought processes: decreased comprehension related to confusion

▶ **Intellectual Dimension—cont'd**

CLIENT DATA	ANALYSIS	NURSING DIAGNOSIS
Regresses	Retreat to a lower level of functioning physically, emotionally, intellectually, socially, and spiritually to protect self and reduce anxiety.	Defensive coping: regression related to confusion
Confabulates	Makes up information to fill in gaps in memory loss.	Altered thought processes: confabulation related to confusion
Uses blocking	Stops in the middle of a thought; may be a painful thought or associated with memory loss.	Altered thought processes: blocking related to confusion
Uses profanities	Lack of ability to control expressions.	Altered thought processes: uses profanities related to confusion
Makes inappropriate responses	Impaired cognitive functioning.	Altered thought processes: inappropriate responses related to confusion
Is easily distracted	Impaired concentration and short attention span.	Altered thought processes: easy distractibility related to confusion
Has rigid responses	Difficulty dealing with new situations and events; sameness is comfortable.	Ineffective individual coping: rigid thinking related to confusion
Lacks tolerance for unusual or unexpected	Impatient and demanding.	Ineffective individual coping: intolerance for the unusual or unexpected related to confusion

▶ **Social Dimension**

CLIENT DATA	ANALYSIS	NURSING DIAGNOSIS
Has lowered self-esteem	Feels worthless and incapable when usual functioning is altered because of confusion.	*Altered self-concept: feels worthless related to confusion
Is cautious, guarded, and suspicious of others	Impaired cognitive functioning.	Impaired social interaction: cautious, guarded, and suspicious relationships with others related to confusion
Has conflicts with family members over perceived injustices	Perceptual disturbances create family conflicts.	Altered family processes: conflicts with family over perceived injustices related to confusion
Is avoided by family members	Regressed behavior alienates and embarrasses family.	Altered family processes: avoidance by family members related to confusion
Decreased independence	Associated with regressed behavior or reinforcement of regressed behavior.	Ineffective individual coping: dependence with regressed behavior or reinforcement of regressed behavior related to confusion
Decreased ability to perform social roles	Impaired cognitive functioning.	Altered role performance: decreased ability to perform social roles related to confusion
Is socially disdained	Impaired social relationships. Behavior is peculiar and bizarre.	Social isolation/withdrawal: scorn and rejection in social relationships related to confusion
Changed social role	Confusion impairs usual role behaviors.	Altered role performance: changed social role related to confusion
Needs light at night	To prevent further confusion.	Ineffective individual coping: confusion related to inadequate lighting
Needs assistance with walking	To prevent wandering.	Impaired home maintenance management: unsafe walking related to confusion

▶ **Social Dimension—cont'd**

CLIENT DATA	ANALYSIS	NURSING DIAGNOSIS
Hardship on family members	Impaired functioning results in hardship on family members who are required to share additional tasks and responsibilities.	Altered family processes: potential for family breakdown related to confusion
Family lacks ability to supervise confused person	Family members' lack of knowledge and skills contributes to inadequate supervision.	Impaired home maintenance management: related to family's inability to supervise confused person
Family is unable to hire help	Lack of finances prevents the family from hiring help.	Impaired home maintenance management: related to family's inability to hire help to meet confused person's needs
Family lacks the knowledge or is unable to use neighbors, churches, and community resources to help with confused client	Alienation from neighbors, churches, and community resources robs family of supportive persons.	Impaired home maintenance management: related to family's inability to use neighborhood resources to help with confused person

▶ **Spiritual Dimension**

CLIENT DATA	ANALYSIS	NURSING DIAGNOSIS
Decreased ability to participate in valued activities and relationships	Impaired cognitive functioning.	Spiritual distress: decreased ability to participate in usual activities and relationships related to confusion
Conflicts when unable to participate in valued activities and relationships	Frustration and anger with self and others.	Spiritual distress: conflicts when unable to participate in valued activities and relationships related to confusion
Has feelings of despair and hopelessness	Confusion prevents participation in valued activities and relationships, with resulting despair and hopelessness	Hopelessness: related to confusion
Unable to learn alternatives or replace valued activities and relationships	Impaired cognitive functioning, difficulty learning.	Spiritual distress: inability to learn alternatives or replace valued activities and relationships related to confusion
Unable to participate in religious activities	Needs assistance in participating.	Spiritual distress: inability to participate in religious activities related to confusion
Impaired sense of achievement, individualism, and productivity	Impaired cognitive functioning.	Spiritual distress: impaired sense of achievement, individualism, and productivity related to confusion
Impaired aesthetic sense	Dependent on caregiver's ability to focus on kinship, loyalty, belonging, mutual dependence, and sense of worth as a person.	Spiritual distress: impaired aesthetic sense related to confusion

PLANNING

Long-Term Goal

To maintain contact with reality and an optimal level of functioning

SHORT-TERM GOALS	OUTCOME CRITERIA
Physical Dimension	
To maintain optimal physical well-being	1. Eats regular meals of nutritious foods 2. Drinks adequate amounts of fluids 3. Has regular bowel movements 4. Exercises daily 5. Sleeps 6 to 8 hours each night without interruption 6. Bathes or showers self regularly
To participate in activities of daily living at an optimal level of functioning	1. Is able to dress and groom self, with assistance if indicated 2. Is able to get to dining room for meals 3. Is able to eat meals, with help if necessary 4. Takes medications as prescribed 5. Spends time in an activity or diversion 6. Uses telephone appropriately
Emotional Dimension	
To demonstrate reduced lability (anger, panic, rage, fear)	1. When feeling upset or frustrated, verbalizes this to a supportive person 2. Responds to instructions for reducing intense feelings 3. Withdraws from others when feelings are out of control 4. Does not injure others or destroy property
To lessen fears/suspiciousness	1. Relates with trust to nurse and others 2. Verbalizes fears and apprehensions 3. Responds appropriately to information about fears and apprehensions
Intellectual Dimension	
To decrease confusion and maintain contact with reality	1. Verbalizes name, date, and place 2. Wears own clothes and jewelry 3. Uses own furniture when possible 4. Wears clothing appropriate for weather 5. Listens to radio, watches TV, and talks with others 6. Shows interest in surroundings and activities 7. Shows increased concentration 8. Shows increased attention span 9. Responds to instructions 10. Participates in decisions 11. Is able to think rationally
Social Dimension	
To demonstrate socially acceptable behavior	1. Tells no risqué or distasteful jokes 2. Eats properly, with help if necessary 3. Urinates and defecates appropriately 4. Controls emotional expressions of anger and hostility 5. Limits own unacceptable behavior 6. Recognizes behavior that stimulates rejection
Spiritual Dimension	
To prevent despair and feelings of hopelessness	1. Humorously accepts own mistakes and limitations 2. Expresses feelings of despair and hopelessness 3. Spends time with others whose company is enjoyed 4. Feels pleasure from involvement in activities

Discharge Planning

The following behaviors demonstrate readiness for discharge:
1. Demonstrates optimal contact with reality
2. Maintains optimal level of functioning in self-care activity
3. Participates in activities and relationships with others at optimal level

IMPLEMENTATION

NURSING ACTIONS	RATIONALE
Physical Dimension	
1. Provide genetic counseling for those in child-rearing ages when there is a genetic predisposition to organic mental disorders.	To provide information about genetic influences for potential parents.
2. Provide familiar objects for client (own clothes, furnishings, bedspread, and family pictures).	To maintain what is familiar to the client and prevent increased confusion.
3. Involve client in simple repetitious activities.	To reduce confusion. Sameness and repetition lessen confusion.
4. Use touch when appropriate.	To provide warm, human contact.
5. Promote activities in which success is achievable.	To increase client's self-esteem.
6. Provide physical exercise alternating with periods of rest.	To prevent confusion associated with physical impairment.
7. Monitor medication regimen.	To gather data regarding side effects of medications that may contribute to confusion.
8. Promote optimal physical well-being: nutrition, rest, activity, sleep, and self-care.	To prevent confusion from increasing when there is general debilitation.
9. Provide care for physiologically induced confusion (drug toxicity, infection, or alcohol withdrawal) as prescribed.	To promote reality and restore client to previous level of functioning.
10. Limit naps in daytime so client will sleep better at night.	To eliminate confusion following daytime naps.
11. Support day-night rhythms.	To follow the body's natural circadian rhythms.
12. Supervise one-to-one if client attempts to wander.	To ensure client's safety.
13. Allow client sufficient time to complete tasks.	To prevent confusion resulting from being hurried.
14. Provide night lights.	To lessen confusion at night.
15. Provide clocks, calendar, direction signs, and daily schedule.	To minimize disorientation, lessen frustration
16. Use color to help client identify room (linen, bedding).	To minimize disorientation.
17. Provide a reality board with date, time, weather, and menu on it.	To minimize disorientation.
18. Provide assistance with self-care when indicated.	To promote personal grooming and increase self-esteem.
19. Keep furniture and possessions in the same place.	To prevent confusion by maintaining sameness.
20. Tape list of daily care activities to bathroom mirror.	To promote self-responsibility.
21. Encourage client to wear and use a watch.	To minimize disorientation and promote independence.
22. Promote use of eyeglasses and hearing aid.	To promote accurate sensory stimulation.
23. Decrease glare from lights or sunlight.	To reduce visual distortions.
24. Speak slowly and face client when conversing with him or her.	To allow client to see and hear clearly.
Emotional Dimension	
1. Be consistent, make few demands, and lessen decision making.	To reduce anxiety and resulting confusion.
2. Refrain from a hurried, harrassed attitude with client.	To avoid increasing confusion.
3. Accept client's irritability, hostility, and anger when expressed as a response to frustration.	To promote client's expression of feelings and provide empathy and understanding.
4. Prevent anxiety from escalating and increasing confusion by anticipating client's needs.	To intervene before client loses control.
5. Provide information about what to expect (nature of tests, hospital policies) briefly and concisely.	To prevent anxiety.

NURSING ACTIONS	RATIONALE
6. Withdraw client physically or psychologically from source of discomfort.	To help client learn to control emotional lability.
7. Assist client in avoiding situations that are anxiety producing.	To prevent increased confusion.
8. Listen attentively to expressions of sadness or loss.	To clarify reality of loss.
9. Empathize with client demands, impatience, and intolerance.	To let client know you understand and to be supportive.
10. Decrease agitation and frustration with comforting, relaxing measures.	To reduce confusion and provide a sense of caring.

Intellectual Dimension

NURSING ACTIONS	RATIONALE
1. Give client specific written instructions for diet, medications, and treatments.	To prevent increased confusion and promote autonomy.
2. Call client by name frequently and identify yourself by name at each interaction.	To present reality.
3. State time and date, as appropriate.	To present reality.
4. Focus on real events, situations, people, and things.	To prevent confusion associated with abstractions and philosophical discussions.
5. Express doubt when reality is disturbed.	To help client question own perception.
6. Avoid direct confrontation when reality is disturbed until a relationship is established.	To prevent disruption of therapeutic relationship. Confrontation before relationship is established may interfere with trust.
7. Set limits for discussing repetitive topics.	To avoid focusing on topics that client is confused about.
8. Explain tasks in short, simple steps and repeat key words.	To reinforce what is said.
9. Tell client expectations directly.	To present information so that it is unlikely to be misinterpreted.
10. Avoid requesting unnecessary decisions.	To prevent increasing anxiety that may be contributing to confusion.
11. Avoid whispered comments that can be misinterpreted.	To prevent increasing confusion.
12. Validate with client your interpretation of what is being communicated.	To clarify communication.
13. Use familiar terminology.	To prevent further confusion.
14. Use communication that maintains client's individuality ("I" instead of "we").	To help client distinguish between self and others.
15. Acknowledge client's presence even if client does not acknowledge your presence.	To present reality.
16. Refrain from belittling or derogating when client misinterprets stimuli or confabulates.	To prevent further decrease in client's self-esteem.
17. Provide magazines, books, newspapers, and television.	To increase intellectual stimulation.
18. Explain any changes in schedules or activities.	To increase tolerance for the unexpected.
19. Give positive feedback when efforts are made to control demands, outrages, and profanities.	To reinforce appropriate behavior.
20. Help client ask for desired outcomes and communicate feelings.	To promote clarity in communication.
21. Be congruent in verbal and nonverbal communication.	To provide consistency. Client will be confused by discrepancy between verbal and nonverbal behavior.
22. Repeat orienting information frequently in a kind tone of voice.	To present reality without demeaning client.
23. Listen closely to client and correct gently in a nonpunitive manner if information is confabulated, if important.	To present reality. Refrain from confrontation if information is insignificant.
24. Teach client to use lists and appointment books.	To minimize forgetfulness.
25. Introduce changes slowly.	To allow client time to integrate new information.
26. Gain client's attention before trying to communicate.	To allow client time to focus on communication.
27. Focus on areas of competent functioning.	To reinforce strengths and promote successful achievements.
28. Motivate client to assume as much responsibility for own health care as appropriate.	To prevent increasing dependence and assist client to function at highest possible level.

IMPLEMENTATION—cont'd

NURSING ACTIONS	RATIONALE
Social Dimension	
1. Identify client's personal space and territory when relocated.	To prevent confusion associated with new environment.
2. Allow client time for self-evaluation (self-understanding and self-identity).	To promote self-awareness and encourage reflection.
3. Promote affection for client from family and friends by role modeling touch and humor.	To provide warmth and caring from familiar persons.
4. Provide social interactions with familiar people.	To prevent further confusion.
5. Walk with the client who wanders aimlessly, providing guidance, safety, and companionship.	To provide safety and help maintain a sense of reality.
6. Refrain from confronting with two or more nurses when client is wandering.	To prevent client from being overwhelmed.
7. Provide group therapy, socialization groups, remotivation groups, reality groups, reminiscent therapy, and groups with a special focus (music, art, poetry, current events, and plants).	To present reality and reinforce appropriate behavior.
8. Provide family of client a way to grieve over client if institutionalized and confusion is increasing or condition is deteriorating.	To promote healthy grieving in family members.
9. Identify family strengths for working with confused client.	To build on the family strengths while intervening.
10. Plan a division of labor using friends, neighbors, and community members.	To relieve family members of total responsibility and allow them time for their own lives.
11. Provide a safe environment; consider lighting, fire hazards, stairs, cooking arrangements, thermostats, and cigarettes.	To protect client from harm.
12. Plan with client if relocation is indicated for hospitalization or nursing home.	To provide anticipatory guidance to client and lessen the confusion associated with new environment.
13. Help family maintain traditions and include client as much as possible.	To promote continuation of family traditions that client is accustomed to.
14. Provide social and cultural experiences with those of similar beliefs.	To prevent confusion associated with new people and experiences.
15. Refrain from promoting change in client within other social or cultural groups.	To prevent anxiety associated with change.
16. Prevent overstimulation by people or environment.	To lessen feelings of being overwhelmed with resulting confusion.
17. Use rewards (smile, touch, nod, praise) to strengthen desired behavior.	To reinforce appropriate behavior.
Spiritual Dimension	
1. Provide for meeting client's physical, emotional, intellectual, social and spiritual needs to form a basis for unconditional acceptance of client.	To promote feelings of value and worth.
2. Promote a caring attitude that does not cause distress: a firm handshake, prompt response to requests, warm voice, unhurried manner.	To lessen anxiety and resulting confusion.
3. Encourage client to continue participation in activities client values and gains pleasure from.	To maintain contact with reality.
4. Help client attend church regularly if appropriate, and sit in the same area.	To lessen confusion from a new seating arrangement.
5. Refrain from requests that client change ideas or beliefs by associating with or participating in experiences that are foreign or intolerable to client.	To prevent confusion resulting from new ideas or experiences.
6. Promote a sense of hope and confidence in client by sharing feelings of affection, concern, small pleasures, and humor.	To help client maintain contact with reality through a relationship with a caring person.
7. Promote attention to beauty of nature with walks outside focusing on sights, smells, and sounds.	To promote reality, to appreciate nature, to lessen self-preoccupation.

EVALUATION

Measurable goals and outcome criteria provide the basis for evaluating progress or lack of progress in the confused client. Nurse observations and family reports provide additional data about the client. The following behaviors indicate a positive evaluation:

1. Maintains contact with reality
2. Functions at an optimal level
3. Participates in usual activities
4. Interacts socially and appropriately with others

BIBLIOGRAPHY

Bolin K: Assisting the states of neurological patients, *Am J Nurs* 77:1478, 1977.

Burnside I: *Psychosocial care of the aged,* New York, 1980, McGraw-Hill Book Co.

Cook E: Is it dementia or depression? *RN* 48(3):40, 1985.

Coyle M: Organic illness mimicking psychiatric episodes, *J Gerontol Nurs* 13(1):31, 1987.

Dacey R et al: Relative effects of brain and non-brain injuries on neuropsychological and psychosocial outcomes, *J Trauma* 31(2):217, 1991.

Frommelt P et al: Familial Alzheimer disease: a large multi-generation of German kindred, *Alzheimer Dis Assoc Dis* 5(1):36, 1991.

Jeste D: *Neuropsychiatric dementias: current perspectives,* Washington, D.C., 1986, American Psychiatric Press, Inc.

Jury M, Jury D: *Gramp: a man ages and dies,* New York, 1976, Grossman Publishers.

Kremer K: Dealing with confused patients, *Nurs '79* 91(11):40, 1979.

Mayers K, Griffin M: The play project: use of stimulus objects with demented patients, *J Gerontol Nurs* 16(1):82, 1990.

Nawakowski L: Disorientation—signal or diagnosis? *J Gerontol Nurs* 6(4):197, 1980.

Pamara N: Memory dysfunction: the benign forgetfulness of age and true dementias, *Consultant* 24(11):136, 1984.

Parva J: Sundown syndrome, *RN* 53(7):46, 1990.

Paterson J: The elderly confused patient, *Aust Nurses J* 14(3):42, 1984.

Richerson K: Right brain—left brain: the nurse consultant and behavior change following stroke, *J Psychiatr Nurs Ment Health Serv* 20(5):37, 1980.

Swanson B, Cronin-Stubbs D, Colletti J: Dementia and depression in persons with AIDS: causes and care, *J Psychosoc Nurs Ment Health Serv* 28(10):33, 1990.

Weiler K, Buckwalter K: Care of the demented client, *J Gerontol Nurs* 14(7):26, 1988.

Wolanin M, Phillips L: *Confusion: prevention and care,* St. Louis, 1981, Mosby—Year Book.

Conversions

Conversions are a type of mental disorder characterized by a loss or alteration in physical functioning, which is an expression of severe psychological conflict. Coping with the conflict is psychological in nature and characterized by physical symptoms (such as paralysis or blindness) that have no organic basis. Conversions, which usually appear suddenly, are not controlled voluntarily. They differ from malingering, a deliberate deception in which the person presents a nonexistent symptom.

The client achieves primary gain by keeping an internal conflict out of awareness, which results in a reduction in anxiety. Secondary gains are achieved by avoiding a distasteful activity and getting support from the environment that otherwise may not be forthcoming. Often the client shows an indifference to the symptoms *(la belle indifference)*, which may produce secondary gains by winning sympathy and relieving the client of unpleasant responsibilities.

Related DSM-III-R disorders

Somatization disorder
Conversion disorder
Somatoform pain disorder
Hypochondriasis
Histrionic personality disorder

Other related conditions

Paralysis
Vomiting
Blindness
Deafness
Seizures

PRINCIPLES

▶ Physical Dimension

1. The symptoms cannot be explained by a known physical disorder or pathological condition.
2. The appearance of a physical symptom without an underlying organic basis leads to a reduction in anxiety.
3. The physical symptom symbolizes the inner conflict.
4. The physical symptom is not under voluntary control.
5. Conversions are mediated by the sensorimotor system.
6. Conversions permit expression of forbidden wishes but are disguised so as not to be recognized by the person having them or by others.

▶ Emotional Dimension

1. Conversions are pathological adaptations to anxiety.
2. The initial conversion episode results in reduction of psychological pain.
3. Conversions arise from conflicts of a sexual nature originating in childhood during the period of sexual identity development (3 to 5 years).

▶ Intellectual Dimension

1. Conversions occur when defense mechanisms are unsuccessful and anxiety remains high.
2. The physical symptoms are viewed as nonverbal body language intended to communicate a message to significant persons.
3. Conversions serve to communicate dependence needs.
4. The conversion expresses conflict that is unconscious.
5. Conversions represent a splitting off from consciousness (dissociation) of painful feelings and their associated ideas.

▶ Social Dimension

1. Repressed sexual drives and dependence may be related to conversions.
2. The symptoms bring certain advantages to the client (secondary gains) and gratify dependence needs.
3. The psychological relief obtained reinforces the conversion response that produced the relief and predisposes the person to repeat the same response each time anxiety and conflict occur; thus

the behavior pattern becomes chronic.

4. Environmental stressors and the client's response to them are considered an important aspect in conversions.
5. Conversions remove a person from threatening or disturbing situations.
6. Conversions provide a new way of relating, through the sick person role.
7. The unconscious goal is to obtain the status of a sick person.
8. The sick person role is not easily relinquished because of associated benefits.
9. Learned helplessness behavior is seen in those whose frail, seductive, or passive behaviors as children were reinforced.

10. Conversion behavior is used to control and manipulate interpersonal relationships.
11. Conversion behavior is shaped and reinforced by environmental circumstances.

▶ **Spiritual Dimension**

1. Sick behavior is valued by the person with conversions.
2. Conversion behavior stifles personal growth by preventing awareness of inner conflicts and by allowing the person to avoid dealing with them directly.
3. The person with conversions has not learned to live in a satisfying manner with self or others.

ASSESSMENT

▶ **Physical Dimension**

I. **History**
  A. Activities of daily living
    1. Physical activities and limitations
      a. Loss of impaired functioning
        (1) Vision
        (2) Hearing
        (3) Speech
        (4) Arm or leg movement
    2. Sexual activity
      a. Impotence
      b. Inorgasmic
  B. Review of systems
    1. Ears
      a. Loss of hearing
    2. Eyes
      a. Loss of vision
    3. Gastrointestinal
      a. Vomiting

    4. Reproductive
      a. False pregnancy
    5. Musculoskeletal
      a. Loss of function in arm or leg
      b. Atrophy
      c. Contracture
    6. Neurological
      a. Seizures
      b. Pain
      c. Loss of sensation

II. **Diagnostic tests**—any diagnostic test to rule out physical basis for symptoms
  A. Vision test
  B. Hearing test
  C. Pregnancy test
  D. X-ray examination
  E. Neurological examination

▶ **Physical Examination**

CLIENT DATA	ANALYSIS	NURSING DIAGNOSIS
Loss of or impaired vision	Physical symptom of converted anxiety; symbolic of inner conflict; unconscious goal is to gain status of sick person.	Ineffective individual coping: conversion related to anxiety with loss of vision
Loss of or impaired hearing	Physical symptom of converted anxiety; symbolic of inner conflict.	Ineffective individual coping: conversion related to anxiety with loss of hearing
Unsteady gait	Physical symptom of converted anxiety; symbolic of inner conflict.	Ineffective individual coping: conversion related to anxiety with unsteady gait
Paralysis (arm or leg)	Physical symptom of converted anxiety; symbolic of inner conflict.	Ineffective individual coping: conversion related to anxiety with paralysis
Loss of sensation	Physical symptom of converted anxiety; symbolic of inner conflict.	Ineffective individual coping: conversion related to anxiety with loss of sensation

▶ **Emotional Dimension**

CLIENT DATA	ANALYSIS	NURSING DIAGNOSIS
Lack of anxiety	Anxiety symbolically displaced to a physical symptom, which symbolizes an inner conflict.	Ineffective individual coping: conversions related to displaced anxiety
Lack of concern regarding severity of symptoms	Exhibits *la belle indifference,* a characteristic of conversions.	Ineffective individual coping: conversions with lack of concern regarding symptoms related to anxiety
Helplessness	Learned helplessness seen in those who received reinforcement for frailty.	Ineffective individual coping: conversions with helplessness related to anxiety

▶ **Intellectual Dimension**

CLIENT DATA	ANALYSIS	NURSING DIAGNOSIS
Conflicts	Unresolved and not in conscious awareness.	Ineffective individual coping: conversions related to unresolved inner conflicts.
Uses repression, reaction formation, and dissociation	To reduce anxiety (defense mechanisms).	Defensive coping: conversions related to anxiety

▶ **Social Dimension**

CLIENT DATA	ANALYSIS	NURSING DIAGNOSIS
Lowered self-esteem	High levels of anxiety contribute to low self-esteem	Self-esteem disturbance: related to anxiety with conversions
Helpless and dependent	Communicates message of "pay attention to me."	Ineffective individual coping: helplessness and dependence related to anxiety with conversions
Manipulative	Uses symptoms to influence others or to play on guilt of others and to control interpersonal relationships	Ineffective individual coping: manipulation related to anxiety with conversions
Impaired social role functioning	Conversions prevent normal life activity; prolonged loss of function produces complications (contractures or disuse atrophy).	Altered role performance: related to anxiety with conversions
Stormy and ungratifying relationships	Chronic sick person role interferes with healthy relationships; sick role is not easily relinquished because of associated benefits.	Impaired social interactions: related to anxiety with conversions
Stress-producing environmental factors	Temporal relationship exists between environmental stimuli and psychological need or conflict and the initiation of symptoms or exacerbation of them.	Ineffective individual coping: conversions related to stress-producing environmental factors

▶ **Spiritual Dimension**

CLIENT DATA	ANALYSIS	NURSING DIAGNOSIS
Believes self to be sick as evidenced in physical symptoms	Psychological invalidism, patterns of behavior difficult to relinquish.	Spiritual distress: psychological invalidism related to anxiety with conversions
Lacks feelings of worth, integrity, and value as a person	Locked into sick person role, which interferes with ability to find pleasurable outlets and to enjoy life.	Spiritual distress: lack of feelings of worth and value related to anxiety with conversions

PLANNING

Long-Term Goals

To develop healthy methods of coping with conflict without conversions
To resolve the conflict producing the physical symptom and resume an optimal
   level of functioning at home and in the community

SHORT-TERM GOALS	OUTCOME CRITERIA
Physical Dimension	
To identify the source of stress	1. Verbalizes conflicts and stressors in life
	2. Talks about what is important in life (persons, work, leisure, and events)
Emotional Dimension	
To express feelings about conflicts	1. Verbalizes feelings of sadness, anger, anxiety, and frustration appropriately
	2. Avoids long discussions on physical symptoms
Intellectual Dimension	
To identify relationship between conflict and physical symptom	1. Identifies conflict situations
	2. Identifies feelings of anxiety related to conflict
	3. Discusses responses to anxiety
	4. Links physical symptom to own response to anxiety
To relieve stress or conflict	1. Removes self from conflict situation; takes time off from work, seeks hospitalization
	2. Uses stress management techniques
To deal with conflict directly and without producing physical symptoms	1. Focuses discussions on feelings rather than physical symptoms
	2. Identifies physical symptoms as a way to cope with conflict
	3. Names other ways to deal with conflict
	4. Uses other ways to deal with conflicts
	5. Expresses feelings of satisfaction and achievement with chosen method of coping
	6. Identifies strategies for coping with future conflicts
Social Dimension	
To decrease secondary gains	1. Expresses feelings to supportive others
	2. Asks directly for what is needed, wanted, or desired
	3. Gives and takes in relationships with others
	4. Identifies helpless, dependent, and manipulative behaviors
	5. Sets limits on helpless, dependent, and manipulative behaviors
Spiritual Dimension	
To experience more pleasure in health and wellness than in sick behaviors	1. Verbalizes good feelings about health
	2. Demonstrates increasing ability to avoid sick role

Discharge Planning

The following client behaviors demonstrate readiness for discharge:
1. Expresses feelings directly
2. Identifies own anxiety
3. Uses stress-reducing measures to lessen anxiety
4. Verbalizes consequences of using physical symptoms to cope with emotional needs

IMPLEMENTATION

NURSING ACTIONS	RATIONALE
Physical Dimension	
1. Refrain from focusing on the symptom. ("Ignore the symptom, but not the person.")	To acknowledge the person and avoid reinforcing the physical symptom.
2. Assist client in focusing on other activities, persons, and environment rather than physical complaints.	To lessen preoccupation with symptoms and help client have relationships with people.
3. Assist with diagnostic tests.	To lessen anxiety and reinforce the information that there is no organic basis for the symptom.
4. Be aware that diagnostic tests themselves are a focus on the physical symptom and may produce secondary gains.	To understand that the test itself may reinforce the symptom.
5. Refrain from responding to client's complaints.	To prevent reinforcing symptoms.
6. Hospitalization of client may be necessary.	To relieve the stress of the conflict situation.
7. Observe and document carefully when symptoms occur.	To gather data and plan interventions.
8. Note precipitating events, effect of the environment, and recovery.	To gather data about onset of symptoms with relationship to what is happening in client's life.
9. Supervise client from a distance for ability to perform activities of daily living and ambulation.	To gather data when client is unaware of being observed.
10. Intervene if client is risking injury to self.	To prevent self-harm.
11. Refrain from allowing special privileges or excusing from expectations because of physical limitations.	To avoid reinforcing symptom and to prevent manipulation.
12. Assign tasks such as watering plants and other housekeeping chores on unit.	To keep client active and busy with useful tasks and in usual roles.
13. Expect client to carry on usual activities, self-care, and eating in dining room as other clients are expected to.	To prevent secondary gains from the symptoms, reduce sick role.
14. Be aware that client usually will not experience physical harm, injury, or deprivation.	To understand that client will not purposefully harm self.
15. Identify inappropriate behavior such as suicide gestures in a matter-of-fact way.	To avoid undue attention. A matter-of-fact approach allows nurse to listen to client without responding emotionally.
16. Encourage client to assume responsibility for own health by an expectation that client can and confidence that client will.	To motivate client towards health not sickness.
17. Be aware that symptoms may indicate organic disease.	To understand that symptom may have an organic basis and plan treatment that rules out any pathology.
Emotional Dimension	
1. Facilitate client's expression of feelings about the conflict, such as anger, resentment, or disappointment.	To help identify feelings and to gather data about possible factors that may contribute to symptoms.
2. Help client experience anxiety directly and identify behaviors associated with it (rapid breathing, dry mouth, and sweaty palms).	To assist client in identifying anxiety, help client acknowledge it as a normal and appropriate feeling in many situations and that it can be managed.
3. Give positive feedback for expressions of anxiety.	To reinforce appropriate expression of anxiety.
4. Focus client's discussion of feelings on home and work situations and relationships with others.	To avoid focusing on physical symptoms.
5. Reduce anxiety and conflicts (restrict visitors or remove from home or work).	To avoid focusing on physical symptoms.
6. Help client find acceptable ways to handle frustrations by physical exercise or talking about them.	To provide client with alternatives for dealing with feelings to promote mental health.

NURSING ACTIONS	RATIONALE
7. Refrain from allowing client to avoid frustrating or unpleasant responsibilities.	To prevent secondary gains.
8. Use empathy.	To convey understanding of burdens on client and facilitate expression of feelings.

Intellectual Dimension

NURSING ACTIONS	RATIONALE
1. Explore with client areas of anxiety and conflict.	To gather data about factors that may contribute to symptoms.
2. Explore with client alternative effective methods of dealing with conflict situations, e.g., problem solving or conflict resolution.	To promote healthy ways to handle conflicts—ways that do not cause behavioral symptoms.
3. Make expectations for client clear.	To specify clearly what you want client to do; for example, "Walk to the dining room," "Carry your own tray."
4. Refrain from arguing about expectations.	To avoid focusing on physical symptoms.
5. Withdraw attention from long discussions of physical symptoms or complaining behavior.	To avoid focusing on physical symptoms.
6. Set limits and stick to them.	To reinforce expectations. It is important that all team members know limits that have been set and consistently enforce them.
7. Focus discussions on home, work, and relationships with others.	To gather data on areas that tend to be problem areas.
8. Offer praise when client is able to discuss use of physical symptoms as a method of coping with conflict.	To reinforce ability to understand the problem.
9. Help client identify strategies to deal with or resolve conflicts.	To strengthen a sense of autonomy and independence.
10. Give feedback in terms of feelings when client is noted to be free of symptoms and looks relaxed.	To role model the expression of feelings in appropriate ways.
11. Listen to complaints to become knowledgeable about scope of complaint.	To avoid making hasty judgments about client's complaint.
12. Teach relaxation techniques (deep breathing, exercises, and visual imagery).	To help client manage anxiety.
13. Identify manipulative behavior such as the use of threats (suicide or fits of temper) in a matter-of-fact way when client is attempting to influence others or play on their guilt.	To increase awareness of client's behavior and ways it affects others.
14. Reinforce assertive behaviors.	To promote client's ability to state own desires and feelings.
15. Foster client's motivation to participate in treatment by being empathic and respectful.	To stimulate client to assume responsibility for maintaining own mental health.
16. Provide information that pain can be psychological as well as physical.	To increase client's understanding of symptoms.

Social Dimension

NURSING ACTIONS	RATIONALE
1. Give feedback to client about effects of complaining, demanding behavior on others.	To increase client's awareness of behavior and prevent alienation and isolation from others.
2. Increase client's ability to face problems directly by enhancing self-esteem.	To feel good about oneself helps a person to look at problem objectively and motivates client to do something about it.
3. Prevent client from obtaining secondary gains from physical symptoms by withdrawing attention to symptoms.	To prevent increased invalidism.
4. Discuss consequences of constant focus on symptoms.	To increase client's awareness of consequences of focusing on symptoms, for example, alienation from others, invalidism.
5. Direct interactions to others or the environment instead of to symptoms.	To promote interactions with others and prevent further invalidism.
6. Promote client's efforts to do something for someone else to divert attention from self.	To help client feel the pleasure that comes with helping others and to feel useful.
7. Provide therapy groups (feeling groups, group therapy, family therapy, occupational therapy, recreational therapy, or activity therapy).	To increase client's understanding of problem, help client change behavior and receive support.
8. Include family in treatment.	To promote awareness of secondary gains and ways family may be contributing to them.

IMPLEMENTATION—cont'd

NURSING ACTIONS	RATIONALE
9. Assist client in identifying relationship between timing of environmental stress or conflict and onset of symptoms or exacerbation of them.	To increase awareness of causative factors of an emotional rather than a physical nature.
10. Promote client's usual social roles; reinforce independent behaviors.	To prevent dependence, helplessness, and a chronic sick role.
11. Remove client from situation where reinforcement for symptoms is received, when appropriate.	To increase health behaviors.
Spiritual Dimension	
1. Help client accept anxiety and conflicts as part of life.	To help client experience life to the fullest and see problems as opportunities to learn and grow.
2. Assist client in gaining self-satisfaction from independent actions and health.	To reduce invalidism.
3. Promote meaningful relationships with others.	To lessen alienation from others.
4. Help client add zest to life with health as a focus rather than illness.	To enhance the quality of client's life.

EVALUATION

Measurable goals and outcomes provide the basis for evaluating the client's progress. The client's self-report, observations by the nurse, and information from family members provide additional data. The following behaviors indicate a positive evaluation:

1. Shows a reduced level of anxiety
2. Expresses feelings directly
3. Identifies conflict situations
4. Has gained insight into responses to stress and their relationship to physical health
5. Uses stress reduction methods to lessen anxiety

BIBLIOGRAPHY

Chodoff P: Hysteria and women, *Am J Psychiatry* 139:545, 1982.

Harm not the hysteric, *Emerg Med* 14(20):262, 1982.

Hudson K: A face-saving formula...conversion disorder..."prescribed sick role," *Nurs Times* 86(24):66, 1990.

Nicassio P: Behavioral treatment of hysterical dysphagia in a hospital setting: a case report, *Gen Hosp Psychiatry* 3:213, 1981.

Stewert T: Hysterical conversion reactions: some patient characteristics and treatment team reactions, *Arch Phys Med Rehabil* 64(7):308, 1983.

Crisis

A crisis is an internal disturbance resulting from a stressful event or a perceived threat. Crisis occurs in the lives of all individuals. The precipitating event, which can be a perceived loss, threat of a loss, or a challenge, can usually be identified. It may have occurred several weeks ago or within the past few days. Crisis situations can be of a situational or developmental nature or both.

An important aspect of crisis is the potential for growth within the individual. The way an individual responds to a crisis determines whether growth or disorganization occurs. During crisis the individual's usual coping skills become ineffective in dealing with the threat, and anxiety increases. Without adequate supports the individual becomes more anxious and tries out new coping skills or redefines the problem so that old coping skills work. If resolution does not occur, the individual goes into a panic level of anxiety and psychological disorganization (crisis). Individuals in crisis are vulnerable and motivated to accept help to relieve the turmoil. For this reason, it is essential that nurses have the knowledge and skills to intervene prior to psychological disorganization.

Related DSM-III-R disorders

Adjustment disorders
Phase of life problem or other life circumstance problem
Marital problem
Parent-child problem

Other related conditions

Situational crisis
Developmental crisis
Suicide attempts
Drug overdose
Alcohol abuse

PRINCIPLES

▶ Physical Dimension

1. Certain inevitable events during the life cycle can be described as crisis situations; resulting adaptive mechanisms may lead to mastery of the new situation or to failure with a more or less lasting impairment to functioning.
2. Crisis reactions are characterized by somatic distress and a change in patterns of activity.
3. A distorted grief reaction to a crisis situation includes overactivity and taking on the symptoms belonging to the last illness of the deceased, as well as the development of health problems such as agitated depression.
4. Crises perceived as challenges mobilize an individual's energy and problem-solving abilities.
5. If the crisis is not relieved, the individual's health status may deteriorate.
6. The state of depleted energy results in the individual's acceptance of assistance.
7. Crisis is sequenced into time periods: the precrisis, the crisis, and the postcrisis.
8. Situations become crises for individuals who by personality, previous experience, or other factors in the present situation are vulnerable to stress and whose emotional resources are taxed beyond their usual adaptive resources.

▶ Emotional Dimension

1. Freud describes crisis as a transition point in his stages of psychosexual development.
2. Erikson describes crisis as a stage every person undergoes in the process of growth and development.
3. Grief and bereavement in response to a loss lead to a crisis in many individuals.
4. When equilibrium is disturbed, the potential for two conditions exists; a crisis is successfully resolved or a crisis is not resolved, the latter leading to development of maladaptive patterns of behavior.

5. When a person faces a problem he or she cannot solve, tension occurs with resulting anxiety, and the person's usual coping mechanisms are activated. If they are effective, a crisis is avoided.
6. With an increase in tension, problem-solving abilities may become ineffective and emergency mechanisms are called upon; these include redefining the problem, discontinuing efforts to achieve the goal, or avoiding the problem by distorting reality.
7. Crisis occurs when the individual has ineffective problem-solving skills, tension continues to increase, and the personality becomes disorganized.
8. Primary concern during crisis is with failures in adaptation "today," what caused them, and what the client can do to learn to overcome them.
9. Crisis is accompanied by increased tension and anxiety.

▶ Intellectual Dimension

1. Perception of the event and coping mechanisms influence outcome of the crisis.
2. Goals of crisis include reducing the impact of the crisis, providing an opportunity for the client to use previous problem-solving skills, and assistance in returning to a precrisis level of functioning or to a higher level of functioning.
3. The event that precipitates the crisis is perceived by the person as stressful before it becomes a crisis.

4. Realistic appraisals of the crisis event provide the arena for problem-solving activities.
5. Preoccupation with the past is a characteristic behavior.

▶ Social Dimension

1. Situational supports influence outcome of crisis.
2. The outcome is governed by the kind of interaction that takes place during the crisis period between the individual and key figures in his or her emotional milieu.

▶ Spiritual Dimension

1. A person in crisis can regain faith in self.
2. A person in crisis is dispirited; hope lies in the release of energies generated by the longing for something better.
3. The capacity for hope gives a person a sense of destination and the energy to get started.
4. A person in crisis can face choices with expectations, not dread.
5. A person in crisis can persuade self that he or she is not a failure.
6. A person in crisis can be helped to have a vision for life.
7. Valuing self provides a person with an ability to accept a failure or mistake and move beyond the crisis.

ASSESSMENT

▶ Physical Dimension

I. **History**
   A. Activities of daily living
      1. Nutrition
         a. Lack of appetite or increased appetite
         b. Weight loss or weight gain
      2. Sleep
         a. Disturbed
      3. Physical activities and limitations
         a. Hyperactive
         b. Psychomotor retardation
      4. Sexual activity
         a. Lack of desire
         b. Impotence
   B. Habits
      1. Alcohol
         a. Increased or excessive intake
      2. Smoking
         a. Increased (chain smoking)
      3. Medications and drugs
         a. Overuse of over-the-counter medications
      4. Caffeine
         a. Increased coffee intake

   C. Destructive behavior
      1. Suicide attempts
      2. High rate of accidents
      3. Threatens harm to others
   D. Health history
      1. Suicide attempt
   E. Review of systems
      1. General
         a. Change in weight
         b. Change in appetite
         c. Change in sleep habits
         d. Malaise with inability to carry out activities of daily living
      2. Cardiovascular
         a. Elevated blood pressure
         b. Palpitations
         c. Tightness in chest
      3. Respiratory
         a. Rapid breathing
      4. Gastrointestinal
         a. Nausea
         b. Diarrhea

c. Indigestion
5. Genitourinary
   a. Frequency
6. Reproductive
   a. Male
      (1) Impotence
   a. Female
      (1) Amenorrhea
      (2) Dysmenorrhea

7. Musculoskeletal
   a. Muscle tension
8. Neurological
   a. Memory impairment
II. Physical examination—findings are similar to those found in Anxiety (see p. 48)
III. Diagnostic tests
   A. Dexamethasone suppression test (for depression)

▶ **Emotional Dimension**

CLIENT DATA	ANALYSIS	NURSING DIAGNOSIS
Overwhelming anxiety	Inability to resolve problem threatens individual and results in severe anxiety.	Anxiety: inability to solve problem related to crisis situation
Helplessness	Thinks no one can help with problem, impaired problem-solving abilities.	Ineffective individual coping: helplessness related to crisis situation.
Hopelessness	Thinks nothing can be done to resolve problem.	Hopelessness: related to crisis situation
Depression	Feels worthless and inadequate.	Ineffective individual coping: depression related to crisis situation
Powerlessness	Feels unable to cope and feels loss of control over own life.	Powerlessness: related to crisis situation
Guilt and shame	No longer feels self-reliant and competent.	*Guilt and shame: related to crisis situation
Anger	Response to stress; may be directed at self or others; intense and out of proportion to situation.	High risk for violence: inability to control anger related to crisis situation
Ambivalence	Struggling to be self-reliant but wants help.	Ineffective individual coping: ambivalence related to crisis situation
Fears of "going crazy"	Increased tension, inability to solve problems, and disorganization in thinking contribute to fear.	Fear: of "going crazy" related to crisis situation
Feeling like everything is going wrong	Increased tension, inability to cope, and disorganization contribute to this feeling.	Anxiety: severe, related to crisis situation

▶ **Intellectual Dimension**

CLIENT DATA	ANALYSIS	NURSING DIAGNOSIS
Distortion of meaning of situation	Misperceives meaning of situation because of high anxiety level, severity of threat, and disorganization in thinking.	Altered thought processes: distorted perception related to crisis situation
Unrealistic perception of problem	Sees situation unrealistically because of high anxiety level and severity of threat.	Altered thought processes: unrealistic perception of the problem related to crisis situation
Inability to recall events	High level of anxiety interferes with memory functioning.	*Altered memory: related to crisis situation
Disorientation	Due to severe anxiety.	Altered thought processes: disorientation related to crisis situation
Tunnel vision	Focuses on small details; narrow focus because of anxiety.	Altered thought processes: tunnel vision related to crisis situation

▶ **Intellectual Dimension—cont'd**

CLIENT DATA	ANALYSIS	NURSING DIAGNOSIS
Selective inattention	Able to hear only parts of conversation or instructions.	Altered thought processes: selective inattention related to crisis situation
Impaired judgment	Anxiety impairs decision making skills.	*Altered judgment: related to crisis situation
Lack of insight	Aware that needs help but fails to recognize own contribution to problem; unable to intervene in own behalf.	Altered thought processes: lack of insight related to crisis situation
Thinking is concrete	Unable to abstract or generalize due to severe anxiety.	Altered thought processes: concrete thinking related to crisis situation
Confused thinking	Disorganization of usual thought processes.	Altered thought processes: confusion related to crisis situation
Ruminations	Preoccupied with crisis event, obsessed with it.	Altered thought processes: ruminations related to crisis situation
Inability to problem solve	Usual coping skills are no longer effective.	Altered thought processes: inability to problem solve related to crisis situation
Inappropriate use of projection, denial, and rationalization	Responses to high levels of anxiety.	Defensive coping: inappropriate use of defense mechanisms related to anxiety
Use of pressured speech	Response to anxiety.	Impaired verbal communication: pressured speech related to crisis situation
Overtalkative and circumstantial	Response to anxiety.	Impaired verbal communication: circumstantial speech related to crisis situation
Rigid thinking	Unable to see other ways to solve problem.	Altered thought processes: rigid thinking related to crisis situation

▶ **Social Dimension**

CLIENT DATA	ANALYSIS	NURSING DIAGNOSIS
Low self-esteem	Threats to self and self-expectations lower opinion of self.	Self-esteem disturbance: related to crisis situation
Lack of a support system	Feelings of helplessness and dependence. Perceives no one to turn to in time of trouble, is alienated from others.	Impaired social interaction: lack of support system related to crisis situation
Impaired functioning in social roles	Reduced ability to perform during period of crisis, unable to carry out usual roles, unable to meet role expectations.	Altered role performance: related to crisis situation
Environmental factors with potential for crisis (illness, death, separation, new baby, divorce, drug trip, arrest, retirement, move, new job, job loss, surgery, hospitalization, Christmas, other family holidays, abortion, assault, rape, body image change, role change, or threat to life goals)	A crisis is dependent on individual's perception of situation, support system, and coping skills. High stress levels in the environment contribute to crisis situations.	Anxiety: related to stressful environmental factors

▶ **Spiritual Dimension**

CLIENT DATA	ANALYSIS	NURSING DIAGNOSIS
Conflict in values (suicide, abortion, divorce, and health intervention in conflict with religion)	Value conflicts are threatening to individual and cause severe anxiety.	Spiritual distress: conflict in values related to crisis situation
Despairs of life situation	Inability to cope, disorganized thinking, and sense that everything is going wrong contribute to despair, depression, and hopelessness.	Hopelessness: related to crisis situation
Thinks God or other religious power has forsaken self	Feels abandoned by religious leaders; is unable to draw on religious or spiritual resources.	Spiritual distress: feeling abandoned by God or other religious power related to crisis situation
Disturbed or distorted perception of faith	May rely unrealistically on faith to solve crisis.	Spiritual distress: unrealistic perception of faith related to crisis situation
Feels death would be a relief	Lacks meaning and purpose for life; unable to see other options for solving problems and living a more fulfilling life.	Spiritual distress: wanting release from problems through death related to crisis situation

PLANNING

Long-Term Goal

To resolve the problem and return to precrisis or higher level of functioning

SHORT-TERM GOALS	OUTCOME CRITERIA
Physical Dimension To identify crisis-producing situation	1. Describes sequence of events that led to crisis situation 2. Identifies problem clearly and realistically 3. Discusses responses to stress and links to present behavior
Emotional Dimension To reduce anxiety over crisis situation	1. Verbalizes anxious feeling 2. Relates feelings of anxiety to specific situation 3. Identifies ways of reducing anxiety in past situations 4. States need for help 5. Is informed about treatment plans 6. Participates in planning care and decision making 7. Gives positive feedback about treatment 8. Verbalizes an increase in comfort level and a decrease in agitation

Intellectual Dimension
To learn effective methods of problem solving
	1. Is able to:
	  a. State problem
	  b. Identify cause
	  c. Discuss thoughts and feelings about problem
	  d. List alternative actions
	  e. Discuss consequences of possible actions
	  f. Choose an option
	  g. Test option
	  h. Evaluate results of chosen option
	2. Demonstrates willingness to participate in treatment planning

To increase repertoire of coping skills	1. Verbalizes new methods to deal with problems 2. Uses new methods to solve problems. 3. Verbalizes positive effects of new coping skills

PLANNING—cont'd.

SHORT-TERM GOALS	OUTCOME CRITERIA
Social Dimension To enlarge support systems	1. Names supportive persons 2. Identifies reasons for lack of supportive persons 3. Initiates approach to a supportive person
Spiritual Dimension To regain a sense of hope and confidence in self	1. Verbalizes feelings of control over own life 2. Acknowledges strength in religious faith 3. Makes statements that reflect confidence in self

Discharge Planning

The following client behaviors demonstrate readiness for discharge:
1. Has realistic perception of problem
2. Has adequate support system
3. Uses increased numbers of effective coping skills
4. Has returned to at least a precrisis level of functioning
5. Knows community resources available for crisis intervention

IMPLEMENTATION

NURSING ACTIONS	RATIONALE
Physical Dimension	
1. Promote sleep with comfort measures or medication.	To promote client's general well-being.
2. Provide physical activities.	To use the energy generated by anxiety.
3. Provide several attractively served, small meals each day.	To stimulate appetite and promote general well-being.
4. Assist with activities of daily living when necessary.	To enhance client's self-respect, to boost esteem.
5. Provide a safe environment if client is suicidal or destructive.	To prevent client from harming self or others.
6. Relieve physical symptoms or complaints.	To promote comfort, to indicate caring and concern.
7. Promote responsibility for self-care with positive feedback.	To encourage independence, autonomy at the precrisis level or higher.
Emotional Dimension	
1. Determine anxiety level.	To plan interventions.
2. Decrease intensity of anxiety to a lesser level.	To promote psychological comfort and readiness to learn new methods for coping with stress.
3. Encourage expression of feelings of anxiety, hopelessness, helplessness, powerlessness, guilt, shame, anger, and ambivalence by being nonjudgmental, accepting.	To determine meaning of event to clients, to plan interventions.
4. Assist client in sorting out feelings and validate them as acceptable and normal.	To help client distinguish between thoughts and feelings and feel comfortable expressing them.
5. Focus on emotionally charged areas.	To determine area of distress, to help client talk about it openly, to explore options for resolving the crisis-producing event.
Intellectual Dimension	
1. Help client clarify problem.	To define problem clearly and eliminate nonessential factors that may contribute to misperception of problem.
2. Help client describe precipitating events in detail.	To obtain a clear history of events of previous 4 to 6 weeks leading up to crisis.
3. Identify present coping skills.	To determine client's problem-solving abilities and build on them.

NURSING ACTIONS	RATIONALE
4. Determine suicide risk.	To plan immediate interventions.
5. Help client sort out thoughts about crisis situation.	To determine if they are rational and if not, to help client question conclusions about crisis situation.
6. Assist client in decreasing blaming of others.	To promote client's consideration of contribution to crisis situation.
7. Promote a realistic perception of problem by questioning, and planting "seeds of doubt."	To present reality.
8. Reinforce coping skills used successfully in past.	To increase client's self-esteem by helping to use past successful coping skills.
9. Explore learning that has taken place in present situation and its application to future situations.	To help client integrate crisis situation into life and grow from it.
10. Offer simple, clear explanations during early crisis period.	To promote clear communication at a time when anxiety is high.
11. Assist client in identifying alternatives for resolving problem.	To help client expand thinking and see other ways to handle problem.
12. Mobilize client's strengths and reinforce them.	To help client use all resources in resolving problem.
13. Teach problem solving.	To increase client's ability to handle problems in the future without precipitating a crisis.
14. Teach stress-reduction measures (e.g., relaxation and imagery).	To reduce anxiety and prevent a crisis.
15. Limit preoccupation with situation.	To prevent continuous self-absorption and promote interaction and involvement with other people and activities.
16. Help with decision making until client is less anxious.	To lessen anxiety associated with making decisions.
17. Foster client's motivation and willingness to participate in treatment planning.	To increase autonomy, independence and feelings of control over own life.
18. Use crisis situation as a therapeutic opportunity.	To increase client's coping skills at a time when usual problem-solving skills are not working, to increase ability to manage stress.
19. Help client use crisis as a learning experience.	To prevent future crisis situations by learning and growing from present situation.
20. Provide crisis intervention to family.	To prevent family disorganization.
21. Refrain from changing or destroying former patterns of coping with stress.	To prevent client from further devaluing self, to use and expand previous patterns for coping.
22. Communicate persistently that client will not be allowed to hurt self or others.	To set limits on impulsive destructive behavior, to assure client that he or she will not be allowed to lose control.
23. Teach client problem-solving self-talk to use in stressful situations (for example, What is the problem? What is the cause? How do I feel? What can I do about it?)	To encourage client to assume responsibility for managing own stress, thereby increasing independence and esteem.
Social Dimension	
1. Help client enlarge support system to include family, friends, and community resources.	To lessen feelings of isolation and rejection.
2. Reduce dependence on others by using assertive skills.	To increase independence and feelings of control over own life.
3. Assist client in meeting role expectations at precrisis level.	To promote client's precrisis level of functioning or a higher level, thereby increasing self-esteem and self-value.
4. Have client participate in usual social activities.	To help client experience pleasure with other persons at client's precrisis level.
5. Discuss environmental factors that are stress-producing.	To identify stressors: learn to avoid, deal with, or accept them.
6. Provide group or supportive therapy if indicated.	To facilitate client's expression of feelings, listen to others' expression of feelings, learn new coping skills, receive feedback and support from others.
7. Provide close supervision if suicidal.	To prevent self-harm.

IMPLEMENTATION—cont'd

NURSING ACTIONS	RATIONALE
Spiritual Dimension	
1. Help client clarify conflicting values using value clarification techniques.	To prevent crisis situation from erupting when there are serious conflicts in values and coping skills are inadequate to handle them.
2. Refer client to clergy.	To provide spiritual support, comfort, and strength.
3. Promote a sense of hope that problem can be resolved.	To bolster client's confidence that problem is solvable with help and time.
4. Restore confidence that client can regain control over own life.	To prevent feelings of hopelessness and helplessness.

EVALUATION

Measurable goals and outcome criteria provide the data for evaluating the resolution of the client's crisis. Client self-reports, nurse observations, and family reports provide additional data. The following behaviors indicate a positive evaluation:

1. Identifies stress-producing situations
2. Perceives the problem realistically
3. Has supportive persons with him or her
4. Uses effective coping skills
5. Knows the telephone numbers of community agencies for crisis intervention

BIBLIOGRAPHY

Capodanno A, Targum S: Assessment of suicide risk: some limitations in the production of infrequent events, *J Psychosoc Nurs Ment Health Serv* 21(5):11, 1983.

Constantino R: Comparison of two group interventions for the bereaved, *Image: J Nurs Schol* 20(2):83, 1988.

Edwards D: Initial psychosocial impact of insulin-dependent diabetes mellitus on the pediatric client and family, *Issues Compr Pediatr Nurs* 10(4):199, 1987.

Flannery J: Guilt: a crisis within a crisis . . . a catastrophic neurologic event, *J Neurosc–Nurs* 22(2):92, 1990.

Foley T, and Davies M: *Rape: nursing care of victims,* St. Louis, 1983, C.V. Mosby.

Halm M: Effects of support groups on anxiety of family members during critical illness, *Heart Lung* 19(1):62, 1990.

Hampson S: Nursing interventions for the first three postpartum months, *J Obstet Gynocol Neonatal Nurs* 18(2):116, 1989.

Judd R: Behavioral and psychological crisis in emergency medical services, *Top Emerg Med* 4(4):1, 1983.

Lindemann E: *Beyond grief: studies in crisis intervention,* New York, 1979, Jason Aronson, Inc.

Morin S: Responding to the psychological crisis of AIDs, *Public Health Rep* 99(1):4, 1984.

Murphy S: After Mt. St. Helens: disaster stress research, *J Psychosoc Nurs Ment Health Serv* 22(7):9, 1984.

Narayan S, Joslin O: *Crisis theory and intervention: a critique of the medical model and proposal of a holistic nursing model, Adv Nurs Sci* 2:27, 1980.

Nyamathi A, van Servellen G: Maladaptive coping in the critically ill population with acquired immunodeficiency syndrome: nursing assessment and treatment, *J Crit Care* 18(2):113, 1989.

Pallikkathayil L, Morgan S: Emergency department encounters with suicide attemptors: a qualitative investigation, *Schol Inq Nurs Pract* 2(3):237, 1988.

Ryan J: The neglected crisis: serious illness can rock the patient's beliefs, *Am J Nurs* 84(10):1257, 1984.

Sirles A, Selleck C: Cardiac disease and the family: impact, assessment, and implications, *J Carciovasc Nurs* 3(2):23, 1989.

Williams H: Social support and social networks: a review of the literature, *J Assoc Pediatric Oncol Nurses* 5(3):6, 1988.

Delusions

Delusions are false beliefs contrary to objective evidence and inconsistent with a person's intelligence and cultural background. They cannot be corrected with reason or logic. The delusional person's thoughts, beliefs, and perceptions are misinterpretations and distortions of reality, although they may be based on a segment of reality within the person's life. Staff members or other persons may be incorporated into the delusional system. Delusions are attempts by the individual to reduce anxiety and make some sense of reality. The person projects his or her own unacceptable thoughts and feelings on the environment and then justifies (rationalizes) the interpretation of reality to self and others.

Delusions represent an exaggerated picture of what the client believes. The following delusions demonstrate different types of exaggerated beliefs: delusions of persecution, delusions of grandeur, delusions of control, delusions of reference, delusions of wealth or poverty, delusions of infidelity, and somatic delusions.

Delusions may be transient or fixed. Transient delusions may develop with an organic illness and disappear when the pathological condition is eliminated. Fixed delusions persist over time or throughout a person's life. Other aspects of the person's personality may function well; only the delusion persists. Fixed delusions are seen in delusional (paranoid) disorders.

To work effectively with delusional clients, the nurse needs an awareness of his or her own anxiety to deal with the anxiety generated by the delusional client. Although the nurse's attempts to establish a relationship may be met with rejection initially, sincerity and persistence are vital and contribute to the client's ability to trust and to have a satisfying relationship with another person. Each success in interpersonal relationships increases the client's self-esteem and sense of worth.

Related DSM-III-R disorders

Schizophrenia
Delusional (paranoid) disorders
Organic mental disorders
Mood disorders

Other related conditions

Delirium
Organic illnesses caused by acute infective or metabolic disturbances
Substance intoxication
Systemic illness

PRINCIPLES

▶ Physical Dimension

1. Infectious or metabolic disturbances, alcohol intoxication, and systemic illness may cause delusional thinking.
2. Loss of hearing contributes to mistrust with the possibility of paranoid (delusional) thinking.

▶ Emotional Dimension

1. An overwhelming sense of anxiety may contribute to delusional thinking.
2. Extreme suspiciousness accompanies paranoid delusions.
3. Feelings of inferiority exist in the person with paranoid delusions.

▶ Intellectual Dimension

1. Delusions determine the presence of a psychosis.
2. Ego functions that maintain contact with reality may be incompletely developed or weakened.
3. Defense mechanisms of denial, projection, and dissociation are used to reduce anxiety and are associated with delusions.
4. A loss of ego boundaries results in an inability to distinguish reality from fantasy.
5. Regression to an infantile state relieves the individual from the overwhelming anxiety contributing to delusional thinking.
6. Attempts to reason or argue with the delusional client increase anxiety and cause the client to hold tighter to the delusion.

7. Delusions may be based on reality. It is this kernel of truth that gives the delusion such convincing power.
8. Delusions may be a means to test others to see if they accept the delusional material at face value or if they are willing to look for the meaning of the material to understand the client.
9. A delusion is an attempt to alter the part of reality that is unacceptable because of a conflict with unconscious needs.

▶ **Social Dimension**

1. Delusions represent Sullivan's "not me" aspect of the personality that is dissociated from reality and is the result of overwhelming anxiety.
2. The "not me" aspect of the personality develops when significant persons fail to acknowledge the existence of a child's thoughts and feelings.
3. A distorted, confused, and vague sense of self contributes to disturbances in evaluating reality and delusional thinking.

4. Unmet needs in real life are met with delusions (for example, needs for aggression, relatedness, dependence, communication, esteem, and sexuality).
5. A delusion is a struggle for adaptation to the environment.
6. Client is not aware of delusional behavior and its effects on others. Client with paranoid delusions places blame on others, relieves anxiety, and raises self-esteem.

▶ **Spiritual Dimension**

1. Delusions prevent the person from living a satisfying life.
2. The goodness of others is misinterpreted and client becomes disconnected from satisfying relationships with others.
3. The delusional client may see self as having little worth and as being without purpose and meaning in life.

ASSESSMENT

▶ **Physical Dimension**

I. History
  A. Activities of daily living
    1. Nutrition
      a. Inadequate with delusions of persecution (food is poisoned)
    2. Sleep
      a. Difficulty with delusions of persecution (fear of being harmed)
    3. Recreation, hobbies, and interests
      a. Lack of interest when preoccupied with delusions
    4. Sexual activity
      a. Dysfunctional (delusions of persecution)
      b. Excessive or inappropriate (delusions of grandeur)
  B. Habits
    1. Medications and drugs
      a. Refuses to take medications and drugs or comply with regimen because fears being harmed or poisoned (delusions of persecution)
  C. Destructive behavior

1. Poor impulse control—may act on delusion
2. Suicide attempts
3. Homicide
  D. Health history
    1. Illnesses
      a. Delusional (paranoid) disorder
      b. Schizophrenia
      c. Organic or systemic illness
      d. Substance intoxication
      e. Brain lesion
      f. Hearing loss
  E. Review of systems—with somatic delusions the client will have complaints in any of the body systems depending on the delusion (for example, client states he or she has no heart or cannot breathe)

II. Diagnostic tests
  A. EEG to rule out organicity
  B. Blood chemistry to rule out biochemical imbalance
  C. Interpretation of proverbs to assess extent of cognitive impairment

▶ **Physical Examination**

CLIENT DATA	ANALYSIS	NURSING DIAGNOSIS
Malnourished appearance	With delusions of persecution, may think food is poisoned and not eat adequately.	*Altered self-care: related to refusal to eat
Poor personal hygiene	Preoccupied with delusions.	Bathing/hygiene self-care deficit: related to preoccupation with delusions

▶ **Emotional Dimension**

CLIENT DATA	ANALYSIS	NURSING DIAGNOSIS
Affect is flat, blunted, inappropriate	If flat or blunted, emotional expression is absent or reduced in intensity; ambivalence is possibly causing this affect. If inappropriate, facts of delusion evoke affect.	*Altered feeling state: flat affect related to delusional thinking
Fears being harmed, rejection, isolation, or mind is being controlled	Unmet needs are expressed in delusions of persecution.	Fears: of being harmed, of rejection, of isolation, or that mind is being controlled related to delusions of persecution
Suspicious	Mistrusting of others, misinterprets others' intentions.	Ineffective individual coping: suspiciousness related to delusions
Hostile or angry	Unmet needs are expressed in delusions. Is a danger to self or others if likely to act on delusions.	High risk for violence: hostility or anger related to delusions
Guilty or embarrassed	Feelings of guilt or embarrassment may follow realization of delusional thinking after treatment is effective and condition is stabilized following a transient episode.	Ineffective individual coping: guilt or embarrassment related to recovery from delusional thinking

▶ **Intellectual Dimension**

CLIENT DATA	ANALYSIS	NURSING DIAGNOSIS
Distorted perception; paranoid, grandiose, sexual, religious, or somatic, delusions	Reality is distorted by overwhelming level of anxiety.	Altered thought processes: distorted perceptions related to delusions.
Impaired judgment and insight	Does not see self as mentally ill or needing treatment; has no insight, sees self as blameless.	Altered thought processes: impaired judgment and insight related to delusions
Inability to think abstractly	Regresses to more primitive (concrete) style of thinking and more comfortable stage of development; is unable to distinguish reality from fantasy.	Altered thought processes: inability to think abstractly related to delusional thinking
Preoccupied with delusions	Delusions are intrusive.	Altered thought processes: preoccupation related to delusions
Suicidal ideas, sexual preoccupation, or homicidal plans	Delusional material. Is a danger to self and others if likely to act on delusions.	Altered thought processes: suicidal ideas, sexual preoccupation, or homicidal plans related to delusions; potential for self-harm and violence related to delusions
Use of defense mechanisms (denial, projection, and regression)	Is a way to cope with and reduce anxiety.	Defensive coping: pathological use of defense mechanisms related to delusions

▶ **Intellectual Dimension—cont'd**

CLIENT DATA	ANALYSIS	NURSING DIAGNOSIS
Fixed delusional system	Is unable to see unreasonableness of delusion; persists over time; other aspects of the personality may function well.	Altered thought processes: related to fixed delusional system

▶ **Social Dimension**

CLIENT DATA	ANALYSIS	NURSING DIAGNOSIS
Lowered self-esteem	Delusions of grandeur compensate for feelings of inferiority; are an attempt to do away with unacceptable aspects of personality.	Self-esteem disturbance: related to delusions of grandeur
Unrealistic perception of self	Sees self as a famous person, leader, or religious or political person with delusions of grandeur.	Self-esteem disturbance: unrealistic perception of self related to delusions of grandeur
Suspiciousness of others and extreme mistrust	Seen with delusions of persecution.	Ineffective individual coping: suspiciousness related to delusions of persecution
Withdrawn and isolated	Alienated from others.	Social isolation: related to delusions
Impaired capacity to perform social roles	Depending on nature of delusion, client struggling to adapt to environment.	Altered role performance: related to delusions
Cultural factors provide basis for delusion	Delusions may be based on reality and influenced by cultural factors such as rural, urban, or metropolitan area of living.	Altered thought processes: delusions related to cultural factors
Lower socioeconomic class	Tendency for more delusional thinking in lower socioeconomic class because of downward mobility.	Altered thought processes: delusions related to environmental factors

▶ **Spiritual Dimension**

CLIENT DATA	ANALYSIS	NURSING DIAGNOSIS
Excessive religiosity	An escape from reality, may represent guilt or low self-esteem.	Spiritual distress: related to excessive religiosity
Lacks ability to enjoy pleasures in life	Delusions prevent a fulfilling quality to life.	Spiritual distress: diminished quality of life related to delusions
May believe self to be Jesus, Queen Victoria, or other powerful person	Delusions of grandeur, efforts to substitute fantasy for real life.	Spiritual distress: related to delusions of grandeur

PLANNING

Long-Term Goal

To cope with anxiety without delusions

SHORT-TERM GOALS	OUTCOME CRITERIA
Physical Dimension To identify threats and stressors	1. Names events and situations in life that are threatening and stressful 2. Identifies subjective experience of anxiety

SHORT-TERM GOALS	OUTCOME CRITERIA
Emotional Dimension	
To reduce fears and anxiety	1. Identifies events, situations that cause anxiety. 2. Verbalizes feelings of anxiety. 3. Uses adaptive methods to reduce anxiety. 4. Seeks help when unable to manage anxiety.
Intellectual Dimension	
To maintain contact with reality	1. Verbalizes what is real and what is fantasy 2. States factual and realistic account of situation 3. Focuses on reality-centered discussions 4. Validates thoughts with others 5. Participates in regularly scheduled activities to decrease time for delusional thinking
To reduce or eliminate delusions	1. Is able to handle anxiety in a healthy manner 2. Recognizes when anxiety is escalating 3. Seeks help from another person when anxiety mounts 4. Takes medicines as prescribed for delusions 5. Can live with delusions; discusses them only in private or with an understanding person 6. Identifies when thoughts become delusional 7. Knows ways to distract delusions 8. Uses stress-reduction methods to relieve anxiety
To gain insight about delusions	1. Identifies stressors in life 2. Identifies feelings of being overwhelmed 3. Verbalizes inability to cope with stressors 4. States relief measures for stressors 5. Relates ways, other than delusions, to cope
Social Dimension	
To interact with other persons	1. Does not isolate self from others 2. Initiates activities and interactions with another person 3. Benefits from group therapy 4. Stays involved with others to lessen time for delusional thinking
Spiritual Dimension	
To accept the real world with its stress and strain	1. Accepts stress and strain in life without being overwhelmed by them
To have confidence and hope that delusions can be controlled	1. Takes prescribed medicine 2. Identifies feelings of anxiety early 3. Sees self as capable person 4. Controls delusions with self-distractions

Discharge Planning

The following client behaviors demonstrate readiness for discharge:
1. Verbalizes importance of taking medications as prescribed
2. Identifies when anxiety is mounting and uses measures to reduce it to avoid delusions
3. Controls delusional thinking by distractions or becoming involved with activities or persons
4. Uses family or significant other for support and to reduce withdrawal and alienation

IMPLEMENTATION

NURSING ACTIONS	RATIONALE
Physical Dimension	
1. Monitor nutritional intake if delusions interfere with food intake.	To ensure adequate nutritional intake.
2. Monitor sleep patterns when delusions interfere with sleep.	To ensure adequate sleep.
3. Promote involvement in activities.	To allow less time for delusional thinking.
4. Give client concrete tasks that he or she can complete successfully.	To promote feelings of achievement and increase self-esteem.
5. Make short, frequent contacts with client.	To build trust and present reality.
6. Be aware of lag time between initiation of medications and relief of symptoms (delusions).	To prevent discouragement when relief of symptoms is slow.
7. Provide safety when client acts impulsively on delusions.	To prevent harm to client or others. A history of impulsive acts helps to determine if client acts on delusions or verbalizes them.
8. Protect client, if suicidal, with one-to-one observation.	To prevent self-harm when client may act on delusion.
9. Refrain from focusing on delusions of a somatic nature.	To avoid reinforcing delusion.
10. Assist with self-care activities and personal hygiene when needed.	To enhance client's appearance and esteem.
11. Be cognizant of potential for self-harm or violence, for example, is client acting on delusions?	To protect client or others from impulsive acts resulting from delusions.
12. Monitor medication regimen.	To be certain client takes medications as prescribed.
13. Protect client from participating in too many new experiences.	To prevent anxiety associated with new experiences.
14. Refrain from touching client.	To prevent client from misinterpreting your intentions.
15. Have client watch food and medication preparation if client thinks it is poisoned.	To prevent suspiciousness and mistrust, to present reality.
16. Avoid tasting medicine to demonstrate safeness.	To prevent client from incorporating you into delusional system.
Emotional Dimension	
1. Identify feelings underlying delusion.	To help client know you understand fears and anxieties.
2. Be aware of what client is saying about feelings with verbal and nonverbal communication.	To decode the message and understand what client is communicating to you.
3. Facilitate client's expression of feelings of fear, rejection, isolation, hostility, of being controlled, or living in an unreal world.	To let client know that it is OK to feel and to express the feeling.
4. Help client explore effective and acceptable ways (painting, writing, talking, or music) to express feelings.	To promote client's expression of feelings in ways that are socially acceptable.
5. Assist client in reducing intensity of feelings with physical activity.	To use the energy generated by strong feelings in an acceptable way.
6. Relieve anxiety by giving information or promoting a predictable environment.	To provide information or promote sameness relieves anxiety, provides security.
7. Promote a sense of safety for client with an attitude of concern and care.	To reduce fears and threats to client.
8. Prevent client from being overwhelmed by monitoring activities.	To lessen anxiety.
9. Help client to identify feeling of anxiety, to label it as anxiety, and to respond to it.	To become aware of feeling of anxiety and plan actions to manage it appropriately.
10. Accept client's right to feel as he or she does, no matter how illogical it seems.	To help client trust and accept own feelings, to accept responsibility for them.
11. Give positive reinforcement to expression of feelings.	To reinforce positive behaviors.
12. Be aware of own frustrations when client is slow to respond or requires readmission to hospital.	To increase understanding of self and responses to client.
13. Be aware that client's hostility and verbal barrages are not a personal affront but inadequate communication of needs.	To prevent taking client's angry tirades personally and responding nontherapeutically.
14. Be aware of your own nonverbal communication (e.g., smiling and nodding head).	To prevent misinterpretation.

NURSING ACTIONS	RATIONALE
Intellectual Dimension	
1. Interpret reality by stating facts clearly and concisely.	To prevent misinterpretation of reality.
2. Refrain from discussing delusional material.	To avoid reinforcing delusional thinking.
3. Avoid being incorporated into delusion by being aware of your verbal and nonverbal communication.	To increase your understanding of your own behavior and ways it affects the client.
4. Respond to delusion by stating feelings that are being expressed symbolically.	To let client know you understand distress.
5. Distract client to other activities when focusing on delusions.	To avoid reinforcing delusions.
6. Explore with client stimuli that cause stress.	To help client identify anxiety and plan other approaches for handling it.
7. Notify client when changes in schedule are made.	To decrease anxiety.
8. Avoid putting client on defensive with threatening or intimidating statements.	To prevent client from feeling that he or she has to protect self and hold on tighter to the delusion.
9. Accept client's need for delusion.	To understand that client's delusions meet otherwise unmet needs in life.
10. Determine what need is being met by delusion.	To plan interventions.
11. Recognize delusion as client's perception of environment.	To understand delusions from the client's viewpoint.
12. Refrain from arguing or reasoning to convince client that delusions are false or unreal.	To prevent client from holding on tighter to delusion.
13. Present factual account of situation.	To avoid agreeing or disagreeing with, approving or disapproving client's delusion.
14. Focus on reality.	To orient to reality.
15. Avoid joking or teasing about delusion.	To promote respect for client, to prevent threatening client.
16. Refrain from conveying to client acceptance of delusion.	To avoid reinforcing delusion.
17. After a relationship has developed, gently question client's delusions.	To interject some doubt about the credibility of the delusion.
18. Interject doubt regarding delusions.	To help client question delusional thinking.
19. Discuss delusional thinking as problem in client's life.	To help client see consequences of behavior and effect on others.
20. Give feedback concerning delusions in terms of feelings (for example, fear or anger).	To help client see relationship of fear or anger to delusions.
21. Refocus conversation to another topic after listening to delusion.	To avoid reinforcing delusions.
22. Avoid nodding head as if in agreement with client.	To prevent misinterpretation of your behavior.
23. State that understanding client is difficult.	To promote honesty in the relationship.
24. Set limits on "crazy talk" and help client say directly what he or she means.	To help client tell you what it is he or she wants.
25. Assist client in learning new ways to deal with stress without delusions such as talking about fears and anxieties with another person.	To improve coping skills.
26. Teach client ways (singing, whistling) to interrupt own delusions.	To prevent alienating self from others who may not understand client's behavior.
27. Respond to feeling tone of delusions.	To let client know you understand fears and uncertainties.
28. Promote intellectual stimulation with items such as crossword puzzles and word games.	To distract from delusional thinking by involving with people and activities.
29. Set limits on discussion of specified delusional material.	To avoid reinforcing the delusions.
30. Enforce limit setting and elicit cooperation of others.	To promote continuity of care by others working with client.
31. Avoid generalizations and use of universal pronouns (for example, "we" or "our").	To help client see self as a distinct individual.
Social Dimension	
1. Provide a busy, structured environment.	To reduce time for delusions and stimulate interest in the real world.
2. Increase self-esteem.	To reduce client's need for delusions of grandeur and orient to reality.

IMPLEMENTATION—cont'd

NURSING ACTIONS	RATIONALE
3. Assure client, if your presence makes client uncomfortable, that he or she can ask you to leave.	To help client identify feelings, to assume responsibility for handling them appropriately.
4. Eliminate whispered comments around client among staff members.	To prevent client from being unduly suspicious.
5. Be aware that laughter may be misinterpreted.	To increase your sensitivity to client.
6. Contact no one about client without letting client know.	To prevent further suspiciousness.
7. Promote client's involvement with others.	To prevent withdrawal, isolation, and alienation.
8. Be knowledgeable about client's cultural background.	To better understand client's behavior. Delusions may be culturally based and may seem bizarre if you lack information about client's cultural background.
9. Provide therapies (group, supportive, family, recreation, activity, reality, and milieu).	To help client maintain a sense of reality, interact with others, feel part of a caring group, understand and change client's behavior, receive feedback, and support.
10. Inform client and family of social agencies that offer help.	To provide supportive services and follow-up care.
11. Elicit support of family to provide a no-demand, low stress level environment.	To prevent a recurrence of symptoms and hospitalization.
Spiritual Dimension	
1. Avoid discussions of religion when delusions are religious in nature.	To prevent reinforcing delusions, to avoid hostile, argumentative behavior.
2. Listen attentively, then refocus conversation when client has religious delusions.	To obtain the feeling tone of the delusion, to distract to reality.
3. Be aware that religion is more an escape than a comfort to client.	To increase understanding of meaning of religiousness.
4. Provide experiences and relationships that are pleasurable to client and enhance quality of life through therapeutic relationship with nurse and fun activities with others.	To help client enjoy the real world more than the unreal world.
5. Instill confidence in client's ability to control delusions with medicine and support with your support and caring.	To increase feelings of control over own life, to live a more satisfying life.

EVALUATION

Measurable goals and outcome criteria provide the data for evaluating the delusional client's progress. Client self-reports, nurse observations, and family reports provide additional data. The following behaviors indicate a positive evaluation:

1. Takes medications as prescribed
2. Identifies anxiety
3. Uses appropriate methods for reducing anxiety
4. Controls delusional thinking with humming, whistling, or other measures
5. Interacts with other people

BIBLIOGRAPHY

Aronson T et al: Relapse in delusional depression: a retrospective study of the course of treatment, *Compr Psychiatry* 29(1):12, 1988.

Barile L: The client who is delusional. In Lego S, editor: *The American handbook of psychiatric nursing*, Philadelphia, 1984, J.B. Lippincott Co.

del Campo E, Carr C, Correa E: Rehospitalized schizophrenics: what they report about illness, treatment, and compliance, *J Psychosoc Nurs Ment Health Serv* 21(6):29, 1983.

Kendler K, Glazer W, Morgenstern H: Dimensions of delusional experience, *Am J Psychiatry* 140:466, 1983.

Meyers B: Late-life depression and delusions, *Hosp Commun Psychiatry* 38:573, 1987.

Rosenthal T, McGuinsess T: Dealing with delusional patients: the distorted truth, *Issues Ment Health Nurs* 8(2):143, 1986.

Rudden M, Sweeney J, Gilmore M: A comparison of delusional disorders in women and men, *Am J Psychiatry* 140:1575, 1983.

Tousley M: The paranoid fortress of David J., *J Psychosoc Nurs Ment Health Serv* 22(2):8, 1984.

Turpin J, Halbreich V, Pena J: *Transient psychosis: diagnosis, management and evaluation*, New York, 1984, Brunner/Mazel, Inc.

Wright L: A symbolic tree, loneliness is the root: delusions are the leaves, *J Psychiatr Nurs* 13:30, 1975.

▼ Denial

Denial is a self-deceptive defense mechanism that protects the individual from a given reality. The process is unconscious on the part of the individual. Occurring in infancy, denial is one of the first protective defense mechanisms that an individual develops. Often expressed as shock or disbelief, denial is a universal initial reaction of most individuals to an anxiety-producing event.

Over a period of time denial may give way to a slowly developing awareness of reality. However, it does not generally lead to problem resolution because an individual cannot analyze a threatening situation when he or she refuses to recognize that situation.

Denial can be a healthy, unhealthy, or destructive defense. It is helpful to evaluate denial according to the purpose it serves at the time. Nurses are involved daily with clients who react to a stressful event with disbelief or persist in using denial to cope with anxiety. A feared diagnosis, an injury resulting in loss of a body part or of functioning, the loss of a loved one, and illness or a disease such as alcoholism are some of the many situations that clients and families face initially with denial. For these reasons it is essential that nurses recognize denial, understand why it occurs in clients and families, and be able to intervene appropriately.

Related DSM-III-R disorders

Psychoactive substance use disorders
Mood disorders

Other related conditions

Losses (body parts or body functions)
Long-term disability
Grief and bereavement
Terminal illness
Dying

PRINCIPLES

▶ Physical Dimension

1. The possibility for denial exists when an individual is faced with stressful situations such as illness, injury, loss, disease, or hospitalization.

▶ Emotional Dimension

1. Denial is a normal way of handling anxiety.
2. Denial allays anxiety by reducing the perception of the threat.

▶ Intellectual Dimension

1. Denial is a protective defense mechanism.
2. Denial is outside of and beyond conscious awareness.
3. Denial achieves its purpose by disowning, rejecting, or ignoring one or more of the elements of the conflict.
4. Denial in the face of reality usually indicates an unhealthy response.
5. Denial of illness can seriously interfere with treatment.
6. Denial of illness protects the ego from becoming overwhelmed by anxiety and averts disorganization.
7. As the stress of the anxiety-producing situation is alleviated, the person's need to deny decreases.
8. Denial is one of the first protective defense mechanisms that an individual develops, occurring first in infancy.
9. Denial (a) applies to every type of conflict, (b) requires no previous learning, (c) distorts reality, and (d) is of little help in solving problems.
10. Denial represents a reaction to fear; attempts to frighten clients with warnings serve to increase fear and denial.
11. Clients who minimize the seriousness of their symptoms are indicating denial.

115

▶ **Social Dimension**

1. Denial may result when an individual is faced with a threat to the self-concept or with a change in role or level of esteem.
2. Denial can serve to alienate the client from supportive interpersonal relationships.

▶ **Spiritual Dimension**

1. Conflicts in values or beliefs may contribute to denial.
2. Guilt or shame over a past act or situation may promote denial of the act or situation.
3. Despairing persons deny themselves life's pleasures and feel unworthy and of little value.
4. Individuals unable to find meaning in suffering may deny the existence of their God or supreme power.
5. Realistic hope provides a base for a beginning awareness of a person's denial.
6. Some world religions emphasize denial of self-pleasures.

ASSESSMENT

▶ **Physical Dimension**

I. History
  A. Activities of daily living
    1. Nutrition
      a. Appetite
        (1) Overeats
        (2) Ignores special diet
      b. Weight
        (1) Gains weight, is obese
    2. Physical activities and limitations
      a. Plunges into activities
      b. Overactive
      c. Compulsive activity
      d. Overly robust or exaggerated activity
  B. Habits
    1. Alcohol
      a. Excessive intake
    2. Smoking
      a. Continues to smoke when stopping is recommended

  3. Medications and drugs
    a. Self-medicates with megavitamins, illegal drugs, or wonder-drugs
    b. May refuse all medications
  C. Destructive behavior
    1. Refuses to follow treatment regimen
    2. Violates medication orders
    3. Shows risk-taking behaviors, such as continuing to drive or exercise
  D. Health history
    1. Refuses to discuss problem
    2. Claims no illnesses, alcoholism, obesity, or chronic disease

II. Physical examination—may reveal illness or disease in any body system, indicating that client disbelieves or minimizes information related to diagnosis, symptoms, or progress of disease or illness

▶ **Emotional Dimension**

CLIENT DATA	ANALYSIS	NURSING DIAGNOSIS
Is anxious	Minimizes seriousness of illness. Sense of adequacy as a person is threatened by illness.	Ineffective individual coping: related to denial of seriousness of illness
Is falsely brave about feeling ill	Pretends vigor and health even though not feeling well; minimizes seriousness of symptoms.	Ineffective individual coping: related to denial of illness
Fears loss of control	Is unable to accept illness because it means losing control of body.	Ineffective individual coping: denial related to fear of losing control
Shows unconcerned, unemotional reaction to illness	Is unable to believe diagnosis of illness.	Ineffective individual coping: related to denial of diagnosis of illness
Has inappropriate emotional reactions (excessive cheerfulness, exaggerated optimism, use of humor, or laughing)	Is unable to accept illness; possibly feels humiliated, embarrassed, or fearful of rejection from loved ones. Response to tension associated with reality of situation.	Ineffective individual coping: excessive cheerfulness, exaggerated optimism, use of humor, or laughing related to denial of illness

▶ **Intellectual Dimension**

CLIENT DATA	ANALYSIS	NURSING DIAGNOSIS
Distorts information about problem	Defense to lessen threat and reduce anxiety.	Defensive coping: distorted perception related to denial of problem
Attributes minor symptoms to serious problems	Minimizing problem and denying its seriousness to reduce anxiety.	Defensive coping: related to denial of seriousness of problem
Minimizes illness, symptoms	Protective defense to lessen threat and reduce anxiety.	Defensive coping: minimizing symptoms related to denial of illness
Avoids discussing denied areas of problem	Response to anxiety. Threat to body system may be too difficult to bear at this time.	Defensive coping: avoiding discussion of problem related to denial of condition
Uses generalities, vagueness	Response to anxiety. Threat may be too difficult to bear at this time.	Defensive coping: use of generalities and vagueness related to denial
Dwells on past, avoids future	Response to anxiety. Threat may be too difficult to bear at this time.	Defensive coping: dwelling on past, avoiding future related to denial
Misunderstands information	Response to anxiety. Threat may be too difficult to bear at this time.	Defensive coping: misunderstanding of problem related to denial
Asks no questions	Response to anxiety. Threat may be too difficult to bear at this time.	Defensive coping: not asking questions related to denial.
Postpones decisions	Response to anxiety. Threat may be too difficult to bear at this time.	Defensive coping: postponement of decisions related to denial
Dismisses medical orders	Response to anxiety. Threat may be too difficult to bear at this time.	Defensive coping: dismissal of medical orders related to denial
Avoids or ignores statements of information	Response to anxiety. Threat may be too difficult to bear at this time.	Defensive coping: avoiding or ignoring statements of information related to denial
Disinterested in progress	Response to anxiety. Threat may be too difficult to bear at this time.	Defensive coping: disinterest in progress related to denial
Jokes and laughs about problem	Discounts significance of condition.	Defensive coping: inappropriate laughing and joking related to denial of problem

▶ **Social Dimension**

CLIENT DATA	ANALYSIS	NURSING DIAGNOSIS
Deceives self	Rejects personal capabilities; fears inability to measure up to own and others' expectations.	Self-esteem disturbance: related to denial of capabilities
Is unable to view self realistically	Threat is producing high level of anxiety.	Self-esteem disturbance: inability to view self realistically related to denial
Has low self-esteem	Minimizes abilities; denies self pleasures and successes that build esteem.	Self-esteem disturbance: related to denial of pleasures and successes
Minimizes or ignores need for dependence on others	Denies need for help from others. Sense of autonomy and independence is threatened.	Self-esteem disturbance: inappropriate independence related to denial of need for help
Is unable to acknowledge problems because of cultural norms	Admitting problems is seen as sign of weakness in some cultures (stoicism, chauvinism).	Self-esteem disturbance: unrealistic perception of self related to denial of symptoms associated with cultural factors

▶ **Spiritual Dimension**

CLIENT DATA	ANALYSIS	NURSING DIAGNOSIS
Believes that illness is weakness	Associated with family or cultural factors.	Spiritual distress: belief that illness is weakness related to denial of symptoms
Becomes overly involved with religion	Is seeking to escape reality.	Spiritual distress: inappropriate religious involvement related to denial of symptoms
Is unable to see realistic hope	Situation too threatening, prevents client from facing reality.	Spiritual distress: unrealistic hope related to denial of situation
Denies self pleasurable experiences	Feels unworthy, of little value; may be based on religious beliefs.	Spiritual distress: inability to experience pleasures related to feeling unworthy
Denies death	Is unable to face reality; death too threatening to discuss.	Spiritual distress: related to denial of death

PLANNING

Long-Term Goal

To accept the reality of the situation without denial

SHORT-TERM GOALS	OUTCOME CRITERIA
Physical Dimension To verbalize that a health problem exists.	1. States that a health problem exists 2. Asks for help with a health problem 3. Identifies consequences of failure to seek treatment for health problem
Emotional Dimension To feel safe expressing thoughts and feelings about situation or illness	1. Discusses situation or illness 2. Looks relaxed 3. Shows interest in learning more about situation or illness 4. Shares anger, fears, grief, and humiliation about situation or illness 5. Asks questions about situation or illness 6. Shares thoughts about seriousness of situation or illness
Intellectual Dimension To identify threat causing denial	1. Verbalizes causes of anxiety 2. Identifies conflicts 3. Admits fears or grief about situation or illness
To decrease need for use of denial	1. Verbalizes accurate information about situation or illness 2. Makes decisions regarding goals for self 3. Discusses specific facts about situation or illness 4. Talks about behavior that indicates denial of situation or illness and behavior that impedes progress 5. Makes statements that imply acceptance of situation or illness: "I ran out of medicine," "I can't function."
Social Dimension To increase self-esteem	1. Statements indicate realistic and positive view of self 2. Identifies self-deception 3. Acknowledges strengths and limitations

SHORT-TERM GOALS	OUTCOME CRITERIA
Spiritual Dimension To rediscover aspects of self that are whole and capable of success	1. Explores impact of situation on own life 2. Identifies areas of self that provide strength 3. Sees self as person of value and worth 4. Statements indicate self confidence 5. Requests to see clergy or religious leader to strengthen religious faith

Discharge Planning

The following client behaviors demonstrate readiness for discharge:
1. Identifies common reactions to threats (anger, denial, or depression)
2. Identifies behaviors that indicate denial of situations or illness
3. Accepts reality of the situation
4. Seeks treatment

IMPLEMENTATION

NURSING ACTIONS	RATIONALE
Physical Dimension	
1. Assist client with self-care when needed.	To help client maintain self-respect.
2. Explore with client consequences of refusal to follow treatment regimen.	To assist client to weigh pros and cons of following treatment.
3. Help client accept responsibility for effects of noncompliance with recommended treatment regimen.	To promote awareness of consequences of not following treatment.
4. Give pain medication when condition is painful.	To relieve pain. Coping with pain and painful awareness at the same time may aggravate the situation.
5. Motivate client to assume responsibility for caring for own health needs (for example, colostomy care, dressing changes, stress reduction) with consistent support and feedback.	To increase independence and autonomy, to increase feelings of control over own life.
Emotional Dimension	
1. Reduce threats that produce anxiety.	To lessen anxiety and need for denial.
2. Promote expression of anger, grief, guilt, fears, and other feelings related to denial using communication techniques of reflection and clarifying.	To help client identify feelings, express them, and plan interventions that will reduce denial.
3. Support client (empathize as client talks, cries, is angry, is embarrassed).	To promote understanding of client's behavior.
4. Connect the discrepancies between client's overly optimistic attitude and physical state.	To promote awareness of inconsistencies in client's behavior.
5. Communicate that the expression of anger and fears (and all emotions) are acceptable and understandable.	To let client know it is OK to feel and provide ways to manage expression of feelings in a mentally healthy manner.
Intellectual Dimension	
1. Provide careful explanations for all procedures, activities.	To reduce anxiety and prevent denial.
2. Present new information when esteem is increased and client is ready to lessen denial.	To use effective timing to work with client. When esteem is low and anxiety high the ability to learn is impaired.
3. Prevent overload of information by using concrete, specific, concise statements.	To enhance accurate comprehension.
4. Present threatening information matter-of-factly.	To prevent misinterpretation.
5. When a relationship is established, plant "seeds of doubt" judiciously.	To lessen possibility of client reacting emotionally. To encourage client to recognize reality.
6. Refrain from chastising client when client uses denial to cope.	To prevent increased feelings of rejection and devaluation.

IMPLEMENTATION—cont'd

NURSING ACTIONS	RATIONALE
7. Identify whether denial is helpful or harmful to client.	To determine the meaning of client's denial and plan interventions.
8. Allow client to develop awareness of reality at own pace.	To provide time for client to face reality and make appropriate adjustments.
9. Refrain from furthering client's denial by agreeing with client.	To avoid reinforcing denial.
10. Use "reality reminders." (Reality reminders accept client's denial, do not encourage or participate in the denial, and remind client of a known reality.)	To avoid a direct attack on client's denial.
11. Understand that client may return to denial at a later time.	To gain awareness of client's need to deny.
12. Identify expressions of anger, frustration, embarrassment, or guilt as signs of progress and encourage expression of them.	Expressions of feelings indicate a lessening of denial and a readiness to face the denial.
13. Allow client's questions to guide presentation of new factors of reality.	To provide accurate information based on client's questions. Questions are an early indication that client is beginning to accept reality.
14. Refocus on subjects that client avoids or sidesteps.	To prevent client from distracting from subject of discussion.
15. Reduce focus when client's anxiety interferes.	To lessen anxiety.
Social Dimension	
1. Provide an environment where client feels free and safe to ask questions by listening actively and using therapeutic communication techniques.	To facilitate client's asking questions that prepare for accepting reality.
2. Plan contacts with family members.	To increase their awareness of client's need to deny.
3. Promote client's self-esteem by emphasizing client's positive attributes and skills.	To increase awareness of client's capabilities and competencies.
4. Assist client in recognizing ways client deceives self by verbalizing observations.	To promote awareness of self-deception.
Spiritual Dimension	
1. Assist client in seeking pleasurable activities.	To assist client in seeking pleasures in life rather than denying them.
2. Question client's belief that weakness is synonymous with illness.	To present client with other explanations for illness.
3. Refer client to religious leader.	To strengthen faith in self and others.
4. Help client accept reality of death when appropriate.	To lessen threat associated with death.

EVALUATION

Denial invariably complicates the evaluation of emotional disorders. Because denial operates to some degree in almost all clients and because it often blocks the goals of nursing therapy, it is essential that nurses:

1. Recognize behavioral clues that suggest client is denying some aspect of reality
2. Understand the need that denial helps client meet
3. Determine when denial is interfering with treatment goals

4. Maintain a supportive relationship as client begins to move toward more reality-based thinking

Measurable goals and outcome criteria provide the data for evaluating clients who deny. Nurse observations and family data also provide data. The following behaviors indicate a positive evaluation:

1. Talks about illness or disability with others
2. Demonstrates hope and optimism about future
3. Follows prescribed treatment regimen

BIBLIOGRAPHY

Cousins N: Denial, *JAMA* 248(2):211, 1982.

Dimsdale J, Hackett T: Effect of denial on cardiac health and psychological assessment, *Am J Psychiatry* 139(11):1477, 1982.

Kiehing M: Denial of illness. In Carlson C, Blackwell B, editors: *Behavioral concepts and nursing interventions*, ed 2, New York, 1978, J.B. Lippincott Co.

Losten T et al: Family denial as a prognostic factor in opiate addict treatment outcome, *J Nerv Ment Dis* 171(10):611, 1983.

McKendry M, Losan R: The recognition and management of denial in patients after myocardial infarction, *Aust N Z J Med* 12(6):607, 1982.

Nyomathi A, van Servellen G: Maladaptive coping in the critically ill population with acquired immunodeficiency syndrome: nursing assessment and treatment, *Heart Lung* 18(2):113, 1989.

O'Mahony P: Psychiatric patient denial of mental illness as a normal process, *Br J Med Psychol* 55.109, 1982.

Robinson K: Denial in myocardial infarction patient, *Crit Care Nurse* 10(5):138, 1990.

Watson M et al: Reaction to a diagnosis of breast cancer: relationship between denial, delay, and rates of psychological morbidity, *Cancer* 53(9):2008, 1984.

Dependence

Dependence is behavior in which one person relies on another for support or aid. The individual seeks (1) physical contact, (2) attention, (3) proximity, (4) physical help, and (5) approval and praise. Other characteristics include resistance to self-care, statements of helplessness, a clinging manner, somatic complaints, demands, ingratiating behavior, attention-seeking behavior, and extreme compliance.

Dependent persons have excessive needs for attention, affection, and approval. Acceptance by others is essential for maintaining security. To achieve security, dependent persons view others as superior and may adopt and function in accord with others' attitudes, beliefs, and opinions rather than their own. Dependence has both healthy and unhealthy aspects. In childhood, in illness and hospitalization, and in chronic disability the individual may experience a dependent role. As the child matures, as the individual becomes well, and as the person who is chronically disabled adapts to the disability, independence increases. Unhealthy dependence is seen in persons with alcohol and drug abuse problems and in those who are emotionally or physically dependent on others.

When independent, the person's behavior is self-motivated and self-directed. Reliance on others to guide behavior is minimal, although the opinion of others is considered. Interdependence is behavior that is balanced between dependence and independence with the individual performing both types of behavior.

It is helpful to recognize the tendency of clients to depend on the nurse for help. Although this may be flattering and help nurses feel important and needed, it is essential that nurses explore underlying dependency needs in themselves and in the client to foster increased independence in the client.

The original content for this section was contributed by Louise Bradford Suit, R.N., Ed.D.

Related DSM-III-R disorders

Dependent personality disorders
Dissociative disorders
Psychoactive substance use disorders

Other related conditions

Injuries
Disabilities
Chronic disease
Hospitalization
Childhood

PRINCIPLES

▶ Physical Dimension

1. Dependence is seen in individuals who abuse drugs and alcohol.
2. Addiction is a manifestation of clients with problems with dependence.
3. Dependent persons may use alcohol and drugs as a coping mechanism.
4. Chemical dependence results in physical damage to the body and may be life threatening.
5. Trauma, hospitalization, disability, illness, and severe emotional disturbances may cause a person to be temporarily dependent on others.
6. Articulate speech and physical maturity help the child become independent.
7. Individuation allows the child to develop as a separate and independent person.
8. Infants are totally dependent on caregivers for physical care.

▶ Emotional Dimension

1. Infants depend on parental figure or caregiver for emotional support.

2. Dependence occurs during the oral phase of development (birth to 18 months).
3. When dependence needs are met, the infant progresses to the next phase of development.
4. When dependence needs are not met, the child may experience difficulties in oral gratification later in life, such as smoking, obesity, and substance abuse.
5. Resolution of separation anxiety in the child results in independent behavior.
6. It is the child's mother or caregiver who provides care and thus satisfies dependence needs, initially.
7. The prolonged period of childhood dependence is a contributing factor in the cause of neuroses.
8. Mastery of the environment depends on the ability to handle outer and inner drives, to delay gratification so that satisfaction and independence are ultimately attained.
9. Achieving independence is moving from environmental support to self-support.
10. Psychological and physical maturation means giving up dependencies on outside support.
11. Maturity does not mean complete self-sufficiency but indicates a sense of responsibility for the self and for support, including asking for help.
12. Maturity and independence may be accompanied by psychological distress when the safety and security of the familiar are left behind.

▶ **Intellectual Dimension**

1. Irrational thoughts may cause a person to maintain self as dependent on others.
2. Self-talk, the way a person sees and thinks about self, is an important factor in maintaining dependent behavior.
3. A person can change irrational thoughts about dependence into rational ones by changing self-talk.
4. A person's acts are consistent with that person's perception of self. If a person sees self as dependent, he or she will act dependently.
5. Learning to fulfill needs with resulting independence begins in infancy and continues throughout life.
6. The ability to fulfill one's needs is to be responsible and act independently.

▶ **Social Dimension**

1. Infants enter the world totally dependent on others for survival.
2. Parents foster independence when they encourage the child to perform age-appropriate behaviors.
3. During the latter part of the infancy phase, children learn to satisfy some of their own needs and separate from caregivers; thus independence begins.
4. Parents or caregivers exert a strong influence on the child's dependent or independent behavior.
5. Parents or caregivers tend to reward independent behavior in children.
6. Positive reinforcement of the child's mastery over the environment is essential for the formation of independent behavior.
7. With successful achievements and positive reinforcements the child develops a positive self-concept and learns independent behaviors.
8. A child with low self-esteem, who seeks excessive attention and help from others, lacks successful achievements and positive reinforcements.
9. Praise and rewards are essential for the development of independent behavior.
10. Secondary gains and reinforcement of dependent behavior may result in difficulty in giving up dependent behavior.
11. Conflicts occur in aging adults, who become increasingly dependent when physical abilities deteriorate.
12. Children are born with basic needs; when children are deprived, they become insecure and dependent.
13. To overcome insecurity, help is sought from others in a dependent way.
14. Overprotective parents do not provide the opportunities needed for learning independence and for the development of necessary skills.
15. Some persons retain infantile patterns of dependency.
16. Dependence on others for satisfaction of needs may result in suppression and repression so that the displeasure of persons being relied on is not incurred.
17. Dependent persons have learned that feelings associated with pleasure are best provided by others.

▶ **Spiritual Dimension**

1. Exposure to beliefs and values of parents or caregivers influences dependence behaviors.
2. Adolescents challenge the beliefs and values of parents or caregivers with their increasing independence.
3. Adolescents not allowed to freely choose beliefs and values as their own incorporate their parents' or caregivers' beliefs and values.
4. Dependence on parents' or caregivers' beliefs and values impairs the individual's sense of autonomy and inhibits growth and self-actualization.

ASSESSMENT

▶ **Physical Dimension**

I. History
  A. Activities of daily living
    1. Waits on others to prepare meals
    2. Waits on others for bedtime preparations
    3. Usually has no recreation, hobbies, or interests
    4. Physical activity may be restricted by physical damage (paralysis)
    5. Sexual activity
      a. Sexual dysfunction
      b. Impotence
      c. Limitations imposed by physical condition
  B. Habits
    1. Physical dependence on alcohol
    2. Physical dependence on smoking
    3. Physical dependence on medications and drugs
  C. Destructive behavior
    1. Lacks self-assertion
    2. Feels victimized
    3. Rescues others as an attention mechanism
  D. Health history
    1. Any acute or chronic illnesses
    2. Traumatic injuries (amputation)
    3. Hospitalization with forced dependence
    4. Temporary dependence following surgery
  E. Review of systems—inquire about physical damage in each body system influencing dependence

II. Diagnostic tests
  A. Neurological
    1. Myelography
    2. Reflexes
    3. Nerve biopsy
  B. Gastrointestinal (GI)
    1. Upper GI
    2. Lower GI
    3. Barium enema
    4. Ultrasonography
    5. Sigmoidoscopy
    6. Esophogastric duodenoscopy (EGD)
    7. Liver function tests
      a. Amylase
      b. Serum glutamic oxaloacetic transaminase (SGOT)
      c. Lactic dehydrogenase (LDH)
      d. Creatine phosphokinase (CPK)
  C. Cardiovascular—ophthalmic examination of blood vessels

▶ **Physical Examination**

CLIENT DATA	ANALYSIS	NURSING DIAGNOSIS
Poor personal hygiene	Waits for others to initiate care.	Bathing/hygiene self-care deficit: related to dependence on others
Overweight, underweight, poor skin turgor, poor muscle tone, pallor, and impaired food and hydration patterns	Poor nutritional habits resulting from waiting passively on others for care.	Altered health maintenance: related to dependence
Peripheral nerve and brain damage	Chronic irritation of the brain from alcohol intake produces irreversible damage.	Altered health maintenance: related to substance abuse
Ulcers, gastroenteritis, esophagitis, colitis, and liver diseases (cirrhosis)	Chemical substances in the gastrointestinal system produce inflammation and damage, especially in the liver. Chemical substances are detoxified by the liver; large quantities over time cause liver damage.	Altered health maintenance: related to substance abuse
Decreased libido; impotence	Chemical substances decrease production of estrogen in women and testosterone in men.	Sexual dysfunction: related to substance abuse
Physical abuse (bruises, burns, bites, injuries, neglect, and malnourishment)	Low frustration tolerance of caregivers when caring for children or the aged contributes to acting-out with physical abuse of dependent person.	Ineffective family coping: compromised, physical abuse related to dependence of family member
Physical injury or disease (spinal cord injury, paraplegia, quadraplegia, amputation, cerebrovascular accident, paralysis, muscular dystrophy, or multiple sclerosis.	Extent to which client can carry out own activities of daily living is determined by nature and location of injury; injury may result in temporary or permanent dependence.	Ineffective individual coping: dependence related to physical injury or disease

▶ **Emotional Dimension**

CLIENT DATA	ANALYSIS	NURSING DIAGNOSIS
Feelings of anger, resentment, depression, loneliness, helplessness, and worthlessness	Low self-esteem and inability to meet own needs leads to variety of feelings.	Ineffective individual coping: anger, resentment, depression, loneliness, helplessness, worthlessness, related to unmet dependence needs
Grief	Grieving occurs in response to physical injury or loss of bodily function, resulting in dependence.	Grief: related to physical injury, loss of functioning with dependence
Depression	Affect may be inappropriate for the situation; excessive sorrow and sadness, cries easily, discusses event or injury as if it were recent, gives out clues that past grief has not been effectively dealt with; failure to grieve influences a person's adjustment and functioning.	Dysfunctional grieving: unresolved loss related to dependence

▶ **Intellectual Dimension**

CLIENT DATA	ANALYSIS	NURSING DIAGNOSIS
Distorted perception	Perception is altered by client's unmet dependency needs or denial of situation.	Altered thought processes: distorted perception related to unmet dependency needs
Impaired communication skills	Dependent person lacks experience with people, may have poor communication skills.	Impaired verbal communication: related to dependence
Denial of dependence	Denial is a defense mechanism, an attempt to deny existence of dependent behavior and protect from anxiety.	Ineffective individual coping: related to denial of dependent behavior
Use of rationalization	Rationalization allows dependent individual to place responsibility for behavior on others.	Defensive coping: use of rationalization related to dependence
Poor decision-making skills	Significant others making decisions for client has not allowed development of decision-making skills.	Knowledge deficit: lack of information on and practice with making decisions related to dependence
Denial of limitations imposed by physical condition	Attempts to do more for self than is physically capable of according to physical status: gets out of bed when bed rest is prescribed; heart attack client exceeds activity order, eats food not on diet, and snacks when advised not to. Unable to assume dependent role.	Defensive coping: denial of physical condition related to need to be independent

▶ **Social Dimension**

CLIENT DATA	ANALYSIS	NURSING DIAGNOSIS
Poor self-concept	Feedback from significant others is inappropriate for establishing positive feelings about self.	Self-esteem disturbance: related to dependence
Low self-esteem	Feedback from significant others is inappropriate for establishing positive feelings about self.	Self-esteem disturbance: related to dependence
Mistrust of self and others	Unmet dependency needs lead to lack of trust in self and caretakers and ultimately in people in general.	Ineffective individual coping: lack of trust in self and others related to dependence

► **Social Dimension—cont'd**

CLIENT DATA	ANALYSIS	NURSING DIAGNOSIS
During weaning does not give up bottle; stays home when young adult; financially dependent on parents; has poor work record	Inappropriate behavior for developmental level; uses dependent behavior when capable of independent behavior. Positive reinforcement from mastery of the environment is essential for formation of independent behavior; secondary gains make it difficult to give up dependent behavior.	Ineffective individual coping: dependence related to inappropriate behavior for developmental level
Inappropriate attention-seeking behaviors; loudness and boisterousness, silence, withdrawal, resistance, need for constant reinforcement; inappropriate touching, bragging, whining	Unmet needs in early development phases combined with reinforcement for inappropriate attention-seeking behavior lead to behavior that gets attention but is not socially acceptable.	Ineffective individual coping: inappropriate attention-seeking behaviors related to dependence Inability to give in a relationship
Inability to give in a relationship	Giving and taking is essential in relationships; dependent person takes from a relationship but is unable to give of self.	Impaired social interactions: inability to give in a relationship related to dependence
Manipulates others	Attempts to get others to do things for self.	Ineffective individual coping: manipulation related to dependence
Family history given of client's injuries does not match the client's injuries	Inconsistencies in explanations of injuries are attempts to cover facts of abuse.	Ineffective family coping: discrepancies in family history history related to injured dependent person
Social acting out; seduction, excessive compliments, helplessness, exploitation, clinging	Attempts to get others to do things for self or to get special privileges since individual does not believe he or she can do things for self. Overconcern for feelings of others, jealousy, expectation of special favors, immature behavior.	Impaired social interaction: related to dependence
Lying, stealing	Behavior alienates others. Indicative of unmet needs, low self-esteem.	Impaired social interactions: socially unacceptable behavior related to dependence
Violence, aggression	May resort to violence or aggression when needs are not met.	High risk for violence: related to dependence
Withdrawal from others, lack of close friends	Reduces anxiety associated with interpersonal contacts.	Impaired social interactions: withdrawal from others related to dependence
Fighting, thefts, illegal occupations, failure to honor debts, reckless driving, abuse of chemical substances, repeated arrests	Characteristics of person abusing substances (drugs, alcohol).	Ineffective individual coping: substance abuse related to dependence needs
Difficulty holding a job, impulsive	Has not learned to rely on self and has difficulty assuming job responsibilities.	Altered role performance: difficulty holding job related to dependence
Fear of independence	Fears that dependence needs will not be met.	Ineffective individual coping: dependence related to fear of independence
Scapegoat	Family conditioning of dependent behavior in one member enables family to direct conflict toward one person and avoid real issues.	Ineffective family coping: related to dependent family member
Excessive dependence on parents; does not cut "apron strings"	Independent behavior is discouraged by parents, who are attempting to meet own needs.	Ineffective family coping: reinforcement of dependence related to parental need for child

▶ **Social Dimension—cont'd**

CLIENT DATA	ANALYSIS	NURSING DIAGNOSIS
Poor occupational functioning	Impulsive, immature, may terminate inappropriately, needs structure on job; dependent person lacks communication skills, decision-making skills, and self-confidence conducive to good occupational functioning.	Altered role performance: poor occupational functioning related to dependence
Procrastination, stubbornness, indecisiveness	Gratification of own needs is central.	Ineffective individual coping: procrastination, stubbornness, indecisiveness related to dependence

▶ **Spiritual Dimension**

CLIENT DATA	ANALYSIS	NURSING DIAGNOSIS
Excessive need for affiliation with religious organization	Internal locus of control produces excessive need for higher power or religious group to externally control self.	Spiritual distress: excessive need for religious organization related to dependence
Impaired self-growth	Lack of trust in self leads to impaired maturity.	Spiritual distress: related to lack of trust in self
Inability to reach full potential	Unresolved dependency needs limit growth in all aspects.	Spiritual distress: related to inability to achieve full potential
Lack of relationship with deity or higher power	Lack of trust and faith in himself and others leads to poor relationship with higher power.	Spiritual distress: related to lack of relationship with deity or higher power
Failure to respect morals and values of others	Lack of self-respect and self-growth produces basic disregard of others. Rigidity and inflexibility lead to inability to see situation from another person's perspective.	Spiritual distress: related to lack of self-respect and respect for others
Failure to adopt own beliefs and values	Through socialization by parents person fails to adopt own beliefs and values; has not internalized own values and beliefs.	Spiritual distress: related to holding on to parental values
Beliefs and values are challenged	Holds on to beliefs and values placed on self. May become inflexible and rigid as result of holding on to others' beliefs and values rather than deciding for self.	Spiritual distress: related to perceived challenge of belief system

PLANNING

Long-Term Goal:

To function at an optimal level of independence

SHORT-TERM GOALS	OUTCOME CRITERIA
Physical Dimension To identify the causes of dependence	1. Discusses manifestation of dependent behavior 2. States sources of dependent behavior 3. Verbalizes role of significant others in maintaining behavior 4. Acknowledges dependent behavior as a part of self 5. Identifies secondary gain for dependent behavior

PLANNING—cont'd

SHORT-TERM GOALS	OUTCOME CRITERIA
To initiate own activities of daily living	1. Attends to own personal grooming needs 2. Attends to own nutritional needs by stating the components of a balanced diet, planning own meals, and maintaining appropriate body weight 3. Initiates an activity 4. Participates in an exercise program
To live free of chemical substances	1. Is admitted for detoxification 2. Complies with treatment program 3. Lives free of chemical substances 4. Attends support group 5. Accepts help and support from family 6. Participates in leisure activities without using chemical substances
Emotional Dimension To deal constructively with own feelings associated with dependence	1. Identifies and explores feelings within self. 2. Verbalizes feelings 3. Acknowledges feelings as acceptable 4. Deals effectively with feelings
Intellectual Dimension To develop a realistic independent style of coping	1. Discusses independent behavior 2. Verbalizes benefits of behaving independently 3. Tries out independent behavior 4. Receives feedback and support for new behavior 5. Consistently acts in an independent fashion 6. Makes independent decisions
To resolve conflicts around unmet dependency	1. Separates and individualizes self from others 2. Identifies associated feelings of anger and resentment 3. Deals effectively with own feelings
Social Dimension To improve self-esteem by developing positive feelings for self	1. Accepts compliments and praise from others without discounting them 2. Verbalizes own positive aspects 3. Makes no self-deprecating remarks
To decrease the need for approval of others	1. Describes own attention-getting behavior 2. Acknowledges attention-seeking behavior as own 3. Verbalizes how behavior affects others 4. Accepts responsibility for own behavior 5. Modifies behavior.
To establish positive relationships with people without manipulation	1. Discusses own manipulative behavior 2. Verbalizes awareness of reaction of others and their feelings 3. Acknowledges behavior as own 4. Accepts limits 5. Complies with treatment and accepts sanctions for noncompliance 6. Communicates openly with others 7. Discusses problem with family or significant others 8. Establishes positive, healthy relationships with others
Spiritual Dimension To accept forced dependence and live a fully enriched life	1. Discusses feelings freely with significant others 2. Identifies assets and physical capabilities 3. Develops additional capabilities 4. Learns skills appropriate for selected career 5. Grieves loss 6. Resolves loss and situation 7. Reenters social world

Discharge Planning

The following client behaviors demonstrate readiness for discharge:
1. Identifies dependent and independent behavior
2. Reenters family system that nurtured and generated dependent behavior with an awareness of situation
3. Demonstrates independent thinking and behavior

IMPLEMENTATION

NURSING ACTIONS	RATIONALE
Physical Dimension	

1. Develop a nursing care plan outlining activities of daily living:
  a. Activities client can perform independently.
  b. Activities client needs help with.
  c. Activities client needs nurse to perform.
	To provide baseline data against which to measure client's progress.

2. Positively reinforce independent behavior in client.	To encourage continuation of appropriate independent behavior.
3. Maintain nurse-client relationship boundaries.	To prevent client from becoming dependent on nurse and nurse from allowing it to happen.
4. In forced dependence assist client in developing remaining body muscles, assets, and capabilities.	To promote an optimal level of functioning.
5. Help client become and remain chemical-free using support groups.	To live an enriched and satisfying life free of chemical substances.
Emotional Dimension	
1. Establish a therapeutic relationship to help client with dependence issues.	To promote independence in the relationship that can carry over with other relationships.
2. Use a nonjudgmental and accepting approach in establishing a trusting relationship to deal with dependent behavior.	To enable client to feel safe as client works on changing behavior.
3. Initially accept client's dependent behavior.	To demonstrate caring about client as a person of worth even though client has a problem with dependence.
4. Help client to set realistic and attainable goals.	To help client feel he or she can change behavior and increase feelings of independence and control of own life.
5. Facilitate client's ventilation of feelings by listening actively and reflecting.	To help client identify feelings associated with dependence on others or chemical substances, both positive and negative.
6. Help client manage feelings surrounding dependent behavior by facilitating the expression of resentment and anger.	To promote healthy ways of handling dependence.
7. Help client acknowledge substance abuse problems by identifying problems associated with substance abuse.	To motivate client to resolve the problem.
8. Help client comprehend self-defeating aspects of dependent behavior.	To promote awareness of consequences of client's behavior.
9. Help client reduce secondary gains associated with dependency by identifying avoided responsibilities.	To promote awareness of client's need for dependence and remove the benefits.
10. Help client grieve loss of use of chemical substances as a coping style through the grieving process.	To prevent maladaptive grieving (depression) and further dependence.
11. Help client identify anger associated with dependence, explore the source, deal effectively with anger, and express it in a socially acceptable manner.	To enable client to be honest with self and acknowledge feelings of anger.
12. Decrease reinforcement of inappropriate attention-seeking behavior by ignoring it and giving attention when not seeking it.	To prevent emphasis on inappropriate attention-seeking behaviors.

IMPLEMENTATION—cont'd

NURSING ACTIONS	RATIONALE
Intellectual Dimension	
1. Assess client's understanding of situation, problems, and behavior related to dependence.	To collect data about client's perception of behavior and plan interventions.
2. Supplement client's learning about mental health issues and decision making using your knowledge of client's intellectual capacity, education, and sociocultural background.	To add to client's knowledge base information that will increase independent functioning in a manner that is sensitive to and compatible with background.
3. Facilitate problem solving by helping client to: Identify problems associated with dependence. Assess problem and how dependence is manifested. Propose solutions. Discuss pros and cons of solutions. Select solution. Apply solution to decrease inappropriate dependent behavior.	To help client learn problem-solving skills, thereby increasing autonomy and independent functioning.
4. Help client set attainable, realistic goals by participating in treatment planning.	To promote independent functioning that is realistic.
5. Intervene directly with denial by: Exploring fears and anxieties of client. Exploring client's perception of situation. Dealing with client's anxiety.	To help client gain awareness of own denial and need for it.
6. Explore with client ways to improve social skills.	To promote comfort in interactions with others and lessen need for dependence on chemical substances.
7. Help client identify behaviors displayed while abusing chemical substances.	To confront client with behavior when abusing substances.
8. Confront client about effects of behavior while abusing chemical substances.	To confront client with the consequences of abuse of substances.
9. Help client who overestimates independence in actual physical condition to identify comfortable and uncomfortable dependency situations.	To present reality and lessen need for independence at a time when it may not be appropriate or in client's best interest.
10. Assign easy-to-complete tasks so client can experience success.	To help client experience the pleasure that accompanies completing a task successfully, thereby motivating client to seek other opportunities to obtain pleasure and increase feelings of autonomy and independence.
11. Teach client to ask for help directly using assertive skills.	To let client know it is appropriate and healthy to ask for help when needed.
12. Interrupt negative self-statements dealing with dependence.	To set limits or negativism about self and help client consider positive self-talk.
13. Assist client in evaluating resources and in learning how to get dependency needs met.	To help client identify who can be relied upon to help meet dependency needs, when appropriate.
14. Allow client as much control over external environment as possible.	To increase autonomy and feelings of control of environment.
15. Reinforce behavior that is consistent with reality.	To give feedback for appropriate behavior.
16. Teach assertiveness skills.	To help client learn to ask for what client wants directly without infringing on the rights of others.
17. Promote decision-making skills.	To provide client with the skill to make decisions on own, thereby increasing independent functioning.
18. Explore conflicts associated with physical limitations.	To gain an understanding of issues related to client's disability and associated dependence and to plan interventions.
Social Dimension	
1. Facilitate client's establishment of appropriate independent relationships with others through nurse-client relationship	To lessen need to rely on others and increase mutually satisfying relationships.
2. Explore with client ways to improve social skills.	To assist client in participating in decisions about treatment and increasing independent functioning.
3. Help client identify manipulative behavior associated with dependence.	To promote awareness about manipulative behavior.
4. Maintain established limits set by staff on dependent behavior or manipulation.	To prevent manipulation.

NURSING ACTIONS	RATIONALE
5. Work with other staff members to present a united front and work through staff problems to consistently approach client.	To provide consistency in setting limits by health care team, thereby preventing manipulation of individual members of the team.
6. Deal with advances of client by stating limitations of nurse-client relationship.	To maintain a nurse-client relationship and prevent client from misinterpreting the nurse's role.
7. Identify attempts by client to be dependent on nurse.	To prevent further dependence.
8. Confront client regarding attempts to be dependent.	To promote client's awareness of behavior indicating dependence.
9. Help client set realistic limits for self.	To promote client's participation in care by developing own limits.
10. Help client accept responsibility for own behavior.	To increase feelings of self-control.
11. Identify unresolved family issues regarding dependency needs.	To gain an understanding of ways family may contribute to client's dependence.
12. Investigate family dynamics that promote development of dependent behavior.	To plan interventions that involve family and increase opportunities for family to be supportive to client's changing behavior.
13. Help family work through tendency to promote client's dependent behavior by identifying dependent behaviors.	To promote more autonomous family functioning for all members.
14. Refer client to appropriate substance abuse treatment programs.	To provide detoxification and rehabilitation.
15. Refer client to self-help groups such as Alcoholics Anonymous, Narcotics Anonymous, and Synanon, as appropriate.	To provide group support for chemically dependent individual. Client cannot resolve problem by self.
16. Reduce secondary gains from dependent behavior by helping client identify them.	To stop all benefits received from dependent behavior.
17. Provide individual, group, or family therapy as needed to intervene in dependent behavior.	To increase self-esteem and foster independent functioning resulting from belonging to a supportive and accepting group.
18. Help client with realistic career planning, taking client's capabilities and assets into consideration.	To increase vocational skills that lead to success at work and improved relationships and lessen the need for dependence.

Spiritual Dimension

1. Help client identify own morals and values related to dependence-independence conflict issues during individual and group counseling sessions.	To gain awareness of conflicts that may contribute to dependence.
2. Have client select and perform values clarification exercises.	To increase awareness of dependence.
3. Facilitate client's adoption of a realistic view toward religious affiliation without overdependence.	To help client question excessive reliance on religion for resolution of problems.
4. Refer to appropriate spiritual leader for spiritual guidance concerning dependence.	To encourage dialogue with a spiritual leader.
5. Facilitate resolution of dependency conflicts related to higher power by increasing self-awareness.	To experience the sense of esteem that comes with resolution of conflicts.
6. Help client adopt own beliefs and values independent of others.	To encourage independent thinking.

EVALUATION

Measurable gains and outcome criteria provide the data for evaluating clients with dependent behavior. Evaluation of dependent behavior is also based on observations made of the client by the nurse, other health professionals, family members, and significant others. The following behaviors indicate a positive evaluation:

1. Identifies dependent behavior
2. Identifies times when dependent behavior is appropriate and accepts it
3. Functions independently and interdependently with others
4. Increases social skills
5. Interacts with others
6. Uses problem-solving skills
7. Uses decision-making skills
8. Stops abusing chemical substances

BIBLIOGRAPHY

Blankfield A: The concept of dependence, *Int J Addict* 22(11):1069, 1986.

Booth T: Institutional regimes and induced dependency in homes for the aged, *Gerontologist* 26:418, 1986.

Carnes B: Concept analysis: dependence, *Crit Care Q* 6(4):29, 1984.

Clough D, Derdiarian A: A behavioral check list to measure dependence and independence, *Nurs Res* 29:55, 1980.

Faugier J: The changing concept of dependence in the drug and alcohol field, *Nurse Pract* 1:253, 1986.

Gorney-Lucerno M: Caring for yourself while caring for others: the issues of codependence, *Perspectives* 6(3):14, 1991.

Hemfelt R, Minirth F, Meier P: *Love is a choice: recovery for codependent relationships,* Nashville, 1989, Thomas Nelson, Inc.

Higley R: Independence vs. dependence: whose decision? *ANNA J* 13:286, 1986.

Homer M, Leonard A, Taylor P: The burden of dependency, *Sociol Rev* (Monograph) 31:77, 1985.

Hutchinson S: Chemically dependent nurses: trajectory toward self-annihilation, *Nurs Res* 35(4):196, 1986.

Hutchinson S: Chemically dependent nurses: implications for nurse executives, *J Nurs Adm* 17(8):23, 1987.

Lenters W: Sick love and sick religion: exposing our dependencies, *J Christ Nurs* 3(1):7, 1986.

Miller A: Nurse/patient dependence—is it iatrogenic? *Adv Nurs Sci* 10:63, 1985.

Murphy R: Patient's advocate: when independence is good medicine, *RN* 47:25, 1984.

Roble D: Interventions: how can we assist our colleagues who may be impaired to seek treatment for chemical dependency? *Fla Nurse* 35(2):4, 1987.

Stride N: An investigation of the dependence of severely disabled people in a hospital. *J Adv Nurs* 13(5):557, 1988.

Willis J: Simple scale for assessing level of dependency of patients in general practice, *Brit Med J (Clin Res,* Ed) 292:1639, 1986.

Zerwekh J, Michaels B: Co-dependency: assessment and recovery, *Nurs Clin North Am* 24(1):109, 1989.

Depression

Depression is a pathological mood disturbance characterized by a wide variety of feelings, attitudes, and beliefs that a person has about self and the world (for example, pessimism, despair, helplessness, hopelessness, low self-esteem, guilt, negative expectancy, and dread of impending disaster). Depression resembles sadness, which is a normal feeling prompted by certain situations such as the death of a loved one. Instead of acknowledging the loss, the person denies the loss and avoids sadness with depressive symptoms.

Depression is also referred to as a symptom, an illness, and a syndrome. When depression is seen as a symptom, various distinguishing characteristics can be identified, including psychomotor retardation or psychomotor agitation. As an illness, depression includes diagnostic categories such as a bipolar disorder, major depression, cyclothymic disorder and dysthymic disorder. As a syndrome, depression is explained by various dynamics, such as anger turned inward or frustrated dependency needs.

A depressive state may be precipitated by many factors. These include a significant loss or disappointment; severe or prolonged stress; perceived inadequacy of personal strivings; unresolved conflicts; inadequate positive reinforcement or excessive negative reinforcement; chronic feelings of anxiety, fear, or anger; disturbances in the structure and function of the brain and nervous system; and toxicity, infection, or injury.

Guilt, hopelessness, and withdrawal are behaviors commonly associated with depression. Guilt is a subjective feeling of remorse and self-reproach. Hopelessness is the belief that no help can be obtained to improve a person's life situation or to solve problems. Withdrawal is an attempt to avoid interaction with others, thus avoiding relationships.

Suicide often is associated with depression and is one of the 10 leading causes of death for all age groups.

The original content for this section was contributed by Peggy Landrum, R.N., Ph. D.

Nursing is thus challenged to recognize and prevent the overwhelming feelings of hopelessness and misery that depressed clients experience.

Related DSM-III-R disorders

Adjustment disorder
Anxiety disorders
Organic mental disorders
Psychoactive substance use disorders
Mood disorders
Schizophrenia

Other related conditions

Chronic disease
Surgery (hysterectomy, mastectomy, amputation)
Divorce
Death
Mid-life crisis
"Empty nest" syndrome
Side effects from medications

PRINCIPLES

▶ Physical Dimension

1. There is a primary disturbance in the structure and function of the brain and nervous system.
2. Physiological chemical changes take place in depression—norepinephrine and serotonin amounts are decreased and steroid output is increased.
3. Metabolism is decreased in depressed persons.
4. Self-care and personal hygiene are neglected in depression.
5. A lack of energy with weakness and fatigue is a classical symptom of depression.
6. Motor activity may be decreased (psychomotor retardation) or increased (psychomotor agitation) in depressed persons.
7. Depressed individuals may abuse or misuse drugs and alcohol as a way to cope with depression.

8. The rate of suicide for depressed persons is high.
9. Cardiovascular symptoms similar to those of anxiety are seen in depression.
10. Heredity plays a role in depression.
11. Depression may be related to a defect in the body's immune system.
12. Abnormalities in cell membranes may contribute to depression.

▶ Emotional Dimension

1. Depression is an attempt to avoid having feelings that the individual has labeled "unacceptable" (anxiety, fear, hostility).
2. Active expression of feelings may ultimately make depression unnecessary.
3. Depression involves unconscious hostility, rage, or anger toward an object of loss; in response to this, guilt and self-punishment arise.
4. An intense need to be loved and approved may predispose a person to depression.
5. Depression is the expression of a state of helplessness and hopelessness.
6. A person's angry feelings are turned inward against the self in depression.

▶ Intellectual Dimension

1. Depression frequently occurs in relation to an unconsciously perceived or imagined loss.
2. The ego is paralyzed because of an inability to cope with the perceived loss.
3. The individual's negative view of events is basic to depression.
4. Irrational thoughts and beliefs about events, rather than the actual events, may precipitate depression.
5. The depressed person develops a negative view of self, the world, and the future that affects subsequent judgments about interactions with others.
6. The negative view may remain dormant until the individual undergoes a major stressful event or a series of stressful events; when activated, negative cognitive patterns dominate thinking and produce affective and motivational phenomena associated with depression.
7. Systematic errors in the thinking of a depressed person include magnification and minimization, personalization, selective abstraction, and arbitrary inference.
8. Individuals are capable of actively replacing irrational thinking with rational thinking, in which case feelings associated with depression will disappear.
9. The person believes that he or she has no control over self or the environment.

▶ Social Dimension

1. Depression is a way of coping with anxiety; anxiety is a response to a feeling of disapproval from a significant other person.
2. Depression may occur in response to an individual's inability to live up to parents' expectations and self-expectations.
3. Relationships of the depressed individual with others are sometimes seen in terms of an excessive dependency.
4. Depressive behavior may be an attempt to manipulate others into fulfilling certain needs.
5. Depression is a self-defeating attempt to repair, reinstate, or revive a relationship.
6. The person who is depressed perceives a lack of support systems.
7. Withdrawal and lack of interest are seen in depression.
8. Particular antecedent events, such as a loss or disappointment, account for the occurrence of depression.
9. Depression results from a low rate of positive outcomes or a high rate of aversive outcomes in person-environment interactions.
10. Reasons for low rates of positive outcomes may include the following: immediate environment has few positive reinforcers or many punishing aspects, person lacks necessary skills to obtain positive reinforcers or to cope with aversive events, and potency of positive events may be reduced or impact of negative events may be heightened.
11. Treatment goals consist of increasing the rate of positive reinforcing interactions with the environment and decreasing the aversive interactions.
12. Social interpersonal behavior, cognitive factors, and self-regulatory mechanisms play important roles in the occurrence of and recovery from depression.
13. Helplessness and depression are learned behaviors.
14. A disruptive, hostile, and generally negative environment constitutes a risk factor for depression.
15. Certain personality characteristics such as introversion, guilt, and dependence are likely to be seen in depressed persons.
16. The precipitating event in depression is the loss of something seen as crucial for maintenance of self-esteem.
17. Risk factors for depression may include lack of an intimate, confiding relationship, lack of employment, and the presence of children in the home.
18. Cultures with a dominant work ethic (e.g., Amish) show little depression.

▶ Spiritual Dimension

1. The individual with a self-concept that includes active participation in activities with others will not need to become depressed.
2. A sense of helplessness and hopelessness pervades the depressed person's life.
3. Separation and withdrawal reinforce the depressed person's negative feelings about his or her miserable life circumstances.
4. The depressed person lacks feelings of worth and value.
5. Hopeless feelings prevent the individual from finding meaning and purpose in life.
6. The depressed person resists feeling pleasure.
7. Depressed persons believe they need to be punished for their behavior.
8. The presence of guilt feelings seems to be related to some religions.

ASSESSMENT

▶ Physical Dimension

I. History
  A. Activities of daily living
    1. Nutrition
       a. Loss of appetite, anorexia
       b. Weight loss
       c. Epigastric distress
    2. Sleep
       a. Early awakening with subsequent inability to sleep
       b. Ability to sleep only for short periods
       c. Fatigue upon awakening
       d. Excessive sleep
       e. Restlessness during sleep
    3. Lack of interest in any recreation, hobbies, or interests
    4. Physical activity
       a. Psychomotor retardation
       b. Lack of interest in exercise
       c. Psychomotor agitation
       d. Restlessness
       e. Hyperactivity
    5. Lack of interest in sexual activity
    6. Average day
       a. Special effort required to get through the day
       b. Withdrawal
       c. Isolation
       d. Lack of interest in usual activities
  B. Habits
    1. Increased use of alcohol
    2. Increased use of medications and drugs
    3. Increased smoking
  C. Destructive behavior
    1. Recent suicide attempts
    2. Increase in number of accidents
    3. Evidence of self-inflicted wounds
    4. Refusal to participate in treatment plans
    5. Malnutrition or overeating
  D. Health history
    1. Serious or chronic illness
    2. Serious disabling injuries
    3. Any hospitalization has potential for causing depression
    4. Loss of body part, such as from amputation or mastectomy
    5. Unresolved grief from previous loss
    6. Suicide attempts
  E. Family health history
    1. Family history of mood disorders, including occurrence of depressive episodes
  F. Review of systems
    1. General
       a. Increased or excessive fatigue
       b. Agitation or restlessness
       c. Weight loss or excessive weight gain
       d. Change in appetite
       e. Change in sleeping patterns
       f. Malaise
       g. Apathy
    2. Skin
       a. Bruises
       b. Scars
    3. Cardiovascular
       a. Chest pain
       b. Dyspnea
       c. Palpitations
    4. Respiratory
       a. Recurrent and frequent infections
    5. Gastrointestinal
       a. Nausea and vomiting
       b. Constipation
       c. Indigestion
       d. Loss of appetite or self-indulgence in non-nutritional foods
       e. Use of laxatives
       f. Anorexia

6. Reproductive
   a. Decreased libido
   b. Impotence
   c. Dysmenorrhea or amenorrhea
   d. Premenstrual tension
7. Musculoskeletal
   a. Muscle tenseness
   b. Decreased motor activity

8. Neurological
   a. Headaches
   b. Dizziness
   c. Blurred vision
   d. Nervousness

II. **Diagnostic tests**
   A. Dexamethasone suppression test (DST)

▶ Physical Examination

CLIENT DATA	ANALYSIS	NURSING DIAGNOSIS
Weight loss	Decrease in metabolism associated with depression contributes to loss of appetite with weight loss.	Altered nutrition: less than body requirements related to depression
Weight gain	Feelings of hopelessness and self-pity may lead to excessive eating.	Altered nutrition: more than body requirements related to depression
Neglect of personal dress and grooming	Feelings of worthlessness associated with depression contribute to lack of interest in personal appearance.	*Altered self-care: neglect of personal dress and grooming related to depression
Slumped posture	Lack of energy with weakness and fatigue.	Altered health maintenance: poor posture related to depression
Extreme slowness in performing any activity	Decrease in motor activity is associated with depression (psychomotor retardation).	Altered health maintenance: psychomotor retardation related to depression
Restlessness, pacing, hand wringing, or other repetitious activity	Possible response to loss with symptoms similar to those of anxiety (psychomotor agitation).	Altered health maintenance: psychomotor agitation related to depression
Odor of alcohol on breath	Possible alcohol abuse.	Altered health maintenance: potential substance abuse related to depression
Bruises, cuts, or scars	Possible self-destructive behavior or abuse by others.	High risk for self-directed violence: related to depression
Dyspnea, palpitations	Possible response to loss with cardiovascular symptoms similar to those of anxiety.	Anxiety: cardiovascular symptoms related to depression
Extreme nervousness	Possible response to loss with symptoms similar to those of anxiety.	Anxiety: neurological symptoms related to depression

▶ Emotional Dimension

CLIENT DATA	ANALYSIS	NURSING DIAGNOSIS
Apathy	Apparent lack of feelings about anything. Feelings of inadequacy and despair contribute to indifference regarding self and surroundings.	Ineffective individual coping: apathy related to depression
Lethargy	Decreased energy reserves for even minimal task accomplishment. Psychomotor retardation or decreased ability to sleep or rest contribute to a sense of fatigue.	Ineffective individual coping: lethargy related to depression
Hostility	Shows irritability, frustration, or negativism toward self and others. Unexpressed anger contributes to maintenance of the depressed state.	Ineffective indivdiual coping: hostility related to depression

► **Emotional Dimension—cont'd**

CLIENT DATA	ANALYSIS	NURSING DIAGNOSIS
Ambivalence	Expresses and feels apparently conflicting emotions (anger and sadness, shame and self-righteousness). Inability to fully experience and express feelings contributes to lack of resolution.	Ineffective individual coping: ambivalence related to depression
Suicidal feelings	Hopelessness contributes to despair.	High risk for self-directed violence: suicidal feelings related to depression
Inability to grieve for loss	Delayed or distorted grief reactions result in depression.	Ineffective individual coping: related to delayed or distorted grief
Excessive guilt	Harsh and punishing superego arouses guilt in depressed persons.	Ineffective individual coping: excessive guilt related to depression

► **Intellectual Dimension**

CLIENT DATA	ANALYSIS	NURSING DIAGNOSIS
Blames self for real or imagined situations	Sense of worthlessness and negativism contribute to self-criticizing and self-blaming thought patterns. Stress contributes to distorted perception of own role in events.	Altered thought processes: self-blame related to depression
Delusions of persecution, guilt, oppression, poverty, unworthiness, or physical illness	Extreme anxiety or guilt contributes to loss of contact with reality.	Altered thought processes: delusions related to depression
Obsessions	Attempts to control extreme anxiety, fears contribute to obsessive thoughts.	Altered thought processes: obsessions related to depression
Impaired remote memory or forgetfulness regarding recent events	Depressed mood contributes to decrease in memory capacity.	Altered thought processes: impaired memory related to depressed mood
Impaired concentration	Apathy and lack of energy contribute to impaired concentration.	Altered thought processes: impaired ability to concentrate related to depressed mood
Confusion or disorientation	Inward direction of attention contributes to lack of contact with surroundings.	Sensory/perceptual alterations: disorientation about time, place, or persons related to depressed mood
Preoccupation with self and disturbing aspects of own situation	Self-oriented, self-absorbed; constantly concerned with self.	Altered thought processes: preoccupation with self related to depression
Diminished fund of information	Impaired concentration and inattentiveness contribute to diminished fund of information. Lacks interest in events and environment.	Altered thought processes: poor concentration and attention span related to depression
Perceived loss of control	Negativism toward self and helplessness contribute to perceived inability to influence current situation. Extreme pessimism regarding own ability to influence outcome.	Altered thought processes: perceived loss of control related to depression
Inability to engage in problem-solving activities	Apathy and perceived helplessness decrease problem-solving capabilities.	Altered thought processes: impaired problem-solving ability related to depression

▶ **Intellectual Dimension—cont'd**

CLIENT DATA	ANALYSIS	NURSING DIAGNOSIS
Inability to make decisions	Depressed mood limits decision-making capacity.	Altered thought processes: impaired decision-making abilities related to depression
Excessive thoughts of self-criticism, self-blame	Low self-esteem and negativism contribute to self-criticizing tendencies.	Altered thought processes: excessive self-criticism related to depression
Suicidal thoughts	Severe depressed mood contributes to self-destructive tendencies.	High risk for self-directed violence: suicidal thoughts related to severely depressed mood
Slowed speech or absence of speech	Poor concentration and general psychomotor retardation contribute to lack of verbal activity.	Impaired verbal communication: slowed speech or absence of speech related to depression
Rigid thinking, ruminations	Relives loss over and over.	Altered thought processes: ruminations related to depression

▶ **Social Dimension**

CLIENT DATA	ANALYSIS	NURSING DIAGNOSIS
Inability to meet standards set for self	Excessively high self-expectations contribute to unrealistic goals, resulting in sense of failure.	Self-esteem disturbance: unrealistic self-expectations related to depression
Inability to recognize strengths or assets	Experiences of perceived failures and negativism contribute to inability to acknowledge positive aspects of self.	Self-esteem disturbance: inability to recognize strengths and assets related to depression
Low self-esteem	Preoccupation with own inadequacies and failures. Low self-esteem contributes to extreme sense of failure.	Self-esteem disturbance: related to depression
Mistrust of others	Failure of others to meet unreasonable demands contributes to mistrust.	Self-esteem disturbance: lack of trust in others related to depression
Withdrawal from contact with family members and friends	Excessive guilt and mistrust or sense of worthlessness contributes to social withdrawal.	Social isolation: withdrawal from others related to depression
Dependent on others, rather than on self, to get own needs met	Sense of helplessness and hopelessness contributes to dependent behavior.	Ineffective individual coping: helplessness and hopelessness related to depression
Alienation of self from friends and family members	Exploitative demands and preoccupation with self contribute to rejection by others.	Social isolation: alienation from others related to depression
Difficulty performing in established social roles	Apathy, anxiety, and decreased self-esteem contribute to decreased motivation for role performance.	Altered role performance: related to depression
Assumption of roles with conflicting functions	Conflicting role expectations contribute to depressed mood.	Altered role performance: role conflicts related to depression
Minimal availability of support	Lack of social support contributes to depressed mood.	Impaired social interactions: related to depressed mood
Excessive or prolonged environmental stress	Extreme stress contributes to decreased effectiveness of usual coping strategies.	Ineffective individual coping: extreme stress related to depression
Sense of worthlessness	Will not acknowledge anything positive about self. Perceived inability to cope contributes to feelings of inadequacy and worthlessness.	Self-esteem disturbance: feelings of worthlessness related to depression

▶ **Spiritual Dimension**

CLIENT DATA	ANALYSIS	NURSING DIAGNOSIS
Conflict in personal values and beliefs	Values conflicts contribute to depressed mood.	Spiritual distress: personal values conflict related to depression
Extreme hopelessness	Believes that it is impossible for life to improve.	Spiritual distress: sense of hopelessness related to depression
Loss of interest in religious activity formerly considered important	Negativism and belief that nothing can help contribute to withdrawal from religious activity.	Spiritual distress: loss of interest in usual religious activities related to depression
View of present condition as punishment for some thought, feeling, or behavior	Overwhelming guilt contributes to perceived need to suffer.	Spiritual distress: overwhelming guilt and need for punishment related to depression
Inability to feel pleasure or joy	Pessimism and inward focus of attention contribute to inability to feel pleasure.	Spiritual distress: inability to feel pleasure related to depression
Sense of meaninglessness and purposelessness in life	Hopelessness and despair contribute to loss of purpose and meaning in life.	Spiritual distress: lack of purpose and meaning in life related to depression

PLANNING

Long-Term Goals

To respond to losses without becoming depressed
To develop a realistic, positive perception of self
To enhance feelings of self-esteem, acceptance by others, and belonging
To establish relationships with significant family members and friends

SHORT-TERM GOALS	OUTCOME CRITERIA
Physical Dimension	
To identify key events precipitating the depressive episode	1. Discusses situations, events, or changes that seem to be associated with the depression 2. Verbalizes depressing nature of key situations, events, or changes 3. Describes relationship between key events and depressive episode 4. Describes general stressors (disappointments, losses, aversive relationships, perceived failures)
To maintain physical health	1. Eats an adequate diet 2. Maintains ideal weight 3. Gets adequate amounts of rest and sleep 4. Exercises regularly 5. Performs activities of daily living 6. Eliminates (bowel and bladder) regularly 7. Takes medications as prescribed
Emotional Dimension	
To identify and express feelings that accompany the depressive episode	1. Identifies feelings such as anger, guilt, fear, sadness, anxiety, and helplessness 2. Verbalizes feelings as they are experienced 3. Identifies source of feelings 4. Makes statements that indicate acceptance of feelings 5. Describes effective ways to express and manage feelings 6. Differentiates between feelings (sadness versus depression, fear versus anger) 7. Acknowledges pain or guilt that may be associated with particular feelings 8. Describes ambivalence associated with particular feelings

PLANNING—cont'd

SHORT-TERM GOALS	OUTCOME CRITERIA
To reduce excessive feelings of guilt	1. Verbalizes feelings of guilt 2. Identifies negative thoughts that contribute to feelings of guilt 3. Identifies attitudes and beliefs that contribute to feelings of guilt 4. Identifies past behavior or events (real or imagined) that contribute to feelings of guilt 5. Identifies meaning of past behavior 6. Rejects feelings of guilt based on irrational beliefs 7. Differentiates between concepts of responsibility and guilt 8. Acknowledges actual consequences of past behavior 9. Verbalizes realistic limitations
To decrease feelings of helplessness	1. Recognizes statements that reflect a sense of helplessness 2. Identifies thoughts and feelings that encourage a helpless position 3. Acknowledges unrealistic or negative expectations 4. Makes statements that reflect positive expectations 5. Identifies personal needs 6. Acknowledges own responsibility for getting needs met 7. Engages in problem solving to identify appropriate ways of getting needs met 8. Makes decisions regarding personal interests 9. Verbalizes relationship between helplessness and manipulation 10. Makes statements that reflect a sense of control 11. Practices assuming control of own behavior
Intellectual Dimension To decrease preoccupation with self	1. Focuses attention on needs rather than catastrophic expectations 2. Shows interest in other people 3. Describes relationship between feelings, thoughts, and behaviors 4. Participates in outside activities 5. Practices alternative ways of coping with anxiety 6. Initiates interaction with other people 7. Practices listening to another person's concerns 8. Participates in some form of exercise
Social Dimension To increase positive feelings about self	1. Identifies irrational thoughts associated with self-criticism 2. Describes relationship between guilt and negative feelings toward self 3. Acknowledges personal strengths, assets, and accomplishments 4. Makes affirming self-statements 5. Describes assertive behaviors that are appropriate in own situation 6. Practices assertive behaviors in present relationships and describes outcomes 7. Accepts compliments from others 8. Makes statements that reflect self-confidence and optimism 9. Successfully completes projects or activities

SHORT-TERM GOALS	OUTCOME CRITERIA
To increase positive responses from other people	1. Describes positive responses from other people 2. Identifies behavior in self that is manipulative (e.g., exploitative, demanding, excessively dependent) 3. Recognizes response that manipulative behavior elicits from other people 4. Verbalizes feelings and thoughts that seem to precede manipulative behavior 5. Verbalizes goals of manipulative behavior 6. Makes statements that reflect an awareness of other people's feelings 7. Describes demands made on other people 8. Distinguishes between reasonable and unreasonable demands 9. Describes appropriate alternatives to manipulative behavior 10. Replaces manipulative behaviors with responsible behaviors 11. Practices nonmanipulative behaviors with nurse, family, and friends, and acknowledges outcomes
Spiritual Dimension To find pleasures in life	1. Renews friendships with others 2. Participates in activities that were previously pleasurable 3. Learns new skills that are pleasurable 4. Does things for others that are self-rewarding 5. Makes statements that indicate pleasure 6. Returns to church or other organized religious activity (if he or she values this) 7. Achieves success in tasks and activities initiated

Discharge Planning

The following client behaviors demonstrate readiness for discharge:
1. Identifies stressors that have contributed to depression
2. Expresses feelings effectively
3. Identifies appropriate ways to meet needs
4. Expresses a sense of control over life situation
5. Initiates relationships with others
6. Minimizes depressive thought patterns

IMPLEMENTATION

NURSING ACTIONS	RATIONALE
Physical Dimension 1. Assist client in activities of daily living when severely depressed.	To help client maintain self-respect and esteem and to meet dependency needs.
2. Encourage cleanliness and neatness.	To promote general health and well-being.
3. Protect against self-destructive tendencies; contract with client not to harm self.	To prevent suicidal attempts, a serious complication of depression.
4. Provide encouragement and opportunity for regular exercise.	To increase energy level, to prevent preoccupation with self.
5. Encourage intake of adequate nourishment.	To promote general health, to increase energy for working on conflicts and problems.
6. Relieve physical symptoms when possible.	To present a caring attitude and alleviate minor discomforts.
7. Encourage physical activity.	To channel agitation, to increase energy level.

IMPLEMENTATION—cont'd

NURSING ACTIONS	RATIONALE
8. Provide structure in the environment with opportunity to participate in meaningful activities.	To keep client busy and prevent preoccupation with self.
9. Show acceptance through touch (within limits acceptable to client).	To demonstrate warmth and caring and promote feelings of self-worth.
10. Reinforce assumption of responsibility for activities of daily living.	To encourage client to continue to take responsibility for activities of daily living.
11. Supervise medication therapy.	To prevent client from hoarding medications, to be assured that client is taking medications as prescribed.
Emotional Dimension	
1. Encourage expression of feelings associated with depression (anger, sadness, guilt, fear, and helplessness) by listening actively, reflecting and clarifying.	To assist client in identifying predominant feelings.
2. Listen carefully and nonjudgmentally to expression of feelings.	To help client feel safe in expressing feelings.
3. Show respect by calling client by name.	To convey that client has worth and value. Depressed clients often feel worthless and of no value.
4. Assist client in identifying source of negative feelings about self.	To determine if negativism about self is a lifelong pattern or a product of depression.
5. Reinforce client's expression of positive feelings about self.	To alter client's negativism about self.
6. Encourage client to identify and verbalize feelings as they are experienced, through active listening and reflecting.	To help client clarify factual information rather than ideas and notions.
7. Encourage client to assume responsibility for own feelings by reinforcing positive behavior.	To prevent dependence on others, to gain a sense of control of own life.
8. Discourage statements that reflect client's lack of control over feelings.	To promote realistic thinking.
9. Use role playing.	To provide opportunity for client to practice expressing feelings in a safe environment.
10. Help client practice exaggerated expression of feelings within therapeutic setting.	To help client express more intense feelings, if appropriate, to get the "feel" of the emotion.
11. Assist client in identifying automatic emotional reactions (fear or anxiety in response to particular events or thoughts).	To promote a rational rather than an emotional reaction.
12. Be available and accessible to client.	To facilitate client's initiation of contact with nurse.
13. Divert attention from preoccupation with painful feelings.	To prevent ruminations.
14. Encourage client to indulge in pleasant sensations (massage, whirlpool, bath, or listening to music).	To increase pleasures in life.
Intellectual Dimension	
1. Provide information about depression.	To help client gain an understanding of depression and see the relationship between events and symptoms.
2. Allow adequate time for client to respond.	To accommodate client's delayed response time.
3. Assist client in distinguishing between thoughts and feelings.	To help client clarify what is fact and what is feeling so that distorted facts (perceptions) can be questioned and feelings can be identified.
4. Help client identify negative thoughts and irrational beliefs.	To clarify misperceptions by supplying accurate information.
5. Explore with client relationship between negative thoughts, irrational beliefs, and the state of depression.	To gain an understanding of client's misperceptions and distortions and link them to client's depression.
6. Help client distinguish ideas from facts.	To help client clarify factual information as opposed to ideas and notions.
7. Assist client in assuming responsibility for own thoughts and beliefs by providing feedback as client expresses thoughts and beliefs.	To prevent dependence on others.
8. Help client identify illogical conclusions and painful feelings.	To promote realistic thinking.
9. Instruct client to set aside a specific and limited time to worry.	To prevent client from spending an inordinate amount of time brooding over plight yet allowing client some time for self-evaluation.

NURSING ACTIONS	RATIONALE
10. Teach client to identify depressive thought patterns and to replace them with task-oriented coping methods.	To prevent recurrence of disabling depression.
11. Help client realistically assess needs and identify those that are not being met.	To gain awareness of emotional status and ask for or seek help.
12. Teach problem solving.	To determine appropriate and effective methods for meeting needs.
13. Teach client to replace self-criticisms and negative thoughts with self-affirmations.	To help client learn to be kind and gentle with self.
14. Teach visualization techniques.	To counteract negative thoughts.
15. Assist client in identifying secondary gains provided by depression.	To identify relationship between benefits received and depression.
16. Orient client to reality when delusions are present.	To present reality.
17. Help client set small achievable goals that are directly relevant to client's needs and develop action plans.	To help client achieve success and increase feelings of competence.
18. Discuss with client situations, events, or changes that seem to be associated with the depression.	To help client identify significance of changes, for example, a precipitating factor. Often this recognition brings relief to client.
19. Encourage verbalization of self-destructive thoughts.	To assess risk for suicide.
20. Make decisions for client when necessary.	To prevent client from making inappropriate decisions because of impaired judgment associated with depression.
21. Encourage and reinforce successful attempts at decision making.	To inform client of progress being made and reinforce appropriate behavior.
22. Minimize importance attached to possible errors in decision making.	To prevent further decrease of self-esteem and competence.
23. Provide only brief explanations when client is severely depressed.	To ensure that client understands message. Severely depressed clients have severely impaired cognitive abilities.
24. Discuss with client how things would be if depression were not a factor.	To help client expand thinking beyond self, to give client something to work toward.
25. Have client identify what he or she can control.	To present reality, to increase feelings of control.
26. Focus attention on daily progress and recognize all performance gains.	To measure daily gains and provide reinforcement for any positive changes.
27. Provide distraction for client when preoccupation with self is evident.	To prevent ruminations over problems.
28. Assist client in focusing on the present.	To encourage client to work on what is troubling self now and what client can do about it now. Cannot change the past, only attitudes about it.
29. Stimulate client's motivation to relieve depression with positive reinforcement.	To help client recognize that methods are available to client to help relieve depression.
30. Help client identify personal strengths, assets, and accomplishments.	To increase client's self-esteem and self-worth.

Social Dimension

1. Initiate contact with client.	To build trust. Depressed clients seldom initiate contact with others.
2. Engage in frequent, brief interactions when client is severely depressed.	To acknowledge client's presence, to prevent overwhelming client with a lengthy interaction.
3. Encourage client to participate in activities with other people.	To increase social interactions.
4. Provide group therapy.	To assist client in interacting with others, to listen and empathize with others' problems, to receive support and encouragement from others.
5. Provide family therapy.	To help client identify conflicts and establish adequate family coping skills.
6. Assist client in identifying typical behaviors in primary relationships, e.g., dependence or negativism.	To promote awareness of typical ways of relating to others.
7. Discuss with client consequences of various behaviors exhibited in relationships.	To help client recognize effects of behavior on others and learn more satisfying ways to relate to people.

IMPLEMENTATION—cont'd

NURSING ACTIONS	RATIONALE
8. Help client identify behaviors that may be more appropriate and effective than present behaviors.	To promote awareness of behaviors that elicit satisfying responses from others.
9. Encourage client to practice alternative behaviors and to discuss responses from others.	To gain confidence in use of new behaviors and determine the effect of new behaviors on others, both positive and negative.
10. Help client set realistic limits in relation to other people.	To encourage assertiveness.
11. Encourage client to verbalize needs.	To lessen predisposition to physical ailments, to promote mental health.
12. Assist client in recognizing that other people will not always be willing to meet needs.	To present reality.
13. Assist client in acknowledging own responsibilities in relationships.	To help client learn the "give and take" in relationships. Depressed clients tend to be "takers."
14. Teach communication skills ("I" messages and empathic listening).	To help client assert self.
15. Give feedback about exploitative or demanding behaviors.	To promote awareness of problematic behaviors.
16. Encourage client to establish specific interaction times with significant other people in which a positive exchange occurs.	To help client seek out social situations that are positive and self-affirming.
17. Encourage client to make and accept positive statements about self and others.	To provide alternatives to negative thinking.
18. Help client identify potential areas of social interest.	To create socially interesting situations.
19. Teach client effective ways to deal with criticism from others.	To prevent client from accepting criticism at face value and reinforcing negative view of self.
20. Use desensitization techniques.	To help client resolve fears associated with social interactions.
21. Encourage client to seek feedback from other people.	To identify impact of client's behavior on others.
Spiritual Dimension	
1. Provide opportunities for client to be creative.	To help client express feelings through creativity, to expand cognitive abilities.
2. Assist client in clarifying values regarding the quality of life.	To determine feelings and beliefs about life and reasons for them.
3. Discuss with client the meaning attributed to suffering and depression.	To understand client's perception of suffering and depression.
4. Help client identify potentially pleasurable experiences.	To increase pleasures in life and feelings of worth and value.
5. Encourage client to feel pleasure; provide opportunities when possible (tell a joke or humorous story).	To enrich quality of client's life.
6. Help client direct attention outside self and immediate concerns.	To prevent self-absorption.
7. Explore with client possibilities for creating meaning or purpose in life.	To promote a will to live a more meaningful and satisfying life.
8. Help client identify realistic ways to participate in meaningful activities.	To provide client with opportunities to make decisions about self, thus increasing sense of worth and value.

EVALUATION

Measurable goals and outcome criteria provide the data for evaluating the depressed client. Client self-reports, nurse observations, and family reports provide additional data. The following behaviors indicate a positive evaluation:

1. Is more animated
2. Has more energy
3. Eats nutritious meals regularly
4. Sleep is refreshing
5. Has no constipation
6. Exercises regularly
7. Includes recreation in daily schedule
8. Has fewer physical ailments
9. Expresses feelings, both positive and negative
10. Has less negative thinking
11. Makes positive statements about self and others
12. Interacts with others socially
13. Is optimistic about future
14. Has a positive self-concept

BIBLIOGRAPHY

Beck A: *The diagnosis and management of depression,* Philadelphia, 1967, University of Pennsylvania Press.

Beeber L: Enacting corrective interpersonal experiences with the depressed client: an intervention model, *Arch Psychiatr Nurs* 3(4):211, 1989.

Berk J: *The down comforter: how to beat depression and pull yourself out of the blues,* New York, 1980, Avon Books.

Davis T, Jenson L: Identifying depression in medical patients, *Image: J Nurs Schol* 20(4):191, 1988.

Drew B: Differentiation of hopelessness, helplessness, and powerlessness using Erik Erikson's "Roots of virtue," *Arch Psychiatr Nurs* 4(5):332, 1990.

Herth K: Laughter, a nursing treatment, *Am J Nurs* 84(8):991, 1984.

Karasu T: Toward a clinical model of psychotherapy for depression 1: systematic comparison of three psychotherapies, *Am J Psychiatry* 147(2):133, 1990.

Kerr N: Signs and symptoms of depression and principles of nursing care, *Perspect Psychiatr Care* 24(2):48, 1988.

Knowles R: Dealing with feelings: handling depression by identifying anger, *Am J Nurs* 81:986, 1981.

Knowles R: Handling depression through activity, *Am J Nurs* 81:1187, 1981.

Mejo S: The use of antidepressant medication: a guide for the primary care nurse practitioner, *J Acad Nurse Practit* 2(4):153, 1990.

Richman C et al: Interventions for nursing practice problems . . . burnout, *J Nurs Staff Dev* 5(4):166, 1989.

Rifkin A: ECT versus tricyclic antidepressants in depression: a review of the evidence, *J Clin Psychiatry* 49(1):3, 1988.

Rosenbaum J: Depression: viewed from a transcultural nursing theoretical perspective, *J Adv Nurs* 14:7, 1989.

Simmons-Alling S: Genetic implications for major affective disorders, *Arch Psychiatr Nurs* 14(1):67, 1990.

Tanner D, Gerstenberger D, Keller C: Guidelines for treatment of chronic depression in the aphasic patient, *Rehab Nurs* 14(2):77, 1989.

Grief

Grief is an alteration in mood or affect consisting of a complex combination of emotions occurring in phases in response to an actual or perceived loss. Phases of grief, although not totally linear, generally include shock and denial, panic and anger, retreat and bargaining, acknowledgement and depression, and acceptance and adaptation. The following emotions are typically associated with the various phases in the grieving process: anxiety, indifference, guilt, hopelessness, helplessness, despair, ambivalence, anger, hostility, and fear of losing control. Grief is often described as a reaction to the death of a significant person; however, a similar reaction may occur in response to other types of loss, such as a change in role, a change in residence, or a change in body image.

Guilt, anger, and depression are concepts commonly associated with grief. Guilt is a subjective feeling of remorse and self-reproach. Anger is a strong feeling of annoyance or displeasure. Depression is a mood disturbance characterized by feelings of sadness, despair, and discouragement resulting from loss or disappointment.

Related DSM-III-R disorders

Uncomplicated bereavement
Mood disorders (depression)
Adjustment disorder

Other related conditions

Losses
    Person
    Object
    Function
    Status
    Relationship
Realization of future loss
    Anticipatory grieving

The original content for this section was contributed by Peggy Landrum, R.N., Ph.D.

PRINCIPLES

▶ Physical Dimension

1. Grief occurs in response to a loss.
2. The circumstances surrounding the loss (e.g., of a loved one by suicide or by violent crime) bear a relationship to an individual's grief response.
3. Physiological changes in grief responses are similar to anxiety responses.
4. A change may occur in self-care, appetite, and weight and sleep patterns during grief.

▶ Emotional Dimension

1. Past unresolved grief creates the potential for grief following a loss later in life.
2. Potential or actual grief evokes anxiety, which signals the ego to engage defense mechanisms.
3. Shock or denial allows the ego to incorporate the loss gradually.
4. Aggression and hostility in love relationships create conflict and ambivalence when loss occurs.
5. A new loss can activate the grieving process for previous losses.
6. Grief is a normal reaction to a perceived or actual loss.
7. Stages of grief related to terminal illness include denial, anger, bargaining, depression, and acceptance.
8. Stages of grief related to a minor loss include shock and disbelief, developing awareness, restitution, and resolution of the loss.
9. Stages of grief following crisis include protest, despair, denial, and resolution.
10. Lack of closure regarding issues associated with the loss may result in psychophysiological manifestations or in depression.
11. Failure to fully express feelings associated with the loss may result in psychophysiological manifestations or in depression.

▶ Intellectual Dimension

1. Identification of effective coping mechanisms facilitates resolution of grief.
2. Irrational beliefs about the object of loss or an individual's own position in relation to the loss prolongs the grief reaction.
3. An individual's experience of grief is shaped largely by learned patterns of thinking.
4. Rational thinking facilitates grief resolution.
5. Awareness of needs created by the loss is a prerequisite to successful resolution.
6. Confrontation of unresolved issues with the object of loss facilitates resolution of grief and future adaptation to similar events.
7. Ineffective coping skills contribute to a failure to resolve the grief reaction.
8. It is not unusual for the grieving person to have transient "unacceptable" thoughts, such as relief (that the death occurred), anger (for being abandoned), or awareness of gains and rewards (possibly accrued from the death).

▶ Social Dimension

1. Transition between stages of development may elicit grief.
2. Emotional energy invested in the object of loss is recouped for investment in new relationships.
3. Significant loss threatens the total self; self-esteem is often lowered.
4. The availability of supportive persons facilitates the resolution of grief.

5. The capacity for an affiliation with another carries with it the potential for grief when the affiliation is broken.
6. Cultural influences and practices aid and support the individual in adjusting to a separation or loss.
7. In the course of growing up a person continuously experiences loss and separation through each stage of maturational development.
8. In western culture the loss of an aged person is more easily accepted than the loss of a child.
9. In some cultures the sex of the child is more significant than age in evaluating the magnitude of the loss.
10. Loss of a spouse alters a person's social role.
11. The recent widow or widower may be ready prey for others to take advantage of, sexually or financially.

▶ Spiritual Dimension

1. Feelings of loss are relative to the value placed on what is lost.
2. The course of grief depends on the meaning an individual attributes to the loss.
3. Underlying assumptions that people have about themselves and regard as unquestionably true can inhibit grief resolution.
4. Denial of the reality of the loss results in an inability to find meaning in the loss.
5. A strong religious faith may assist in accepting an untimely death.
6. Grief and bereavement can be a creative experience, spurring significant contributions to productive and worthwhile endeavors.

ASSESSMENT

▶ Physical Dimension

I. **History**
   A. Activities of daily living
     1. Nutrition
       a. Decreased appetite
       b. Anorexia
       c. Gluttony
       d. Weight loss or gain
     2. Sleep
       a. Insomnia
       b. Excessive sleep
       c. Attitude toward sleep (fear, relief)
     3. Recreation and hobbies
       a. Decrease in outside interests
     4. Physical activities and limitations
       a. Decrease
       b. Excessive
       c. Restlessness
     5. Sexual activity
       a. Abstinence
       b. Increase
       c. Impotence
     6. Average day
       a. Isolated from others
       b. Disorganized
       c. Exhausting
   B. Habits
     1. Alcohol
       a. Increased use
     2. Medications and drugs
       a. Increased use
     3. Caffeine
       a. Increased use
     4. Nicotine
       a. Increased smoking
   C. Destructive behavior
     1. Suicide attempts
     2. Increase in accidents
   D. Review of systems

1. General
   a. Increased fatigue
   b. Change in appetite
   c. Change in sleep patterns
   d. Malaise
   e. Restlessness
2. Cardiovascular
   a. Tightness in chest
   b. Tachycardia
   c. Palpitations
   d. Syncope
   e. High blood pressure
3. Respiratory
   a. Shortness of breath
   b. Sighing respirations
4. Gastrointestinal
   a. Nausea and vomiting
   b. Diarrhea or constipation
   c. Stomach or abdominal pain
   d. Loss of appetite
5. Reproductive
   a. Decreased libido
   b. Impotence
   c. Amenorrhea or dysmenorrhea
6. Musculoskeletal
   a. Muscle tenseness
   b. Decreased muscle strength
7. Neurological
   a. Difficulty in remembering
   b. Nervousness
   c. Mood changes
   d. Disorientation

▶ **Physical Examination**

CLIENT DATA	ANALYSIS	NURSING DIAGNOSIS
Weight loss or gain	Feelings of indifference or helplessness may result in appetite changes.	Altered nutrition: less than or more than body requirements related to grief
Neglect of personal dress and grooming	May have feelings of despair, lack of energy for personal grooming.	*Altered self-care: unclean and untidy grooming related to despair
Restlessness	May result from anxiety, inability to relax, or tension.	Altered health maintenance: excessive restlessness related to grief
Tightness in chest, palpitations, tachycardia, and shortness of breath	Physiological response, which may result from anxiety associated with loss.	Anxiety: cardiovascular symptoms related to grief
Muscle tenseness	Physiological response may result from anxiety associated with loss.	Anxiety: muscle tenseness related to grief
Stomach upset	Physiological response may result from anxiety associated with loss.	Anxiety: gastrointestinal symptoms related to grief
Inactivity	Weakness, fatigue, and loss of energy may contribute to inactivity.	Altered protection: related to grief

▶ **Emotional Dimension**

CLIENT DATA	ANALYSIS	NURSING DIAGNOSIS
Fear	Fear of inability to cope with future or of losing control. Uncertainty about future contributes to personal insecurity.	Fear: personal insecurity related to anticipated inability to cope with loss
Remorse	Remorseful about missed opportunities prior to the loss. Feelings of inadequacy to change situation contribute to focus on unresolved issues.	Ineffective individual coping: remorse related to unresolved grief
Anger	Angry that loss is imminent or has occurred. Forced alteration in expectations of future contribute to uncertainty that needs will be met.	Ineffective individual coping: anger related to loss of loved one
Sadness	Awareness of reality of loss contributes to feelings of sadness.	*Sadness: related to inability to accept loss as final
Excessive feelings of guilt regarding the loss	Anxiety and remorse may contribute to distorted perception.	*Guilt: related to distorted perception associated with loss

▶ **Intellectual Dimension**

CLIENT DATA	ANALYSIS	NURSING DIAGNOSIS
Distortion of reality of some aspect of loss	Intense emotional response contributes to distorted perception.	Altered thought processes: impaired perception related to intense feelings of grief
Perceived loss of control	Extreme fear and anxiety associated with loss contribute to a sense of powerlessness.	Powerlessness: related to grief
Impaired memory	Severe anxiety or depression associated with loss interferes with memory.	*Altered memory: related to grief
Impaired concentration	Severe anxiety associated with loss contributes to impaired concentration.	Altered thought processes: impaired ability to concentrate related to grief
Preoccupation with image representing loss (person, role, or opportunity)	Unreadiness to accept reality of loss contributes to focus of attention on object of loss.	Altered thought processes: preoccupation with image of loss related to grief
Inability to solve problems	Intense emotional response and perceived helplessness can limit problem-solving abilities.	Altered thought processes: impaired problem-solving ability related to grief
Decreased ability to decide about small matters	Intense emotional response can limit decision-making abilities.	*Altered decision-making: related to grief
Denial	Perceived inability to tolerate intense feelings and to cope with loss contribute to distortion of reality.	High risk for ineffective individual coping: denial of loss related to grief
Excessive crying, sobbing, screaming, or muteness	Intense feelings may impair verbal communications. May signify unresolved conflict.	Impaired verbal communication: related to grief

▶ **Social Dimension**

CLIENT DATA	ANALYSIS	NURSING DIAGNOSIS
Inability to imagine self without object of loss	Thought of functioning without object of loss causes fear and anxiety.	Self-esteem disturbance: perceived future inadequacy related to grief
Diminished self-worth	Blaming self for loss contributes to a sense of failure and low self-esteem. Social value attached to loss.	Self-esteem disturbance: diminished self-worth related to grief
Excessive dependence in remaining relationships	Lowered self-esteem and diminished problem-solving ability contribute to sense of helplessness.	Ineffective individual coping: helplessness related to grief
Sense of loneliness	Social network may have been altered by loss.	*Altered social interaction: lack of contact with significant others related to grief
Excessive drug or alcohol use	May be attempt to avoid intense feelings of grief.	Ineffective individual coping: excessive drug or alcohol use related to grief
Difficulty functioning in social roles	Preoccupation with loss can decrease energy or motivation to perform in social roles.	Altered role performance: inability to perform usual social roles related to grief
Difficulty adjusting to or defining new roles and relinquishing old roles	Anxiety associated with change can impair adaptation to new situation defined by loss.	Ineffective individual coping: role dysfunction related to anxiety associated with change in role

▶ **Spiritual Dimension**

CLIENT DATA	ANALYSIS	NURSING DIAGNOSIS
Conflicting values regarding aspects of loss	Conflict in personal values contributes to anxiety, ambivalence, or guilt.	Spiritual distress: values conflict related to loss
Despair over loss	Feelings of hopelessness contribute to sense of despair about future.	Spiritual distress: despair and hopelessness related to grief
Excessive involvement in religious activities	Attempt to alleviate intense feeling of grief through religious practice.	Spiritual distress: excessive religious activity related to grief
Belief that loss is punishment for some behavior	Guilt may be lessened by distorted perception of loss as punishment.	Spiritual distress: belief that loss is punishment related to grief
Inability to participate in pleasurable experiences	Feelings of grief prevent experiences of pleasure.	Spiritual distress: inability to experience pleasure related to grief.
Interpersonal conflicts in beliefs about meaning of loss	Conflicting beliefs with significant others increase discomfort and experience of stress; can encourage isolation.	Spiritual distress: inability to resolve interpersonal conflicts in beliefs related to grief
Loss of purpose or meaning in life	Hopelessness and despair contribute to decreased interest in anything outside self.	Spiritual distress: loss of purpose in life related to grief

PLANNING

Long-Term Goals

To acknowledge and accept the loss
To express and resolve feelings associated with each stage of the grieving process
To identify and use resources to cope effectively with the loss

SHORT-TERM GOALS	OUTCOME CRITERIA
Physical Dimension	
To identify the actual loss that precipitated feelings of grief	1. Discusses object of loss (person, role, opportunity, or image) 2. Discusses when, where, and how loss occurred 3. Discusses significance of the object of loss
Emotional Dimension	
To recognize and express various feelings precipitated by loss	1. Verbalizes feelings, such as anger, guilt, resentment, sadness, loneliness, relief, and hopelessness 2. Discusses beliefs and attitudes held toward such feelings 3. States that such feelings are a normal aspect of the grieving process 4. Makes statements that reflect acceptance of own feelings even though they may create discomfort and pain
To reduce anxiety associated with the loss	1. Describes physical manifestations of anxiety 2. Discusses feelings of anxiety 3. Recognizes thoughts, feelings, or events that lead to anxiety 4. Exhibits control even when anxious 5. Focuses on present 6. Engages in activities other than ruminating or worrying 7. Identifies ways to increase sense of control over life situation 8. Makes fewer statements that reflect helplessness 9. Is able to sleep

SHORT-TERM GOALS	OUTCOME CRITERIA
To examine fears associated with loss	1. Verbalizes anticipated results of loss 2. Discusses perceived loss of control over particular aspects of life situation 3. Examines needs that will be more difficult to meet as a result of the loss 4. Identifies how past losses have been experienced and what coping mechanisms were used
To reduce excessive feelings of guilt	1. Verbalizes feelings of guilt 2. Identifies thoughts that contribute to feelings of guilt 3. Identifies attitudes and beliefs that contribute to guilt feelings 4. Rejects feelings of guilt based on irrational beliefs 5. Differentiates between concepts of responsibilities and guilt
Intellectual Dimension To develop a sense of control regarding present and future	1. Identifies personal strengths and assets 2. Makes and accepts positive statements about self 3. Practices assertive behaviors 4. Makes fewer statements that reflect helplessness 5. Engages in problem solving about obstacles to meeting goals 6. Identifies new ways to meet goals 7. Identifies new goals to replace those that are now unattainable 8. Sets goals and develops action plans 9. Practices new behaviors designed to facilitate goal attainment
Social Dimension To use available social support system	1. Describes role changes resulting from the loss 2. Expresses feelings associated with loss of old roles or creation of new ones 3. Identifies current sources of support among family members and friends 4. Describes how each source can be helpful 5. Associates need fulfillment with each identified source 6. Makes statements that indicate individual is comfortable when asking for assistance in meeting needs 7. Identifies potential new sources of support (self-help groups) 8. Expresses interest in other people
Spiritual Dimension To identify the meaning of the loss	1. Discuss life goals as they existed before the loss 2. Describes how loss has affected goal attainment 3. Verbalizes feelings associated with goal alterations resulting from the loss 4. Describes secondary losses that may result from primary loss 5. Contributes to or participates in a worthwhile endeavor

Discharge Planning

The following client behaviors demonstrate readiness for discharge:
1. Identifies and discusses personal meaning of the loss
2. Expresses feelings precipitated by the loss
3. Expresses a sense of control over life situation
4. Has set new goals and developed action plans
5. Experiences pleasure for at least brief periods of time

IMPLEMENTATION

NURSING ACTIONS	RATIONALE
Physical Dimension	
1. Protect client from harm if in initial phase of shock.	Some disorganization or disequilibrium often accompanies shock. The individual becomes numb or dazed as a defense.
2. Provide guidance in routine activities or in specific activities that are necessary as a result of the loss.	To maintain self-respect, to convey attitude that life goes on, and to prevent helplessness.
3. Discuss any symptoms of physical distress that client is currently having.	Somatic complaints are associated with grief.
4. Limit activity if client is overactive.	To prevent exhaustion. Overactivity may be manifestation of resistance to deal with emotions.
5. Instruct in self-help measures (exercise, relaxation techniques, warm bath).	To decrease anxiety and enhance ability to relax.
6. Assure client that physical symptoms are self-limiting.	To offer hope for relief and to provide comfort.
7. Motivate client to assume responsibility for own health care.	To reduce dependency and to assist in focusing on self rather than on loss.
Emotional Dimension	
1. Use effective communication techniques (e.g., empathy) and role playing.	To encourage awareness and expression of emotions associated with loss.
2. Encourage reminiscing.	To facilitate expression of feelings.
3. Encourage acceptance of feelings by statements that acknowledge it is normal to feel sad, angry.	To convey the idea that they are a normal part of the grieving process.
4. Encourage discussion of feelings associated with any previous loss that may now be reactivated.	To allow client to compare and clarify meaning of present loss. Past unresolved grief may evoke grieving process.
5. Explore with client fears associated with the loss, particularly regarding loss of control.	Exploration of fears provides a means for identifying potential coping mechanisms.
6. Encourage awareness of aspects of future that are now perceived as threatening.	To help client confront the loss and plan interventions.
7. Discuss feelings of guilt.	To prevent maladaptive emotional responses. Provides opportunity for gaining a new perspective. Excessive guilt is an indication of ambivalence toward the loss.
8. Explore alternative ways of expressing feelings (e.g., by exercising, playing piano, or painting).	To strengthen coping ability.
Intellectual Dimension	
1. Discuss actual or anticipated loss.	Awareness of needs created by the loss aids in grief resolution. Discussing the details of a loss before its occurrence helps people cope by reducing anxiety.
2. Discuss secondary losses that may result from primary loss.	Same as #1.
3. Explain typical phases of grief.	To acknowledge that grief is a universal human experience and to convey the idea that it is a self-limiting process.
4. Assist client in decision making if appropriate.	In the initial phase of grief, shock and disbelief prevent decision making.
5. Help client to identify goals that are unattainable because of the loss.	To reduce feelings of helplessness and to assist client in gaining a new perspective.
6. Help client to identify needs associated with goals now perceived as unattainable.	To plan interventions and promote feelings of control by having client participate in decision making.
7. Assist client in finding new ways to meet needs.	To reduce feelings of helplessness.
8. Provide examples of areas in which client still exerts control and is not helpless.	To reinforce strengths and assets.
9. Discuss ways to increase a sense of control over life situation.	To strengthen coping abilities and a sense of personal competence.
10. Teach problem solving.	To strengthen coping abilities.
11. Teach assertiveness.	To strengthen coping abilities.
12. Encourage realistic goal setting.	To reduce distortions of reality associated with loss and mobilize energy for constructive actions.
13. Assist client in developing action plans to reach new goals.	To encourage responsibility and to provide direction for goal achievement. Reduces feelings of helplessness.
14. Explore conflicts associated with excessive guilt.	Excessive feelings of guilt prolong the grief process and increase the potential for maladaptive behavior.

NURSING ACTIONS	RATIONALE
15. Discuss meaning of previous losses.	To explore beliefs and attitudes that may be relevant to client's experience of the loss.
16. Assure client that the grieving process is self-limiting.	To provide hope and comfort.
17. Assist client in identifying positive aspects of relationship with object of loss that can be carried into future.	Uses positive aspects of the relationship as a means for coping with the loss.
18. Discuss unfinished business client may have with object of loss.	To help resolve conflict.
19. Encourage realistic statements about current situation that reflect acknowledgement of reality of loss.	To help to face the reality of the loss.
20. Encourage focus on the present.	To promote resolution of the grief process.
Social Dimension	
1. Encourage client to focus on assets and strengths.	To promote self-esteem and aid coping.
2. Teach family members how to offer support effectively.	To facilitate the resolution of grief through nurturing and ensuring that role functions are met.
3. Help client identify sources of support currently available and potential new sources of support.	To strengthen coping. Moves the client in the direction of investing self in new relationships.
4. Explore perceived risks of initiating social contacts.	To reduce client's resistance to forming new social contacts.
5. Support client in initiation of contact with sources of support.	To provide positive reinforcement.
6. Explore ways in which social support system has changed as a result of loss.	Loss often results in changes in social roles, and identification of changes can facilitate adaptation to the new situation.
7. Explore effect of loss on client's self-esteem.	Self-esteem is often lowered with a loss.
8. Have client practice self-affirmations.	To increase self-esteem.
9. Assist client in identifying specific needs that can be met by family members and friends.	To reduce feelings of helplessness.
10. Refer client to self-help groups such as Widowed Persons, Parents Without Partners, Compassionate Friends (for parents who have lost a child).	Support groups prevent the complications of prolonged grief.
Spiritual Dimension	
1. Explore beliefs and attitudes that may be relevant to client's experience of loss.	To encourage the grief work necessary for adjustment to the loss.
2. Assist client in clarifying beliefs and values related to loss.	To decrease confusion about beliefs and values.
3. Encourage expression of feelings of hopelessness or meaninglessness precipitated by loss by increasing self-awareness.	To acknowledge that feelings are normal and appropriate.
4. Encourage client to find ways to experience pleasure.	Grief inhibits the experience of pleasure.
5. As grief subsides, reinforce any experiences of pleasure.	Positive reinforcement helps client to continue behavior.
6. Promote client's awareness of options for creating meaning in life.	To reduce helplessness and despair.
7. Encourage client to participate in activities that are directed outside self and that bring pleasure.	To help client refocus and to direct energy from self to others and to new situations.
8. Support and reinforce creative efforts.	To help client discover a new purpose in life.

EVALUATION

Evaluation is based on the client's self-reports and on observations by the nurse, other health professionals, family members, and significant individuals in the client's life. Measurable goals and outcomes provide the data for evaluating the degree to which the client has accepted and adapted to the loss. Outcomes are seen as favorable if soon after the loss, the grieving person:

1. Has positive interactions with others
2. Participates in support groups with others similarly bereaved to share expressions of loss and offer companionship
3. Establishes goals and works to achieve them
4. Discusses the meaning of the loss and its effect on the person's life

BIBLIOGRAPHY

Baumer J, Wadsworth J, Taylor B: Family recovery after death of a child, *Arch Dis Child* 63(9):42, 1988.

Carter S: Themes of grief, *Nurs Res* 38(6):354, 1989.

Cody W: Grieving a personal loss, *Nurs Sci Q* 4(2):61, 1991.

Franks L: When a patient dies—grief—the patient's, the family's and your own, *RN* 47(2):24, 1984.

Gifford B, Cleary B: Supporting the bereaved, *Am J Nurs* 90(2):49, 1990.

Horsley G: Baggage from the past, *Am J Nurs* 88:60, 1988.

Hutti M: A quick reference table of interventions to assist families with pregnancy loss or neonatal loss, *Birth* 15(11):33, 1988.

Ivery J: No code: why won't middle-aged children consent? *J Gerontol Nurs* 10(5):17, 1984.

Jones M, Peacock M: Nursing interventions with continuous loss, *Focus Crit Care* 15(3):26, 1988.

Kubler-Ross E: *On death and dying,* New York, 1969, Macmillan Publishing Co., Inc.

Morris D: Management of perinatal bereavement, *Arch Dis Child* 68:870, 1988.

Neeld E: *Seven choices: taking the steps to new life after losing someone you love,* New York, 1990, Clarkson N. Potter, Inc.

Sheald T: Dealing with the nurse's grief caring for the terminally ill, *Nurs Forum* 21(1):43, 1984.

Simonton O, Mathews-Simonton S, Creighton J: *Getting well again,* New York, 1978, Bantam Books.

Strother A: Drawing the line between life and death, *Am J Nurs* 91(4):24, 1991.

Wordon J: *Grief counseling and grief therapy: a handbook for the mental health practitioner,* New York, 1982, Springer Publishing Co.

Guilt

Guilt is a subjective feeling of remorse and self-reproach resulting from a person's belief that he or she has done something wrong and is possibly going to be punished or has evoked someone's displeasure. The feeling of guilt is central to all humans, and like anxiety, it can be both healthy and unhealthy. Effectively handled, guilt acts as a motivator to keep our behavior in line with our value systems; it signals a violation of conscience. Inappropriately handled, guilt may have far-reaching and devastating consequences; it can emotionally cripple a person. Guilt ranges from the absence of guilt, as in clients with some personality disorders, to severe guilt, as is frequently found in depressed clients.

Shame and embarrassment are behaviors commonly associated with guilt. Shame is a feeling of disgrace or regret resulting from one's real or perceived transgressions being exposed to another person. Embarrassment is a feeling of insecurity, a lack of self-assurance, or a self-conscious distress in response to a specific observed behavior.

The behavioral characteristics of guilt closely resemble those of anxiety, which is a reaction to guilt. The individual then uses defense mechanisms to handle this anxiety.

Nurses are in a vital position to help clients recognize and manage feelings of guilt in an effective manner, thereby preventing the crippling effects of severe guilt.

Related DSM-III-R disorders

Anxiety disorders
Uncomplicated bereavement
Mood disorders
Psychoactive substance-use disorders

Other related conditions

Depression
Violations of personal moral code
Violations of the law

PRINCIPLES

▶ Physical Dimension

1. An individual who injures another may feel guilt.
2. Guilt is a normal response to wrongdoing.
3. The physical sensations of guilt are similar to those of anxiety.

▶ Emotional Dimension

1. The person with a harsh or punitive superego (conscience) may experience excessive guilt.
2. Feelings of guilt may result in an unconscious need for punishment.
3. Guilt feelings may be eased by suffering or punishment.
4. Adolescents may feel guilt when they challenge parental values.

▶ Intellectual Dimension

1. Irrational thoughts may cause a person to feel guilt.
2. Rational thinking can free a person from guilt.
3. An individual can choose to reject the irrational thoughts resulting in guilt feelings.
4. Individuals have the ability to change irrational thoughts (guilt) to rational ones.
5. Overly critical parental messages create feelings of guilt and become a person's internalized standard, which guides behavior.
6. The person who represses and does not confront guilt may experience "neurotic" guilt.

▶ Social Dimension

1. Childhood training has a strong influence on promoting guilt.
2. Misconduct requires confession, contrition, and restitution.

155

3. If parental standards are unrealistic (not age appropriate), the child tends to feel guilt.
4. If society's or parent's standards are not internalized during childhood, feelings of guilt may be absent, resulting in antisocial behavior.
5. Achievement of the developmental stage of initiative versus guilt leads to the abilities to express curiosity and to experience pleasure in achievement.
6. Failure to achieve the developmental stage of initiative versus guilt leads to imitation of others, embarrassment over small mistakes, inability to forgive oneself, and resentment toward authority.
7. Guilt may result when a person feels responsible for others' behavior.

▶ Spiritual Dimension

1. Infractions of a person's moral code or cultural norm may result in guilt feelings.
2. The person who is able to attain idealized values and standards may experience guilt.
3. Individuals inherently feel guilt because they are aware of the potential for many life experiences but find it impossible to carry out all opportunities for living.
4. Individuals who deny their human and spiritual potentialities may feel guilt.
5. The person who conforms and fails to be genuine may feel guilt.
6. Freedom from guilt occurs when individuals confront and bear their own guilt.
7. Individuals are continually committing transgressions, feeling guilt, repenting, and receiving forgiveness.
8. Self-forgiveness is an important component for reducing guilt.
9. Religion may intensify the need for punishment to relieve guilt.

ASSESSMENT

▶ Physical Dimension

I. History
  A. Activities of daily living
    1. Nutrition
      a. Appetite
        (1) Lacks interest in eating
        (2) Overeats
      b. Weight
        (1) Loss
        (2) Gain
    2. Sleep
      a. Insomnia
      b. Excessive sleep
    3. Physical activities
      a. Little or none
        b. Excessive
    4. Sexual activity
      a. Indiscriminant sexual behavior
      b. Abstinence from sex
  B. Destructive behavior
    1. Attempts suicide
  C. Health history
    1. Illnesses
      a. Sexually transmitted disease (STDs, AIDS)
      b. Abuse of alcohol or drugs
    2. Abortion
  D. Review of systems—cardiovascular
    1. Palpitations
    2. Tachycardia

▶ Physical Examination

CLIENT DATA	ANALYSIS	NURSING DIAGNOSIS
Neglect of personal dress and grooming	Excessive guilt contributes to lack of concern for personal appearance.	Bathing/hygiene self-care deficit: neglect of personal dress and grooming related to guilt feelings
Bradycardia, tachycardia, and palpitations	Physiological response suggestive of anxiety.	High risk for anxiety: related to guilt feelings
Weight loss or gain	Feelings of unworthiness may result in lack of appetite and weight loss or in overeating and weight gain.	Altered nutrition: more than body requirements related to guilt feelings
		Altered nutrition: less than body requirements related to guilt feelings

▶ **Emotional Dimension**

CLIENT DATA	ANALYSIS	NURSING DIAGNOSIS
Shame	Disgrace at having behavior exposed to others. Lack of self-esteem and personal insecurity contribute to unrealistic perceptions of behavior.	Ineffective individual coping: shame related to guilt about behavior
Embarrassment	Overly concerned about being perfect. Excessive embarrassment over small mistakes; has difficulty accepting mistakes.	Ineffective individual coping: embarrassment related to guilt about making a mistake
Remorse	Overly reactive. Disproportionate amount of remorse for past conduct.	Ineffective individual coping: excessive remorse related to guilt
Inferiority	Feeling of worthlessness; belief that feeling is deserved. Low self-esteem contributes to feelings of inadequacy and worthlessness; is possible symptom of depression.	Self-esteem disturbance: feelings of inferiority related to guilt
Inability to experience pleasure	Preoccupation with guilt and excessive remorse prevent participation in pleasurable experiences. Client may have unconscious need for punishment.	Diversional activity deficit: related to preoccupation with guilt

▶ **Intellectual Dimension**

CLIENT DATA	ANALYSIS	NURSING DIAGNOSIS
Unrealistic, bizarre, or imagined guilt	Disturbed perceptions can be response to stress.	Altered thought processes: related to unrealistic, bizarre, or imagined guilt feelings
Delusions of worthlessness	Out of touch with reality; possible response to overwhelming guilt.	Altered thought processes: delusions of worthlessness related to guilt feelings
Preoccupation with "shoulds" and "oughts"	Reliance on early parent messages or idealized values; own value system not developed.	*Guilt: related to lack of own value system
Self-deprecation, belittling self when unable to meet own and other's expectations	Parental messages dominate when expectations are not met, resulting in self-deprecation.	Self-esteem disturbance: self-deprecation related to guilt
Blame placed on self for not living up to standards of perfection	Low self-esteem and unrealistic self-expectations contribute to self-blame and self-punishment.	Self-esteem disturbance: self-blame related to guilt
Excessive thoughts about past guilt-producing events	Rumination over events in past, unable to forgive and forget past event.	Altered thought processes: ruminating over past events related to guilt
Inability to concentrate and recall information	Preoccupation with guilt diminishes fund of information; attention span is decreased.	Altered thought processes: inability to concentrate related to guilt
Rigid interpretation of moral code and standards of behavior	Insecurity and lack of clear values and beliefs contribute to rigid interpretation of moral code.	Altered thought processes: rigid interpretation of moral code related to guilt

▶ Social Dimension

CLIENT DATA	ANALYSIS	NURSING DIAGNOSIS
Inability to live up to ideals for self	Standards for self set excessively high; feels guilt when these goals and expectations not met.	Self-esteem disturbance: related to guilt over unmet ideals for self
Disappointment in others who fail to live up to client's expectations	Assumption of responsibility for others' behavior and feels guilt when expectations not met. Projects own expectations on others. May attempt to induce guilt in others.	Self-esteem disturbance: related to guilt over expectations of others that are not met
Inability to live up to high standards set for self	Feeling of guilt when unable to achieve high standards.	Self-esteem disturbance: related to guilt over unmet ideals for self
Inability to accept achievements	Low self-esteem contributes to difficulty in accepting success; denies successes and minimizes achievements.	Self-esteem disturbance: related to guilt over nonacceptance of achievements
Dependence in family relationships	Guilt feeling may result from denial of potentialities.	Ineffective individual coping: guilt related to dependence on family
Seeking of approval and acceptance from others	Lowered self-esteem causes client to seek approval and acceptance from others; results in guilt feelings when not recognized.	Ineffective individual coping: guilt related to lack of approval and acceptance from others
Reduced ability to perform social roles	Preoccupation with guilt may impair ability to perform usual roles.	Altered role performance: related to guilt

▶ Spiritual Dimension

CLIENT DATA	ANALYSIS	NURSING DIAGNOSIS
Opposition of some personal values with society's values	Possibility of values conflict creates guilt.	Spiritual distress: conflict in values related to guilt
Belief that one has to suffer and be punished	Based on religious and cultural beliefs, client believes suffering and punishment may reduce guilt.	Spiritual distress: need to suffer and be punished related to guilt
Despair over guilt	Lack of hope that life will improve.	Spiritual distress: lack of hope related to guilt
Lack of participation in religious activities	Separation from religious activities may cause guilt.	Spiritual distress: inability to participate in religious activities related to guilt
Overinvolvement in religious activities	Seeking forgiveness for guilt with overinvolvement	Spiritual distress: overinvolvement in religious activities related to guilt
Belief that God or superior power is vengeful and unforgiving	Own characteristics attributed to God.	Spiritual distress: anger with God or superior power related to guilt
Difficulty forgiving self and others	Engaging in blame toward self and others.	Spiritual distress: inability to forgive self and others related to guilt
Inability to make restitution for past action	Possible reinforcement of continued guilt feelings.	Spiritual distress: inability to make restitution related to guilt
Inability to be creative	Energy used to promote or prolong guilt.	Spiritual distress: inability to be creative related to guilt
Inability to enjoy life	Preoccupation with guilt keeps client from experiencing life pleasures.	Spiritual distress: inability to enjoy life related to guilt

PLANNING

Long-Term Goal

To express guilt feelings and learn effective ways of coping with situations that
cause guilt

SHORT TERM GOALS	OUTCOME CRITERIA
Physical Dimension	
To identify the physical sensations of guilt	1. See Anxiety, p. 48
Emotional Dimension	
To express feelings of guilt, remorse, shame, and embarrassment	1. Expresses feelings of guilt, shame, remorse, and embarrassment
	2. Acknowledges irrationality when feelings are excessive
	3. Explores reasons for feelings of guilt, shame, remorse, and embarrassment
	4. Learns new ways to manage stress that causes guilt
Intellectual Dimension	
To identify the source of guilt	1. Discusses situations or events that precipitated feelings of guilt
	2. Verbalizes feelings of guilt that are related to critical parental or authority messages
	3. Verbalizes feelings of guilt that are related to cultural standards
	4. Verbalizes feelings of guilt that are related to failure to achieve potential
To alter client's irrational beliefs	1. Acknowledges futility of idealized, unrealistic standards
	2. Verbalizes ability to alter self-expectations.
Social Dimension	
To explore ways to relieve guilt	1. Apologizes for wrongdoing
	2. Makes restitution for actions
	3. Seeks support from others
Spiritual Dimension	
To examine beliefs and values in past situations for which client is feeling guilty	1. Discusses beliefs and values
	2. States beliefs and values that were violated in past situations
	3. Verbalizes how behavior fits into value system
	4. Engages in problem solving about beliefs and values to determine their relevance
	5. Verbalizes rational and irrational aspects of beliefs associated with behavior
	6. Acknowledges responsibility for behavior
	7. Acknowledges ability to learn new values, beliefs, and behaviors
	8. Acknowledges consequences of behavior
	9. States behavior is part of self
	10. Acknowledges wrongs that have been done
To forgive self for past behavior	1. Verbalizes acceptance of personal limitations
	2. Makes statements that reflect self-acceptance

Discharge Planning

The following client behaviors demonstrate readiness for discharge:
1. Identifies situations that cause guilt
2. Uses effective ways to cope with guilt feelings
3. Explores own values and moral code and adjusts expectations to a healthy, realistic level

IMPLEMENTATION

NURSING ACTIONS	RATIONALE
Physical Dimension	
1. Help client attend to physical sensations to get a sense of how guilt feels.	To discover bodily awareness of guilt.
2. Promote client's involvement in an activity that is avoided.	To encourage initiative, mastery, and sense of achievement.
3. Encourage client's awareness of physical pleasure derived from activity or creative efforts.	To increase client's awareness of the mind/body interaction.
4. Prevent destructive behavior.	Guilt feelings may be eased by suffering or punishment.
Emotional Dimension	
1. Encourage expression of feelings of guilt by active listening, reflecting, and clarifying.	Verbal expression of guilt feelings indicates client's recognition of those feelings and helps client choose other feelings.
2. Assist client in accepting realistic and responsible feelings of guilt, (let client know it is a "normal" feeling).	Feelings of guilt are disproportionate to past conduct.
3. Encourage acceptance of forgiveness offered by others.	To accept forgiveness by others is to forgive oneself.
4. Encourage acceptance of self-limitations.	Expectations of self are unrealistically high; strives for perfection and has difficulty accepting mistakes.
5. Encourage awareness of pleasure felt in achievements.	Preoccupation with guilt and excessive remorse interfere with capacity to experience pleasure.
6. Help client assume responsibility for relieving own guilt feelings, for example, by saying "I'm sorry" or talking with a supportive person.	To increase sense of achievement and self-esteem.
Intellectual Dimension	
1. Discuss sources of client's guilt.	Guilt may not have a rational basis but exists because the individual has a harsh conscience. Examining the source of guilt and its irrational aspects provides opportunity for change.
2. Explore rational and irrational aspects of client's beliefs.	To plan interventions.
3. Encourage recognition of client's responsibility for behavior.	To acknowledge responsibility assists the client in understanding that people have choices and one can choose to change one's behavior.
4. Encourage admission of wrongdoing.	Wrongdoing may be denied and there may be no conscious awareness of guilt. Knowing and accepting responsibility for behavior is a means of dealing with guilt in an appropiate manner.
5. Help client assume responsibility for wrongs that have been done.	To promote awareness of behavior and assume responsibility for it.
6. Limit self-punishing statements.	To interrupt irrational aspects of excessive self-reproach.
7. Promote rejection of irrational thoughts and actions that result in guilt feelings.	To help to establish rational thinking and encourage reality testing.
8. Divert attention from preoccupation with guilt feelings.	To redirect focus of attention and interrupt behavior.
9. Explore client's reasons for self-criticism.	To help the client discover the irrational or rational aspect of self-criticism.
10. Explore guilt-producing situations in which client rescues others and assumes responsibility for their irresponsibility.	When client becomes aware of own behavior, client can develop new strategies for change.
11. Help client develop and implement a practical solution to feelings of guilt.	To provide support and encouragement needed to test new behaviors.
12. Encourage reevaluation of idealized, unrealistic standards.	Standards that are too high cannot be met and may produce guilt.

NURSING ACTIONS	RATIONALE
13. Encourage development of exploration, curiosity, and spontaneity.	Excessive guilt interferes with initiative and reduces the capacity to take pleasure in these activities.
14. Give feedback about appropriateness of guilt feelings.	Feelings of guilt may be appropriate or inappropriate.
15. Support realistic assessment of the guilt-producing situation.	To reinforce reality testing.
16. Refrain from negative criticism related to client's feelings of guilt.	Negative criticism may increase feelings of guilt.
17. Discuss consequences of not dealing with guilt.	To establish a cause and effect relationship.
18. Refrain from giving or agreeing with "should" or "should not" statements.	"Should" and "ought" statements indicate that client's value system is poorly developed. Such statements often reflect irrational thinking.
19. Help client accept own actions without devaluing self.	To learn to praise self in a realistic and an accepting manner. Unrealistic self-expectations contribute to self-blame and self-punishment.
20. Be aware of others' need to tell client to "forget it" or "be quiet."	To prevent increased feelings of guilt, since client is unable to "forget it" or "be quiet."
21. Discuss consequences of seeking perfection and approval of others.	To establish a cause and effect relationship between attempts at perfectionism and guilt feelings.
22. Assist client in resolving underlying conflict and using a realistic assessment to deal with self-accusatory delusion.	Irrational thoughts and beliefs may lead to unrealistic, bizarre, or imagined guilt.
23. Assist client in identifying "should" or "should not" statements that may produce guilt.	To help the client gain insight.
Social Dimension	
1. Encourage restitution if appropriate	To relieve guilt feelings and to gain forgiveness from others and for self.
2. Provide family therapy, group therapy, or individual therapy for client.	To help client discover realistic expectations for self and others, to receive support.
3. Encourage sharing of guilt feelings with others (in group therapy)	To provide catharsis and opportunity to express feelings.
4. Encourage sharing with others' experiences of handling guilt.	To provide opportunity to help others with their guilt and allow group members to help client resolve guilt feelings.
5. Refer to self-help groups.	Self-help groups provide social support and are therapeutic.
6. Include family in the treatment if appropriate.	Family involvement increases cooperation with treatment plan.
Spiritual Dimension	
1. Refer client to appropriate clergy or supportive person.	Forgiveness is an important component in reducing guilt.
2. Help client forgive self.	Self-forgiveness is an important component in reducing guilt.
3. Examine moral codes or value systems transgressed.	To determine rational and irrational aspects of beliefs about guilt.
4. Refrain from arguing over moral issues.	Arguing discourages a rational examination of beliefs.
5. Promote client's awareness of reasons for living.	Preoccupation with guilt interferes with life's pleasures.
6. Avoid reinforcing client's belief of guilt.	Reinforcement of belief of guilt will increase feelings of guilt.
7. Encourage client to recognize, confront, and bear his or her guilt.	Confrontation and bearing of guilt serves to decrease it.
8. Encourage client to pursue, challenge, and create.	To provide a means of relieving guilt; provides an alternative to guilt.
9. Promote self-awareness, a sense of being without guilt.	Self-awareness facilitates self-actualization.
10. Promote self-worth.	Acceptance of self and limitations helps remove irrational sources of guilt.

EVALUATION

Evaluation is based on observations by the nurse, other health professionals, members of the family, and significant persons in the individual's life. Measurable goals and outcomes provide the data for evaluating the amount of life disruption the client's guilt is producing and adaptive ways client has learned to cope with guilt. Interventions are successful when the client:

1. Becomes less preoccupied with guilt
2. Makes fewer self-critical statements
3. Indicates acceptance of self and imperfections
4. Forgives self
5. Recognizes feelings of guilt as client's own and manages them in a positive way

Guilt is a separating experience, and when the estrangement can be reconciled the client can move forward to become a more spontaneous, creative, and fully functioning person.

BIBLIOGRAPHY

Berger L: Parental guilt, *Clin Pediatr* 19:499, 1980.

Borysenko J: *Guilt is the teacher, love is the lesson,* New York, 1990, Warner Books.

Bradshaw J: *Healing the shame that binds you,* Deerfield Beach, Fla, 1988, Health Communications.

Engle L, Ferguson T: *Hidden guilt: how to stop punishing yourself and enjoy the happiness you deserve,* New York, 1990, Pocket Books.

Firestone R: The "voice": the dual nature of guilt reactions, *Am J Psychoanal* 47:210, 1987.

Flannery J: Guilt: a crisis within a crisis . . . a catastrophic neurologic event, *J Neurosci Nursing* 22(2):92, 1990.

Gaylin W: *Feelings: our vital signs,* New York, 1988, Ballentine Books.

Grassl S: A special guilt, a special grief: my mother-in-law had a mastectomy, *Nurs '84* 14(4):88, 1984.

Johnson M: We had no choice: a study in families' guilt feelings surrounding nursing home care, *J Gerontol Nurs* 8(11):641, 1982.

Johnson S: The guilt trip: why parents blame themselves or others, *J Pract Nurs* 31(1):25, 1981.

Johnson S: Counseling families experiencing guilt, *Dimens Crit Care Nurs* 3(4):238, 1984.

Knowles R: Managing guilt, *Am J Nurs* 81:1850, 1981.

Knowles RD: Dealing with feelings: overcoming guilt and worry, *Am J Nurs* 81:1663, 1981.

Krozek C: Free yourself from guilt, *Nurs* 20:88, 1990.

Labun E: Spiritual care: an element in nursing care planning, *J Adv Nurs* 13:314, 1988.

Limandri B: Disclosure of stygmatizing conditions: the disclosers' perspective, *Arch Psychiatr Nurs* 3(2):69, 1989.

Menninger K: *Whatever became of sin?* New York, 1988, Hawthorn Publishing Co.

Peterson E, Nelson K: How to meet your patients' spiritual needs, *J Psychosoc Nurs Ment Health Serv* 25(5):34, 1987.

Potter-Efron R, Potter-Efron P: *Letting go of shame,* New York, 1989, Harper & Row, Publishers.

Smith M: *When I say no I feel guilty,* New York, 1975, Dial Press.

Wilkinson J: Moral distress in nursing practice: experience and effect, *Nurs Forum* 23(1):16, 1988.

Hallucinations

Hallucinations are perceptions of an external stimulus when no such stimulus is present. They may involve any of the senses: sight, sound, smell, taste, and touch. Hallucinations are associated with disturbances that may have an organic basis, for example, delirium, dementia, intoxication, or organic mental disorders. They may also have a nonorganic basis, such as in schizophrenia and mood disorders.

Nonorganic hallucinations usually occur as a result of stressful events that cause severe anxiety. The individual lacks a supportive person with whom to share feelings and becomes lonely and isolated. As anxiety increases and hallucinations continue, the ability to focus attention and maintain self-control lessens. Comments and criticisms from others about the client's hallucinatory experience further increase anxiety and isolation and reinforce the client's low self-esteem.

With hallucinations an individual attempts to meet some need that he cannot meet in the real world (for example, relatedness, communication, dependence, or aggression). Delusions frequently accompany hallucinations. The person appears to be listening and watching, or appears preoccupied and unaware of the surroundings. The individual may mutter, mumble, or laugh to himself. He may simply listen to the hallucinations, or may act on them, creating a potentially harmful situation if the nature of the hallucinations is threatening to the individual or others.

Responding with fear, anger, or confrontation or avoiding the client who hallucinates are common responses when the nurse does not understand the hallucinatory process. It is essential that nurses understand the dynamics of hallucinations and feel competent working with the client in order to intervene effectively.

Related DSM-III-R disorders

Schizophrenia
Bipolar disorders
Organic mental diseases
Psychoactive substance use disorders

Other related conditions

Amphetamine psychosis
Digitalis toxicity
Hallucinogenic agents
  Cocaine
  LSD
  Phencyclidine (PCP)
Thyrotoxicosis
Intensive care unit (ICU) psychosis
Brain lesions

PRINCIPLES

▶ Physical Dimension

1. Hallucinations may involve any of the five senses; auditory hallucinations are the most common.
2. In some hallucinations several voices may be talking at once and discussing the client in the third person.
3. Hallucinations may result from metabolic responses to stress that release hallucinogenic neurochemicals.
4. Hallucinations may result from a variety of conditions: extreme fatigue, drugs, delirium accompanying fever, alcohol intoxication, and sleep deprivation.
5. The person may be inattentive to personal hygiene and self-care when hallucinations dominate life.

▶ Emotional Dimension

1. An overwhelming sense of anxiety contributes to the hallucinatory experience.
2. Hallucinations can be of a frightening nature and cause the client to act on the fear.

▶ Intellectual Dimension

1. Hallucinations indicate a break with reality and an attempt to restructure reality in such a way as to protect psychological integrity.

2. The ego functions that maintain contact with reality may be incompletely developed or weakened in the person who hallucinates.

3. The client with overwhelming anxiety uses regression to reduce anxiety to a tolerable level.

4. Hallucinations are an attempt by the ego to defend against impulses that have been repressed but are threatening to enter awareness.

5. Projection allows the ego to deal with the impulses from outside, thus decreasing anxiety.

6. Hallucinations may be of an obscene or threatening nature.

7. Hallucinations may absorb all of a client's attention and control the client's behavior to a great extent.

8. The client gains some control over the hallucinations by telling the voices to go away.

▶ Social Dimension

1. Hallucinations meet needs (relatedness, communication, control, and self-esteem) that the client cannot meet in the real world.

2. Hallucinations form a substitute for human relationships.

3. The client will relinquish hallucinations when he is able to replace them with reality-based interactions that are more satisfying.

4. Hearing voices prevents loneliness, and the client needs real people to fill the void.

5. Hallucinations evolve from the dissociated components of the self-system and have an uncanny quality of reality for the person having them.

6. The person who hallucinates tends to isolate himself from others.

7. Hallucinations are a powerful influence on behavior, for example, hallucinations that tell a person to hurt himself or another person.

8. Hallucinations involve anxiety and then withdrawal from people to relieve the anxiety.

▶ Spiritual Dimension

1. A client who hallucinates has lost control over his own life.

2. Hallucinations are frequently perceived as the voice of God, the devil, or a powerful being.

3. The search for personal meaning to life is contingent on a relatedness to others, which results in a sense of involvement and belonging with others and the universe. The person who is hallucinating is denied this experience.

4. People who hallucinate may not be consciously aware of their daily existence, but the quality of their daily existence contributes to their sense of worth and well-being.

5. Those who hallucinate are cut off from opportunities to reestablish a sense of relatedness with others, who are resources for maintaining hope and confidence.

ASSESSMENT

▶ Physical Dimension

I. **History**
  A. Activities of daily living
    1. Nutrition
      a. Inadequate when voices command client not to eat
    2. Sleep
      a. Deprivation
    3. Recreation, hobbies, and interests
      a. Withdrawal and failure to participate
    4. Physical activities and limitations
      a. Restless
      b. Agitated
      c. Pacing
      d. Strange gestures
      e. Odd actions
      f. Stereotyped mannerisms
  B. Habits
    1. Withdrawal from alcohol (delirium tremens)
    2. Medications and drugs
      a. Uses amphetamines
      b. Uses digitalis
      c. Uses hallucinogens
    3. Destructive behavior
      a. Self-mutilation
      b. Suicide attempts
      c. Impulsive, violent acts
  C. Health history
    1. Illnesses
      a. Schizophrenia
      b. Delirium accompanying fever
      c. Substance abuse
      d. Sleep deprivation
  D. Family history of schizophrenia
  E. Review of systems
    1. General
      a. Weight change
      b. Fever
    2. Neurological
      a. Mood changes
      b. Disorientation
    3. Endocrine
      a. Unaffected by extremes in temperature
II. **Diagnostic tests**—to determine if client is taking medications or has metabolic imbalance
  A. Urinalysis
  B. Blood levels

▶ **Physical Examination**

CLIENT DATA	ANALYSIS	NURSING DIAGNOSIS
Inappropriate dress	Inattentive to dress; may forget to tie shoes, zip zipper, wears sweater in warm weather or no sweater when cold.	Dressing/grooming self-care deficit: inappropriate dress related to hallucinations
Neglects personal hygiene	Inattentive to personal hygiene; fails to brush teeth, shower, comb hair, change clothes; a general untidiness.	Bathing/hygiene self-care deficit: neglects personal hygiene related to hallucinations
Deterioration in self-care	Fails to attend to own usual self-care activities.	*Altered self-care: related to hallucinations

▶ **Emotional Dimension**

CLIENT DATA	ANALYSIS	NURSING DIAGNOSIS
Inappropriate affect	Incongruent for situation.	Ineffective individual coping: inappropriate affect related to hallucinations
Severe or panic level of anxiety	Inability to cope with anxiety, may have extreme apprehension with no apparent cause; leads to hallucinations.	Sensory/perceptual alterations: hallucinations related to severe level of anxiety
Belligerent, negative, or hostile	Low frustration tolerance, easily angered. Content of hallucinations is often threatening.	High risk for violence directed at others: belligerent, negative, or hostile behavior related to hallucinations
Guilt or embarrassment	Occurrence upon recovery, when client realizes impact of behavior.	*Guilt: related to hallucinations

▶ **Intellectual Dimension**

CLIENT DATA	ANALYSIS	NURSING DIAGNOSIS
Distorted perceptions; hallucinations are auditory, visual, tactile, olfactory, and gustatory	Inability to discriminate between real and unreal events or situations. Hallucinations are an attempt to restructure reality so as to protect psychological integrity.	Sensory/perceptual alterations: related to hallucinations
Impaired judgment and insight	Hallucinations may be of commanding, threatening nature.	Sensory/perceptual alterations: impaired judgment (insight) related to hallucinations
Thought content is bizarre, unrealistic, illogical, and difficult to follow	Associations are loose; thinking is disorganized.	Sensory/perceptual alterations: bizarre, unrealistic, illogical, or difficult-to-follow thinking related to hallucinations
Lack of motivation	Ambivalence regarding alternative courses of action may lead client to cease most activities.	Sensory/perceptual alterations: impaired motivation related to hallucinations
Use of defense mechanisms (repression, regression, and denial)	Coping mechanisms that reduce anxiety to more tolerable levels.	Defensive coping: related to hallucinations
Communication (talks to self, mumbles, mutters, and uses third person pronouns; uses neologisms and echolalia; is digressive, vague, circumstantial, and metaphorical; uses symbolic communication; makes loose associations)	Disorganization in thinking.	Impaired verbal communication: related to hallucinations

▶ **Intellectual Dimension—cont'd**

CLIENT DATA	ANALYSIS	NURSING DIAGNOSIS
Poverty of speech	Diminished speech because of withdrawal and alienation from others and from vagueness, concreteness, and repetition.	Impaired verbal communication: poverty of speech related to hallucinations
Rigid thinking	Changes in routines and schedules are anxiety producing; sameness is security.	Anxiety: related to hallucinations

▶ **Social Dimension**

CLIENT DATA	ANALYSIS	NURSING DIAGNOSIS
Disturbed identity	Loss of ego boundaries; is perplexed about self; has incompletely developed or weak ego.	*Altered self-concept: confused identity related to hallucinations
Withdrawal and alienation from others	Preoccupation with own world and emotional detachment from others. Hallucinations form substitute for other human relationships.	Social isolation: withdrawal and alienation from others related to hallucinations
Mistrust of others	Others thought to be controlling client's mind or inserting thoughts into mind. Expression of dissociated parts of self-system.	Altered thought processes: mistrust related to hallucinations
Impaired capacity to function socially	Deterioration in routine daily functioning (work, social relations, and self-care).	Self-esteem disturbance: deterioration in social functioning related to hallucinations

▶ **Spiritual Dimension**

CLIENT DATA	ANALYSIS	NURSING DIAGNOSIS
Despair	Lack of sense of hope and faith. Disconnection from others leads to loss of vital resources for maintaining hope.	Spiritual distress: despair related to hallucinations
Diminished quality of life; incapacitation from stress and anxiety	Little gratification in life; lack of motivation to change.	Spiritual distress: diminished quality of life related to hallucinations

PLANNING

Long-Term Goals

To function at an optimal level with fewer or no hallucinations

To experience satisfying relationships with real persons without reverting to hallucinations

To understand the hallucinatory experience and its relationship to stress and anxiety

SHORT-TERM GOALS	OUTCOME CRITERIA
Physical Dimension	
To identify stressors in life	1. Verbalizes events and situations that cause stress and anxiety
To decrease impulsivity and protect self and others	1. Accepts close supervision for protection of self and others.
	2. Shows less frequent impulsive acts
	3. Verbalizes feelings of anxiety, anger, being overwhelmed, hostility, and rejection rather than acting out
	4. Expresses feelings appropriately
	5. Knows when angry feelings are building up
	6. Uses physical energy to release tension
	7. Takes responsibility for self and feelings
Emotional Dimension	
To decrease fears and anxiety	1. Verbalizes feeling afraid or anxious
	2. States events, desires, impulses, needs, or situations causing fear and anxieties
	3. Shows ability to manage anxiety in a healthy manner
	4. Knows when anxiety is increasing and seeks help from appropriate others
	5. See Anxiety, p. 48
Intellectual Dimension	
To reduce or eliminate hallucinations by staying in contact with reality	1. Takes medications as prescribed
	2. Stays in contact with reality
	3. Identifies clues that trigger hallucinations and takes measures to interrupt them
	4. Seeks out a staff person when upset or has strong feelings
	5. Uses projection less often
To identify need served by the hallucination	1. Verbalizes decreased anxiety
	2. States that fears of rejection are reduced
	3. States that fears of loneliness and abandonment are decreased
	4. States that uncomfortable, fearful impulses are less threatening
	5. States a desire to relate to others
	6. States a desire to communicate with others
	7. States a desire to be independent
	8. States a desire to feel better about self
Social Dimension	
To interact with others satisfactorily without hallucinating	1. Responds to others in a realistic, socially acceptable way
	2. States satisfactions in relationships with others
	3. Tells appropriate person when hallucinations occur and interfere with conversation and activities with others
	4. Touches others appropriately and allows others to touch him to establish reality
	5. Learns social skills
Spiritual Dimension	
To be less incapacitated by stress and anxiety	1. Seeks out others when anxious
	2. Controls hallucinations with effective methods
	3. Receives pleasure from experiences with others
	4. Becomes self-motivated and initiates actions when anxious

Discharge Planning

The following client behaviors demonstrate readiness for discharge:
1. Sees hallucinations as a part of mental illness
2. Manages anxiety constructively
3. Refrains from responding to voices when in the presence of others
4. Explains importance of taking medications even when feeling better and not hallucinating
5. Has a significant person with whom he can share feelings and from whom he can receive support
6. Anticipates difficulties on returning home or to community and knows where to get help

IMPLEMENTATION

NURSING ACTIONS	RATIONALE
Physical Dimension	
1. Treat physical symptoms or harm resulting from self-mutilating actions.	To maintain biological integrity, to demonstrate caring.
2. Assist with self-care when needed.	Disorganization and lack of self-care are seen in persons who hallucinate.
3. Have client assume responsibility for self-care.	The hallucinating client is inattentive to usual self-care activities.
4. Provide protective supervision for client to prevent impulsive acts that would harm self or others.	Hallucinations may be commanding or threatening and client may act on them.
5. Be aware of high risk of suicide when client's hallucinations are of a threatening, cruel, or terrorizing nature.	Same as #4.
6. Supervise closely when client is taking medications to be sure client has swallowed them.	Client may fear that medication will harm him or may be so disorganized that he does not know to swallow them.
7. Check lab reports if you are not certain that client is taking medications.	To verify that client is taking medications.
8. Give medications in liquid form if client does not swallow tablets.	Liquids cannot be hidden in the mouth or hoarded.
9. Offer appropriate prescribed medications when hallucinations are threatening and client is in danger of losing control.	To assure client's safety.
10. Provide routine daily schedule of activities.	The client will know what to expect and can prepare, thus reducing anxiety.
11. Refrain from touching client.	To prevent misinterpretation or lashing out.
12. Monitor situations that increase anxiety, which results in hallucinations, and intervene immediately.	Anxiety or stressful situations precede the hallucinatory experience.
Emotional Dimension	
1. Help client identify feelings of anxiety by active listening, reflecting, and clarifying.	Anxiety precedes the hallucinatory experience.
2. Share observations of nonverbal expression of feelings with client ("you look annoyed").	To focus on underlying feelings rather than on content of the hallucination.
3. Explore with client his feelings about hallucinations when appropriate and when client demonstrates readiness.	When recovered, client may feel guilt or embarrassment about his behavior.
4. Accept client's feelings of anxiety, anger, and sadness.	The nurse's acceptance of the client's feelings will enable the client to accept them.
5. When feelings are inappropriate for situation, gently confront client (after a relationship has been established).	To help to learn appropriate behavior.
6. Explore with client ways to express anxiety, for example, talking with another person.	To help discover more effective ways to manage anxiety.
7. Provide tasks and activities that client is familiar with and capable of doing.	This client often has a low tolerance for frustration.

NURSING ACTIONS	RATIONALE
8. Refrain from joking about or judging client's hallucinations.	The nurse may relieve her own anxiety concerning her ability to interrupt client's hallucination or concerning the content of the hallucination and joke or make judgments.
9. Be alert for signs of increasing anxiety.	To intervene before client hallucinates.
10. Accept client's belligerent, negative, and hostile behavior without taking it personally.	Hostile and negative behavior is a reflection of how client feels and is not directly related to the nurse.
11. Provide quiet area or restraints if client is unable to control impulsive responses to voices.	To ensure client's safety.
12. Be aware of fear, pain, and sadness underlying client's hallucinations.	To communicate an empathic response that engenders trust.
13. Ask for help if personally frightened by client's distorted perceptions.	To increase the nurse's feeling of security. Fear may be transmitted to client and he may not be able to distinguish it from his own.
14. Be aware that even though client seems remote, detached, and distant, your behavior, both verbal and nonverbal, is influential.	The client still observes and hears what is occurring around him.

Intellectual Dimension

1. Interrupt the hallucination by calling client by name and focusing attention on real things, events, or activities.	To provide competing stimuli that are real.
2. Avoid conveying the belief that hallucinations are real, verbally or nonverbally (as with head nodding).	Verbal or nonverbal behavior can act to validate client's distortions.
3. Refrain from discussing hallucinations, except to find out whose voice is talking and what is being said.	To avoid reinforcing the behavior.
4. Communicate in direct, specific terms.	Because thinking is disorganized, client may have difficulty understanding communications.
5. Avoid gestures and abstract ideas that client may not understand and that may increase client's anxiety.	Same as #4.
6. Respond verbally to anything real client talks about.	To reinforce ability to focus on reality. Behavior that is reinforced tends to be repeated.
7. Give positive feedback when client focuses on reality.	Same as #6.
8. Use broad openings when approaching hallucinating client ("Tell me what is happening").	To decrease anxiety.
9. Ask client what the voice seems to be saying.	To avoid conveying the idea that the voices are real.
10. Use a calm, consistent, and unhurried approach.	To convey your availability and concern.
11. Teach client relationship between increased anxiety levels and hallucinations.	To establish the cause and effect relationship.
12. Explain carefully what is happening and what you are doing to reduce anxiety.	Client's perceptions are distorted and he may misinterpret or not understand what you are saying or your actions.
13. Verbalize actions; do not rely on nonverbal communication.	Same as #12.
14. Ask client to seek help from staff to control voices.	To teach client to ask for help and to encourage client to take constructive steps to get rid of voices.
15. Teach stress-reduction and problem-solving skills.	To teach alternative behaviors for managing anxiety.
16. Teach client to test reality by seeking validation for perceptions.	Client is unable to distinguish between real and unreal situations or events. Consensual validation from another person reinforces reality testing.
17. Indicate doubt about the reality of the hallucinations.	To convey the idea that the hallucinatory experience is not real.
18. Offer other explanations for conclusions that client develops in support of hallucinations.	To increase reality testing.
19. Indicate in a direct manner that hallucinations may seem real to client but they are not real to you.	Indicates acceptance of client and his experience but not of his reality.
20. Respond to the feeling content of the hallucination ("It's scary to hear voices no one else hears").	To acknowledge client's experience.
21. Use direct responses if client hallucinates while talking with you ("Listen to me, look at me, do not listen to the voices now").	Redirects the focus of attention.
22. Teach client to intervene when hallucinating (Say "go away" or sing or whistle).	To teach client to focus on other competing stimuli.

IMPLEMENTATION—cont'd

NURSING ACTIONS	RATIONALE
23. Give positive feedback when client begins to tell voice to go way or leave him alone and consciously participates in activities as a way to cope with them.	Behavior that is reinforced tends to be repeated.
Social Dimension	
1. Promote a realistic perception of self: a person of worth, value, and respect.	To increase self-esteem.
2. Provide a safe environment, especially at night when hallucinations may occur.	To increase client's sense of security and ensure safety.
3. Stay with client to ensure safety.	Same as #2.
4. Assist client in becoming more involved in activities with others.	Client is lonely and uses hallucinations as a substitute for human relationships.
5. Offer a consistent, no-demand, supportive relationship.	To reduce anxiety.
6. Notify persons whom client may endanger because of what the voices say.	To ensure their safety. Professionals have a "duty to warn" potential victims.
7. Assist client in meeting needs of dependency, self-esteem, communication, and relatedness in real life that hallucinations meet.	To meet needs and encourage effective coping.
8. Teach social skills.	To increase self-esteem and feelings of adequacy.
9. Assist client in increasing social interactions gradually, starting one-to-one and then moving to small groups.	Since interpersonal contacts create anxiety, provide the opportunity for client to become desensitized.
10. Provide group therapy, conversation, remotivation, reality groups, or occupational therapy.	To encourage social interaction.
11. Enlist help of family to reduce demands on client and lessen stress level at home.	Family or significant others are an important part of the treatment plan.
12. Inform client and family of social agencies available for help.	To assist the family in developing community resources. Client's illness tends to be chronic and may require further treatment in a community setting.
13. Help develop plans for appropriate social activities in the community.	Same as #12.
Spiritual Dimension	
1. Assist client in managing despair and alienation by exploring effects of client's behavior on others.	The client has isolated himself from others. Help him understand why.
2. Promote realistic hope that hallucinations can be controlled by reducing stress and taking medications as prescribed.	To reduce hopelessness and despair.
3. Assist client in achieving satisfying relationships with others by learning to listen to others' concerns and sharing own concerns with others.	To encourage relatedness with others who can improve client's hope and confidence.
4. Help client find pleasures in life.	To enhance the quality of his life.

EVALUATION

Measurable goals and outcome criteria provide a basis for evaluating the client's progress and the effectiveness of his treatment. As the client's condition stabilizes and the hallucinations decrease in frequency, the following behaviors indicate successful intervention:

1. Verbalizes events and situations that cause anxiety
2. Assumes responsibility for self and feelings
3. Demonstrates the ability to manage anxiety in a more effective manner
4. Takes medications
5. Explores needs served by the hallucinatory experience
6. Improves social skills and increases relatedness with others

When hallucinations are of a more chronic nature, psychological deterioration progresses and increased supervision is important to help the client function at an optimal level.

BIBLIOGRAPHY

Asaad G, Shapiro B: Hallucinations: theoretical and clinical overview, *Am J Psychiatry* 143:1088, 1986.

Bick P, Kinsbourne M: Auditory hallucinations and subvocal speech in schizophrenic patients, *Am J Psychiatry* 144:222, 1987.

Easton C, MacKenzie F: Sensory-perceptual alterations: delirium in the intesive care unit, *Heart Lungs: J Crit Care* 17(3):229, 1988.

Feder R: Auditory hallucinations treated by radio headphones, *Am J Psychiatry* 139:1188, 1982.

Field W: Hearing voices, *J Psychosoc Nurs Ment Health Serv* 23(1):9, 1985.

Field W, Ruelke W: Hallucinations and how to deal with them. *Am J Nurs* 73:638, 1973.

Green H: *I never promised you a rose garden,* New York, 1964, Holt, Rinehart & Winston.

Hellerstein D, Frosch W, Koenigsberg H: The clinical significance of command hallucinations, *Am J Psychiatry* 144:219, 1987.

Schwartzman S: The hallucinating patient and nursing interventions, *J Psychiatr Nurs* 13(6):23, 1975.

Siegal F: Hostage hallucinations: visual imagery induced by isolation and life-threatening stress, *J Nerv Ment Dis* 172:264, 1984.

Wasow M: *Coping with schizophrenia: a survival manual for parents, relatives and friends,* Palo Alto, Calif., 1982, Science & Behavior Books.

Williams C: Perspectives on the hallucinatory process, *Issues Ment Health Nurs* 10(2):99, 1989.

Hyperactivity in Children

Hyperactivity is a developmental disorder in children characterized by inappropriate inattention, restlessness, and impulsivity. It begins in childhood and may diminish during adolescence. In the past a number of names, including hyperkinesis, minimal brain damage, and minimal brain dysfunction (MBD), have been assigned to this disorder. According to the DSM III-R, the disorder is now called *attention-deficit hyperactivity disorder (ADHD)* because attention difficulties are prominent and nearly always present in children with these diagnoses. It is the hyperactivity associated with ADHD that this chapter addresses.

The child's inappropriate attention, impulsivity, and restlessness create problems for him. In the classroom the child has difficulty staying with tasks and organizing and completing work. The child gives the impression of not listening to what has been said. The child's work is sloppy and impulsively done; careless errors are made. Group situations are particularly difficult, and attention problems are even more pronounced when sustained attention is expected.

At home the child has trouble following parental requests and instructions. Ability to stick to activities and play is inappropriate for the child's age. Thus the child suffers in academic achievement and social functioning.

Symptoms vary in children and with situations and time. A child may be well organized and appropriate on a one-to-one basis and become disruptive in a group. The child may adjust satisfactorily at home and have problems at school.

The disorder is seen in 3% of prepubertal children in the United States. Understanding the behavior and having the knowledge and skills to effect change in these children have tremendous potential for relieving the anxiety of the child and his family and for helping the child become a well-adjusted and functional adult.

Related DSM-III-R disorders

Attention-deficit hyperactivity disorder (ADHD)
Mental retardation
Conduct disorders

Other related conditions

School failure
Antisocial behavior
Hypoglycemia
Hyperthyroidism
Secondary reaction to lack of achievement in school
Acting-out of pathological family dynamics
Depression

PRINCIPLES

▶ Physical Dimension

1. There is a chemical imbalance caused by neurological dysfunction.
2. Damage to the central nervous system structures being formed or already formed (such as in trauma, infection, hemorrhage, and hypoxia) has been known to cause hyperactivity.
3. Prenatal causes of central nervous system dysfunction include infections and metabolic, genetic, toxic, and psychogenic factors.
4. Perinatal causes include prematurity, postmaturity, prolonged labor, abnormal labor, induction of labor, effects of medications, immunological incompatibility, and normal mechanics of labor.
5. During the postnatal period (to 5 years) causes include infections, injuries, medications, toxins, metabolic or vascular disturbances, environmental factors, neoplasms, and convulsive disorders.
6. Maternal smoking, exposure to carbon monoxide, and x-ray examinations are related to hyperactivity.
7. A higher percentage of boys than girls suffer from hyperactivity.
8. A high incidence of physical anomalies (epicanthus, widely spaced eyes, curved fifth finger, adherent ear lobes) may be seen.
9. A higher than expected incidence of psychiatric diagnoses among parents of hyperactive children is seen.
10. There is some research evidence of higher rates of the following in parents of hyperactive children:

history of alcoholism in mothers and fathers, hysterical behavior in mothers, and antisocial behavior in fathers.
11. Hyperactive children often have relatives who were hyperactive.

▶ Emotional Dimension

1. The repercussions of physical or mental illness of the mother make a child at risk for hyperactivity.
2. Overreaction to minor stimulation results in explosive emotional outbursts.
3. Overreaction is organically based and pervasive.
4. The child is unable to appropriately stop emotional outburst in reaction to stimuli.
5. The child is emotionally labile, moving easily from tears to temper tantrums.
6. Emotional responses to the environment are unpredictable and aversive.
7. The continual frustration leads to frequent responses of irritability and anger.
8. Acting-out behavior reflects a child's miserableness.

▶ Intellectual Dimension

1. Some hyperactive children have specific learning disabilities.
2. Rigid, unrealistic, and imposed curricular requirements and expectations increase the torment and tension in the hyperactive child.
3. Ineffective teaching and role modeling (a role model is tense, loud, and anxious) may contribute to hyperactivity.
4. An inability to sort out stimuli from the environment and determine which one(s) to respond to results in attempts to respond to them all.
5. The hyperactive child is unable to focus on more than one stimulus at a time.
6. An inability to delay immediate gratification of needs leads to inappropriate responses and impulsive acts.
7. The hyperactive child becomes preoccupied with an object or task and resists efforts to distract him from it.
8. Hyperactive, impulsive children lack proficiency in verbal control tasks.
9. Hyperactive, impulsive children have less verbal control of nonverbal behavior. (For example, when learning a new task, they do not give themselves verbal instructions on the sequential steps necessary for task completion, as most children do.)

▶ Social Dimension

1. Hyperactivity is normal behavior in certain ages and stages of growth.
2. A noisy, distracting, and chaotic environment may contribute to hyperactivity and inattention.

3. Overly crowded homes near airpor[...] streets, or high crime areas, improper [...] cooling, and hunger contribute to acting-o[...] sonal frustrations.
4. Chronic marital problems with angry emotional [...] bursts contribute to a tense family relationship, which results in the child acting out.
5. Distractions result from school and classroom conditions (poor, drab, overcrowded, and noisy conditions, uncomfortable seats, and inadequate lunch arrangements).
6. Low economic status with its problems of poor nutrition and lack of prenatal care is related to learning and behavior problems.
7. Order and routine in the home, rather than unpredictability, favorably influence learning and behavior.
8. A barren physical environment without appropriate toys and opportunities for variety influences behavior and learning.
9. The prolonged absence of the father (desertion, divorce, separation, or extended military service) is associated with behavior and learning problems.
10. The effects of family instability, obstetrical complications, and low birth weight increase susceptibility to hyperactivity.
11. Diminished contact with a premature baby decreases the mother-child attachment and is related to hyperactivity.
12. Mothers of hyperactive children demonstrate lower expectations for independence and achievement than mothers of other children.
13. Fathers demonstrate more rewarding behaviors and less punishment to hyperactive children than mothers demonstrate.
14. Being labeled hyperactive and confronted with it daily, the child acts in a hyperactive fashion.
15. The hyperactive child may become the family scapegoat, which prevents the child from behaving in socially acceptable ways.
16. Hyperactivity in a cultural context emerges from a particular social situation (school) where the child's behavior is distressing to others.
17. In industrial societies with compulsory education all children with varying degrees of perception, language capabilities, attention span, and tolerance for immobility are asked to sit still, not talk or make trouble, and focus on learning.
18. There are cultural variations in perception of hyperactivity and in management of socially different behavior.

▶ Spiritual Dimension

1. Hyperactive behavior results in negative responses from others and contributes to the child's feelings of isolation and sometimes despair.

rth are intensified by the
re.
d and lack the warmth and
r healthy personal growth.

4. Perceived differentness from other children is seen as not good and contributes to the child's devaluation of self.

Physical Dimension

I. History
A. Activities of daily living
  1. Requires little sleep
  2. Physical activities
    a. Constantly active
    b. Shifts from one activity to another
    c. Handles and fingers things
    d. Fascinated with spinning objects
    e. Plays excessively with water
    f. Lacks coordination with eye-hand movement (breaks things easily)
  3. Destructive behavior
    a. Acts impulsively, is a danger to self and others
    b. Is accident-prone
B. Health history
  1. Illnesses
    a. Encephalitis
    b. Lead ingestion
    c. Hypoglycemia
  2. Injuries
    a. Birth trauma
  3. Allergies
    a. Food allergies
C. Family health history
  1. Psychiatric diagnoses of alcoholism, hysteria, and antisocial behavior in parents and relatives of hyperactive children

II. Physical examination—generally physically healthy

III. Diagnostic tests
A. EEG
B. Psychological testing
C. Allergy testing
D. Glucose tolerance test

▶ Emotional Dimension

CLIENT DATA	ANALYSIS	NURSING DIAGNOSIS
Explosive irritability	May be set off by minor stimuli; child dismayed and puzzled.	Ineffective individual coping: explosive irritability related to hyperactivity
Anxiety and inner tension	Organically based; basic and pervading.	Anxiety: related to hyperactivity
Overreaction	Inability to turn off inappropriate reactions (in school or church).	Ineffective individual coping: overreaction related to hyperactivity
Emotional lability	Easily set off to laughter or tears.	Ineffective individual coping: lability related to hyperactivity
Unpredictable moods	Unpredictable aversive response to environment.	Ineffective individual coping: unpredictable moods related to hyperactivity
Hostility, anger, aggression	Easily frustrated when needs unmet or gratification delayed; or there is continual frustration and failure in social interactions and academic endeavors.	Ineffective individual coping: hostility and anger related to hyperactivity
Excitability	Tendency to become overexcited and more active in stimulating situations, particularly in groups with other children.	Ineffective individual coping: excitability related to hyperactivity
Depression	Miserableness reflected in acting out behavior, which may be symptom of underlying depression.	Ineffective individual coping: depression related to hyperactivity

▶ **Intellectual Dimension**

CLIENT DATA	ANALYSIS	NURSING DIAGNOSIS
Short attention span, easily distracted, and unable to concentrate	Incapable of attending to more than one stimulus at a time. Unable to inhibit response to any stimulus that comes along.	*Altered learning processes: short attention span, easily distractible, and inability to concentrate related to hyperactivity
Inability to delay gratification	Acts impulsively; is unable to wait or be put off for even a short time.	Ineffective individual coping: inability to delay gratification related to hyperactivity
Difficulty organizing school work	Acts without thinking.	Altered thought processes: inability to organize work related to hyperactivity
Inconsistency in responses	May do well at a task one day and have trouble doing it the next day.	Altered thought processes: inconsistency in responses related to hyperactivity
Unpredictability and variability in thinking	Fluctuation in performance.	Ineffective individual coping: unpredictability and variability in performance related to hyperactivity
Academic failure or underachievement	Inattention, poor concentration, and extreme restlessness interfere with achievement.	Ineffective individual coping: academic failure or underachievement related to hyperactivity

▶ **Social Dimension**

CLIENT DATA	ANALYSIS	NURSING DIAGNOSIS
Negative self-concept	General nuisance value and lack of explanation for behavior leads to parental dissatisfaction and pressures. Hostility is worsened by the child thinking "I'm bad, I'm dumb."	Self-esteem disturbance: related to negative effects of hyperactive behavior
Proneness to failure	Receives low level of positive reinforcement from others; gives up quickly because of long failure record.	Self-esteem disturbance: proneness to failure related to hyperactivity
Lack of order and stability in family	Disorganized family structure and unpredictability create anxiety, which exacerbates hyperactivity. Predictable structure and experiences in family minimize anxiety and reduce hyperactivity.	Altered parenting: lack of family stability related to hyperactivity
Poor performance in school	Impaired ego functions both create and worsen difficulties, causing criticism and pressures.	Self-esteem disturbance: poor school performance related to hyperactivity
Lack of social skills	Misconduct, antisocial behavior, social isolation, and rejection impair relationships with others.	Self-esteem disturbance: impaired social skills related to hyperactivity
Immature personality	Biological development delayed. Underachieves.	Altered thought processes: underachieves related to hyperactivity associated with immature personality

▶ **Spiritual Dimension**

CLIENT DATA	ANALYSIS	NURSING DIAGNOSIS
Despairing; enslaved by illness (according to family)	Hyperactive behavior results in negative responses from others and contributes to child's feelings of despair and worthlessness.	Spiritual distress: despair related to hyperactivity
Sees self as different from other children, of less value	Inability to be like other children contributes to feelings of low self-worth; being different is not good or is bad.	Spiritual distress: low self-worth related to hyperactivity

PLANNING

Long-Term Goal

To reduce activity level so that social interactions and academic achievements are attained at the child's optimal level

SHORT-TERM GOALS	OUTCOME CRITERIA
Physical Dimension To channel impulsiveness so that it can be controlled	1. Incorporates acceptable control devices that delay or prevent impulsive actions 2. Can talk out a situation rather than act out 3. Is able to wait and delay gratification 4. Deliberately controls specific behavior 5. Recognizes consequences of impulsive acts
Emotional Dimension To reduce responsiveness to the environment	1. Sits still for increasing periods of time 2. Concentrates on a task for increasing periods of time 3. Completes a task 4. Identifies stress and anxiety within the environment 5. Removes self to another area when distracted by stimuli 6. Watches self on videotapes and shows awareness of behavior
Intellectual Dimension To develop language skills through which frustration, disappointment, rage, and ideas can be expressed	1. Verbalizes thoughts and feelings about specific problem situations (fights or taking toys from other children) 2. Discusses age-appropriate issues of power, control, and persons in authority (parents and teachers) 3. Discusses reputation, status in relation to peers, parents, and teachers 4. Discusses anger, guilt, and shame 5. Discusses uselessness, hopelessness, and discouragement
Social Dimension To participate in groups without distracting others	1. Participates in group activities without distracting others 2. Requests permission to leave group if restless and becoming overresponsive 3. Walks around quietly when restless without provoking others 4. Completes a group activity
To develop social skills	1. Eats properly 2. Waits turn 3. Engages in conversation 4. Says "please" and "thank you"

SHORT-TERM GOALS	OUTCOME CRITERIA
Spiritual Dimension To increase self-worth	1. Talks about self with positive statements 2. Uses fewer self-derisive statements ("I'm bad, dumb") 3. Participates in family activities that result in positive reinforcements for appropriate behavior 4. Achieves goals at school (as appropriate for age and child) 5. Plays with other children (as appropriate for age and child)

Discharge Planning

The following client behaviors demonstrate readiness for discharge:
1. Controls or limits impulsive behavior
2. Parents comply with dates for follow-up visits
3. Parents contact school or other agency that child will encounter
4. Parents know names of appropriate agencies to call on for assistance with child

IMPLEMENTATION

NURSING ACTIONS	RATIONALE
Physical Dimension	
1. Help child identify specific problem behaviors (handling, touching, fighting, or taking toys).	Discussing problem areas brings them to conscious awareness so that instructions can be implemented.
2. Monitor conditions under which problem behaviors occur.	To identify situations which provoke problem behaviors.
3. Note duration and frequency of the behavior.	Baseline data are needed to determine the effect of treatment interventions.
4. Explore with child the consequences of behavior.	To assist child in recognizing the cause-and-effect relationship that arises with impulsive acts and problem behaviors.
5. Reward behaviors not acted on impulsively.	To increase self-esteem. Behavior that is rewarded is more likely to be repeated.
6. Administer medications as prescribed and monitor closely for behavior effects.	Medications are often administered to reduce hyperactive behavior and are prescribed on the basis of an effective range rather than by body weight.
7. Reduce impulsive behavior with negative reinforcement.	Behaviors that are not rewarded (i.e., ignored, given "time out") are less likely to be repeated.
8. Provide relaxation exercises, deep breathing, and biofeedback.	To learn alternative behaviors. Child learns to focus and reduce tension.
9. Provide activities child can complete in short periods of time.	Attention span is short. Completion of a task increases self-esteem.
10. Provide safe recreation for child.	Acts impulsively and can be of danger to self and others. Is accident-prone.
11. Use learning tasks and exercises to reduce hyperactivity (see box, p. 178)	To increase muscular inhibition and self-control.
Emotional Dimension	
1. Help identify feelings of frustration, anger, rage, and discouragement by listening actively, and empathizing.	To help child begin to recognize the cause (feelings) and effect (acting out) relationship of his behavior.
2. Facilitate expression of feelings of frustration, anger, rage, and discouragement in an appropriate manner; talk about them, use physical energy to express them.	To provide alternatives to problematic behaviors.
3. Explore alternative methods of expressing feelings ("What could you have done to express yourself without _____?" or "What were you feeling when you _____?").	To teach alternative responses.

MIRROR STARE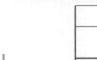

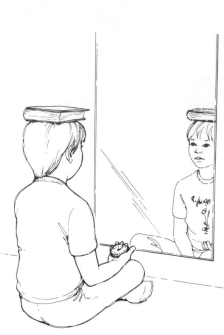

My Time Record	
Date	Time

Objective: To increase the ability to sit still.

Materials: Mirror; book; stopwatch; recording chart.

Procedure: Say to the child, "Start the watch. Now sit comfortably cross-legged on the floor (or pillow) in front of the mirror. Carefully sit up straight and place a book on your head. Balance the book and watch yourself in the mirror as long as you can without moving. When you move or when the book falls, record your time."

The child continues to try this and see if he can remain still for longer periods of time.

Extended Activities: The child can try to balance old records, bean bags, rulers, toy animals, pillows, and other objects without moving.

From Valett R.: The psychoeducational treatment of hyperactive children, Belmont, Calif, 1974, Fearon Publishers, p 40.

IMPLEMENTATION—cont'd

NURSING ACTIONS	RATIONALE
4. Ask for clarification when behavioral expression of feelings is not understood.	A function of the nurse-client relationship is to clarify feelings and to relate them to behavior.
5. Use empathy abundantly ("Throwing chairs is frightening, isn't it?" or "You get angry when _____.").	Responding to feelings conveys caring, understanding.
6. Decrease pressure to conform to peers. Avoid comparisons with others.	Recognizes the individuality of the child and also reduces tension that may be associated with demands to conform.
Intellectual Dimension	
1. Solicit from child reason for specific behavior.	Provide a means for child to examine his behavior.
2. Help child increase attention span by providing a less stimulating environment.	Helps childs learn self-control.
3. Use positive reinforcement to help child delay immediate gratification to learn to wait, to take turns.	Helps child learn self-control.

NURSING ACTIONS	RATIONALE
4. Give brief, concise directions and assignments.	Attention span is short and child has difficulty concentrating. Too many stimuli are distracting to child.
5. Allow child to work at own pace within reasonable limits.	Reduces tension associated with pressure to complete a task. Completing task increases child's self-esteem.
6. Provide for repetition.	To promote learning and consistency in response.
7. Help child abstain from making derogatory remarks about self.	To increase self-esteem.
8. With support and encouragement, promote the attitude that being different is not bad.	Indicates acceptance and aids self-acceptance.
9. Read allegorical stories such as "The Ugly Duckling" and discuss metaphorical meaning.	To decrease feelings of isolation and failure and point out acceptability and rewards of being different.
10. Increase awareness of problem behavior and causes.	Reduces misinterpretation and distortions of child's experience.
11. Provide alternatives for problem behaviors (e.g., "punch pillows when you are frustrated rather than hit Susie").	To strengthen coping ability.
12. Increase verbal skills that allow for expression of feelings.	To reduce the need to act out.
13. Provide training in self-control, for example, using pennies, privileges for rewards.	To assist child in learning to internalize self-control.
14. Teach self-reinforcement with positive self-talk: "I did it!"	To increase self-esteem. Self-reinforcement is a means of rewarding desirable behavior.
15. Provide immediate feedback.	Child can know quickly how well he is doing.
16. Discipline with short-term actions (grounding for two weeks is ineffective).	Child can immediately learn the relationship between his behavior and discipline. Excessive punitiveness lowers self-esteem and defeats the purpose of intervention.
17. Ask child to restate negative statements so that they become positive.	To increase self-esteem; to decrease criticism.
18. Teach child to use self-directed verbal statements such as, "I will stop, look, listen, think, before I answer . . . before I move."	To learn to control nonverbal behavior verbally.
Social Dimension	
1. Improve child's self-concept by increasing social skills.	The capacity to relate to others will increase self-esteem and reduce isolation.
2. Provide opportunities for child to have successful interactions with peers by supervising play.	To learn to be successful in social exchanges.
3. Include family in the treatment.	The family is the primary source of care and discipline. Involvement increases cooperation in treatment.
4. Provide family therapy.	Dysfunction in a family member indicates dysfunction in the family system. The family needs to examine their response to the child, ways in which they contribute to the child's behavior, and ways in which they can assist the child in adapting.
5. Provide opportunities for child to play with other children.	To increase socialization.
6. Supervise play with other children.	Child is impulsive and may need assistance to control his behavior.
7. Provide safe environment for child to play with others.	Impulsive actions create danger to self and others.
8. Determine factors in parents' behavior (alcohol, drugs, mental illness) that may be disruptive to child.	Dysfunction in a family member indicates dysfunction in the whole family.
9. Determine methods of discipline and limit-setting in the family.	Family discipline and limit-setting may be inconsistent, too harsh, or too lenient.
10. Explore with parents appropriate discipline and limit-setting.	To learn new ways of disciplining child.
11. Determine family's ability to allow verbal expression of conflicts, fears, and disappointments.	Intolerance for verbal expression may provoke acting-out behavior.
12. Discuss with parents effects of overstimulation and sensory deprivation that precede rage, fright, and temper tantrums.	Helps family gain insight and provides a means for intervention.
13. Refer to social agency in community for additional therapy and counseling.	To assist family in using community resources.

SAMPLE PARENT OBSERVATION SHEET

" + " Behaviors		" − " Behaviors
1. Saying thank you		1. Pushing or shoving
2. Helping others		2.
3.		3.

Observation:

Date	Time Start	No. " + " Behaviors	No. " − " Behaviors	Time Stop	Total Time	No. + /Time	No. − /Time

IMPLEMENTATION—cont'd

NURSING ACTIONS	RATIONALE
14. Have parents monitor and chart behavior at home (see box, above).	To increase family's awareness of child's behavior and circumstances associated with positive or negative behavior. Provides a means for intervention.
15. Encourage parents to plan activities without the child.	To provide relief from responsibilities of caring for hyperactive child.
Spiritual Dimension	
1. Provide a nurturing, supportive relationship.	Child can experience a sense of security and trust in others.
2. Provide an attitude that child is unique and special and is valued as a person with rights and is capable of respecting others' rights.	To convey message that child is OK and expectation that child can control behavior. Increases child's self-esteem.
3. Promote child's sense of love and belonging within the family. a. Teach child to demonstrate affection. b. Respond to child in a warm and caring way. c. Show child that satisfaction can be gained from helping parents and siblings.	To reduce isolation.
4. Promote parents' sense of acceptance of the child as different and a valued member of the family. a. Encourage parents to demonstrate affection. b. Discuss benefits of playing, shopping together, spending more time with child. c. Teach parents to communicate praise effectively. d. Discuss positive aspects of being different.	To reduce parental rejection and to increase their response to child's needs.
5. Promote cooperation with treatment.	To prevent further deterioration of behavior and to enhance satisfaction and pleasure in relationships and life in general.

EVALUATION

Evaluation of the effectiveness of treatment is based on measurable goals and outcome criteria. Measuring progress using a multidiscipline approach enhances the evaluation process because team members can contribute information specific to their areas of expertise. Including the family and school personnel adds an additional dimension to the evaluation process. It is essential that parents have supportive relationships and frequent time-outs from the heavy responsibilities of caring for the child who is hyperactive.

The following behaviors indicate a positive evaluation:

1. Develops some recognition of the consequences of impulsive acts
2. Is able to start and complete simple tasks
3. Begins to talk about a situation rather than act out
4. Learns to leave a situation when it becomes too stimulating
5. Begins to use language to express frustration, disappointment, rage, despair
6. Listens attentively to others
7. Makes positive statements about self
8. Plays with other children, demonstrating less volatile behavior.
9. Demonstrates warmth and affection for parents
10. Is polite (e.g., says please, thank you)

BIBLIOGRAPHY

Barkley R: What is the role of group parent training in the treatment of ADD children? *J Child Contemp Soc* 19(1/2):143, 1986.

Cantwell D, Baker L: Attention-deficit disorder in children: the role of the nurse practitioner, *Nurse Pract* 12(7):38, 1987.

Cherry B, Hayes J, Feeg V: Temperament and cognitive style in early childhood, *Pediatr Nurs* 13(5):347, 1987.

Clunn P: *Child psychiatric nursing,* St. Louis, 1991, Mosby—Year Book.

Kramer J: What are hyperactive children like as young adults? *J Child Contemp Soc* 19(1/2):89, 1986.

Moss N: Child therapy groups in the real world, *J Psychosoc Nurs Ment Health Serv* 22(3):43, 1984.

Pond E, Gilbert C: A support group offers help for parents of hyperactive children, *Child Today* 16(6):23, 1987.

Pothier P: Child psychiatric nursing, *J Psychosoc Nurs Ment Health Serv* 22(3):10, 1984.

Rie H, Rie E: *Handbook of minimal brain dysfunctions: a critical view,* New York, 1980, John Wiley & Sons.

Walker M et al: Effects of methylphenidate hydrochloride on the subjective reporting of mood in children with attention deficit disorder, *Issues Ment Health Nurs* 9(4):373, 1988.

Whalen C, Henker B: Cognitive behavior therapy for hyperactive children: what do we know? *J Child Contemp Soc* 19(1/2):123, 1986.

Hypochondriacal Behavior

Hypochondriasis is a disorder characterized by an exaggerated concern for physical health, which is accompanied by a multitude of physical complaints. Unrealistic interpretations of physical sensations as abnormal result in preoccupation with those sensations and the fear of having a serious disease. Somatic complaints have no logical symptom pattern, and a thorough physical examination reveals no organic or physiological disorders. The individual is not malingering and is sincere in the belief that symptoms represent real illness.

Hypochondriasis is a type of somatoform disorder under the DSM-III-R classification system. Somatoform disorders involve physical symptoms that suggest underlying physical disorders. Somatization disorder is a chronic disorder that begins early in life and involves multiple symptoms. Secondary hypochrondriacal symptoms occur in a variety of psychiatric conditions. Another of these disorders, somatoform pain disorder, is characterized by complaints of pain that have no organic basis and is attributed to psychological factors. Another type, conversion disorder, involves a loss or alteration of physical function, which is attributed to psychological conflict. Health anxiety, excessive fear of having a disease, also occurs in a number of nonpsychiatric patients including the physically ill.

The person with hypochondriasis is often referred to in derogatory terms and is the source of much derision, which may be engendered by the capacity of the client to tap into the caregiver's own conflicts about dependency and anger. Since the client is well known to medical personnel, real physical illness may be overlooked.

The original content for this section was contributed in part by Rosalynn Wise, R.N., M.N.Sc.

Related DSM-III-R disorders

Schizophrenia
Major depression
Dysthymic disorder
Panic disorder
Generalized anxiety disorder
Obsessive-compulsive disorder
Somatization disorder
Narcissistic personality disorder

Other related conditions

Chronic physical illness
Grief and bereavement
Developmental crises of adolescence and aging
Guilt
Anger
Stress

PRINCIPLES

▶ Physical Dimension

1. Early childhood experiences may predispose an individual to the later development of hypochondriacal behavior.
2. The parent who is inclined to be hypochondriacal may be a model for the child to learn to be overly sensitive to and concerned with bodily functions.
3. Overconcern by the parent for the child's every sneeze, cough, rash, or other illness manifestation may teach the child to place undue significance on such manifestations.
4. An actual early illness or injury that focused attention on the child may predispose that person to the later development of hypochondriasis.

▶ Emotional Dimension

1. The hypochondriacal phenomenon involves the desire to be nurtured and is manifested in the form of self-gratifying secondary gain, which is derived from the attention of others.
2. The symptoms of hypochondriasis are compromise solutions of unconscious conflicts.
3. Somatization is a defensive function and may be the expiation of guilt about anger and dependency.
4. In some cultures and subcultures emotional experiences may be devalued, and persons learn to attend to somatic components of affective experiences.
5. Persons with alexithymia (without words for mood) do not use words to communicate their emotional feelings and may be prone to hypochondriasis.
6. Hypochondriacal symptoms are a defense against depression through displacement of depressive affect onto somatic symptoms.
7. Hypochondriasis is an expression of emotional distress in somatic terms.

▶ Intellectual Dimension

1. An individual's beliefs and thoughts can create distress such as physical symptoms.
2. Hypochondriasis can be conceptualized as a disorder of perception and cognition in which somatic sensation is experienced as abnormally intense.
3. Bodily signs and symptoms are perceived as more dangerous than they really are.

▶ Social Dimension

1. Hypochondriasis is seen in individuals with a negative, pessimistic view of themselves, low self-esteem, and feelings of social inferiority and worthlessness.

a. Such individuals restructure all interpersonal relationships on the level of continual discussions of bodily sensation, symptoms, and possible disease.
b. Hypochondriasis is a shift of emotional interest from disturbing interpersonal relationships to an intense preoccupation with body function.
2. As an occupant of the sick role, the person with hypochrondriasis may be exempted from normal role responsibilities and role expectations.
3. The sick role may represent an attempt to provide for oneself the care not adequately obtained from others and justifies the gratification of dependency needs.
4. The sick role may provide justification of the failure to live up to one's potential.
5. Hypochondriasis may excuse the individual from tasks or roles that are unpleasant or that the individual feels incompetent to perform.
6. Hypochondriacal individuals use their symptoms to control the behavior of others.
7. Sympathy and support reinforces hypochondriacal behavior.
8. Attitudes toward being sick are culturally determined.
9. Certain ethnic, religious, or cultural groups may more readily engage in illness behavior.

▶ Spiritual Dimension

1. The person with hypochondriasis is unable to relate to others in a genuine, warm, and caring way.
2. Hypochondriasis interferes with the ability to make decisions regarding the discovery of one's own nature.
3. The hypochondriacal individual is restricted in the choice for openness to human development and is exercising less freedom.

ASSESSMENT

▶ Physical Dimension

I. History
  A. Identifying information
    1. Age
      a. Usually begins between 20 and 30 years
  B. Activities of daily living
    1. Nutrition
      a. Appetite—loss
      b. Weight—minor changes in weight
    2. Sleep—insomnia
    3. Recreation, hobbies, interests
      a. Narrow interests
    4. Physical activities and limitations
      a. Perceived physical problems interfere with physical activities

  C. Habits
    1. Medications and drugs
      a. Frequent use of over-the-counter medications
      b. May have variety of prescribed drugs as a result of doctor-shopping and may show a reluctance to give up formerly prescribed medications
  D. Health history
    1. History of chronic recurring problems
    2. Many hospitalizations for observation and diagnostic procedures with temporary symptom relief

3. May have had one or more exploratory surgical procedures, which temporarily relieved symptoms

E. Review of systems—relates history in an obsessive manner, sometimes maintains log book detailing daily events
   1. General
      a. Complaints of generalized body fatigue
      b. Generalized malaise
   2. Skin—acutely aware of rashes, bites, lesions, bruises, or perspiration
   3. Complaints of frequent sore throats, irritations, and scratchiness
   4. Cardiovascular
      a. Complaints of chest pain
      b. Palpitations
   5. Respiratory
      a. Shortness of breath
      b. Wheezing
   6. Gastrointestinal—frequent complaints
      a. Nausea
      b. Vomiting
      c. Diarrhea—notes minor abnormality
      d. Constipation
      e. Heartburn
      f. Gas
      g. Indigestion
      h. Loss of appetite and taste
      i. Frequent use of laxatives
      j. Cramping pain
   7. Genitourinary—frequent complaints
      a. Pain
      b. Burning or stinging
      c. Urgency
      d. Frequency
      e. Hesitancy
      f. Infections
   8. Musculoskeletal—frequent vague complaints
      a. Joint pain
      b. Muscle pain or cramps
      c. Muscle tenseness
      d. Muscle rigidity
      e. Stiffness
      f. Deformity
      g. Back problems
   9. Neurological—frequent complaints of sensory and motor dysfunctioning

II. **Physical examination**—because of chronic complaints, true organic disease may be missed. Thorough physical is required with presentation of new symptoms. New symptoms may be indicative of early stages of neurological disorders, thyroid or parathyroid disease, or systemic disease. Organic disease may coexist with hypochondriasis.

III. **Diagnostic tests**
   A. Minnesota Multiphasic Personality Inventory (MMPI)—elevated hypochondriasis scale
   B. Projective tests—Rorschach test or Thematic Apperception Test (TAT)
   C. Myelography
   D. Nerve biopsy
   E. CAT scan
   F. Upper and lower GI
   G. Blood chemistry tests

▶ **Emotional Dimension**

CLIENT DATA	ANALYSIS	NURSING DIAGNOSIS
Anxious	Fears of illness manifestations are disproportionate to actual organic disease. Constantly vigilant for new illness manifestations.	Anxiety: related to somatic complaints and beliefs of having a disease
Looks worried	Symptoms described with urgency and intensity. Overconcern for self is transformed into somatic changes, which are felt as anxiety.	Anxiety: related to inability to express emotional needs directly
Depressed (masked)	May have typical physical symptoms of depression but denies psychological awareness of depressed state. Hypochondriasis and depression are related. Some persons learn to attend to somatic components of affective experience rather than to their emotional state.	

▶ **Emotional Dimension—cont'd**

CLIENT DATA	ANALYSIS	NURSING DIAGNOSIS
Angry	Hypochondriacal symptoms are defense against depression through displacement of depressive affect on to somatic symptoms. Expression toward physicians or health care system for inability to relieve symptoms or for uncaring attitude. Client may be shuffled from clinic to clinic. Caregivers may attempt to stifle complaints by ignoring them. Anger may result when dependency needs are not met.	Ineffective individual coping: excessive physical complaints related to depression *Anger: related to inability to meet dependency needs through excessive complaints and demands on health care providers

▶ **Intellectual Dimension**

CLIENT DATA	ANALYSIS	NURSING DIAGNOSIS
Belief that disease is present despite medical reassurance that it is not.	Beliefs are fixed, difficult to change.	Altered thought processes: related to inability to evaluate reality because of fixed and rigid beliefs about physical basis of somatic complaints
Morbidly preoccupied with digestive and excretory functions; obsessively detailed	Symptoms of hypochondriasis are compromise solutions of unconscious conflicts.	Altered thought processes: related to morbid preoccupation with digestive and excretory functions
Is usually avid reader of popular magazines or avid watcher of TV programs on medical topics	Self-diagnosis based on that information. Believes he has every new disease read or heard about.	Ineffective individual coping: related to self-diagnosis based on magazine articles and programs
Continues or increases complaints when reassured	Client communicates need to maintain symptoms. Knowledge that he is healthy or that new treatment will be used provokes anxiety rather than reassurance.	Anxiety: related to irrational need for symptom maintenance
Complains more intensely with sudden change in treatment	Giving up beliefs about illness may result in overwhelming anxiety. Irrational beliefs result in irrational or inappropriate consequences.	Anxiety: related to sudden change in treatment plan
Denies emotional basis of problems	Reluctant or refuses to participate in psychiatric treatment program or activities. Defense mechanism, which reduces anxiety.	Ineffective denial: related to psychological conflicts
Displaces depressive affect to somatic symptoms	Defense mechanism, which reduces anxiety. Symptoms of hypochondriasis are compromise solutions of unconscious conflicts.	Ineffective individual coping: related to excessive use of displacement
Regresses to more dependent level	As fears of illness intensify and anxiety increases, individual retreats and becomes more dependent and less anxious.	Ineffective individual coping: regressed behavior related to anxiety about illness
Obsessed with fears of illness	Although gives a detailed history of physical complaints, gives very little personal information.	*Obsessions: related to physical complaints and fears of illness
Rigid and inflexible in thinking	Unable to consider alternatives.	Altered thought processes: related to rigid and inflexible thinking

▶ **Social Dimension**

CLIENT DATA	ANALYSIS	NURSING DIAGNOSIS
Preoccupied with illness	Hypochondriasis is shift of emotional interest from disturbing interpersonal relationships to an intense preoccupation with body. Does not recognize effect on others; insensitive to others because of preoccupation with concerns about illness.	Impaired social interaction: related to preoccupation with illness
Bores others with litany of complaints	Individual restructures all interpersonal relationships to the level of continual discussions of bodily sensations, symptoms, and possible disease.	Impaired social interaction: related to preoccupation with illness, bores others with continuous complaints
Overconcern about health interferes with expressions of intimacy	Inability to relate to others on a warm and personal basis.	Impaired social interaction: related to inability to share emotional or intimate feelings or thoughts related to overconcern with health
Unexpected intensification of symptoms when asked to participate in undesirable activities	Symptoms used to control the behavior of others. Hypochondriacal pattern enables individual to avoid stressful life situations while gaining sympathy from others.	Altered role performance: related to increase in symptoms to avoid responsibilities
Feels worthless, inferior, and like a failure	Hypochondriasis is seen in individuals with negative-pessimistic view of themselves. Sick role may provide justification of the failure to live up to one's potential; it may excuse individual from roles he feels incompetent to perform.	Self-esteem disturbance: chronic, related to feelings of worthlessness and failure
Is dependent and clinging	Dependency is manifested with attitude of, "I can't care for myself, someone else will have to care for me." Somatization is defensive function and can be expiation of guilt about anger and dependency.	Ineffective individual coping: related to dependency
Is demanding of spouse and others	Symptoms enable client to gain added support. Individual finds self-gratifying secondary gain from attention of others. Sick role may represent attempt to provide for oneself nurturing care not adequately obtained from others, and it justifies gratification of dependency needs.	Ineffective individual coping: related to demands made of spouse. Impaired social interaction: related to demanding behavior and effects of multiple somatic complaints on relationships
Misses work or unable to maintain employment	Symptoms interfere with work. "Sick" persons not responsible for same level of achievement as well persons.	Altered role performance: related to multiple somatic complaints and belief that he has illness
Unable to fulfill family role responsibilities	Symptoms provide legitimate excuse and hinder fulfillment of family role responsibilities.	*Altered family role: related to multiple somatic complaints and beliefs that he has illness
Has exacerbation of symptoms with stressful situations	Illness and hospitalizations are related to stress. In sick role the hypochondriac is exempted from normal role responsibilities and expectations.	Ineffective individual coping: related to increase in symptoms when in stressful situation

▶ **Social Dimension—cont'd**

CLIENT DATA	ANALYSIS	NURSING DIAGNOSIS
Alienates others	Clinging, demanding behavior. Easily angered when dependency needs not met. Provokes dislike from others.	Impaired social interaction: related to clinging, demanding behavior and anger

▶ **Spiritual Dimension**

CLIENT DATA	ANALYSIS	NURSING DIAGNOSIS
Illness is of paramount value in life	Obsessed with fears of illness. Unwilling and unable to give up claim to illness.	Spiritual distress: related to inability to find meaning in life beyond illness and somatic complaints
Dwells on and is proud of sacrifice, suffering, and bodily illnesses	Illness serves unknown or unconscious value in client's life.	Spiritual distress: pride in sacrifice, suffering, and bodily illness related to inability to find meaning in life beyond illness and somatic complaints
Unable to find comfort in religious beliefs	Focus almost exclusively on illness perceptions.	Spiritual distress: related to inability to find comfort in religion
Unable to accept and transcend discomforts of everyday life	Contact lost with self, others, and the environment; focus on symptoms.	Spiritual distress: related to inability to transcend daily discomforts
Life experience severely limited	Experience of aliveness and involvement in life severely limited. Focus is on self. Inability to think or act in creative manner. Egocentricity prevents the individual from relating to others in a genuine manner.	Spiritual distress: severely limited life experiences related to egocentricity
Has phobia-like fears of death and disease	Hypochondriasis interferes in a person's ability to discover his own nature, to accept mortality. Anxiety associated with denial of mortality results in phobia-like fears of death and disease. Hypochondriacal person is restricted in choice to "be" and is exercising less freedom.	Spiritual distress: related to phobia-like fears of death and disease

PLANNING

Long-Term Goals

To decrease preoccupation with and frequency of somatic complaints

To increase the capacity to form more satisfying relationships so that emotional energy is vested in others rather than in physical symptoms

To begin to develop pleasure in being healthy rather than unhealthy

SHORT-TERM GOALS	OUTCOME CRITERIA
Physical Dimension To decrease the number of somatic complaints	1. Identifies relationship between anxiety and somatic complaints 2. Reduces reference to somatic and sensory complaints 3. Discusses topics other than aches, pains, and illnesses 4. Participates in more physical activities 5. Uses fewer medications 6. Uses less detail when discussing bodily functioning

PLANNING—cont'd

SHORT-TERM GOALS	OUTCOME CRITERIA
Emotional Dimension	
To relieve anxiety associated with somatic complaints and belief that he has an illness	1. Verbalizes fewer fears of illness 2. Discusses fewer symptoms and with less urgency and intensity
To identify and distinguish the emotional (affective) experience from somatic (physical) components of experience	1. Uses more words conveying emotional feelings (sad, happy, blue, upset, angry, and caring) 2. Discusses pain and differences in physical and emotional origins
To acknowledge and reduce anger related to inability to meet dependency needs	1. Assumes more responsibility for own behavior and for making own independent choices 2. Lists possible options in problematic situations to guide more independent actions in problem resolution 3. Expresses self in more assertive manner
Intellectual Dimension	
To increase capacity to make reality-based judgments regarding physical bases of somatic complaints	1. Is able to make more accurate discrimination of differences between affect and physical symptoms 2. States that some physical complaints are associated with stress and that they may have psychological basis
Social Dimension	
To become more attentive to spouse, relatives, and friends and less dependent on them	1. Shares thoughts and feelings with others 2. Increases association with others 3. Focuses more on others and less on somatic complaints 4. States that others tire of hearing complaints 5. Expresses willingness to become more responsible for actions and not so demanding of others
To increase self-esteem	1. See Negative Self-concept, p. 231
Spiritual Dimension	
To increase the experience of aliveness and reduce alienation of self from others	1. Expresses willingness to experiment and try out new ideas and things 2. Becomes more spontaneous 3. Indicates verbally more awareness of world 4. Becomes involved in more self-nurturing activities such as a hot sudsy bath, a quiet walk in the woods, going to a movie, enjoying the solitude of a beautiful sunset
To discover purpose in life to replace need for illness	1. Verbalizes those things that are personally meaningful 2. Questions and seeks answers to meaning of life 3. Examines ways others have coped with adversity in their lives 4. Begins to discuss values and philosophy of life 5. Searches for an explanation of own experience in the world 6. Uses suffering as a means to get in touch with deeper meaning of life and nature
To resolve fears of death and disease	1. Views life and death as destiny of human beings 2. Establishes goals to be achieved in life 3. Develops an awareness of living in the present

Discharge Planning

The following client behaviors demonstrate a readiness for discharge:
1. Displays less anxiety regarding physical well-being
2. Has decreased frequency of somatic complaints
3. Has assumed more responsibility for self
4. Exhibits ability to establish beginning relationships

IMPLEMENTATION

NURSING ACTIONS	RATIONALE
Physical Dimension	
1. Promote general health habits to reduce use of medications.	Medications are symbols of illness and reinforce sick role behavior. Changes focus from illness to health.
a. Explain importance of diet, bulk-producing foods, and adequate fluid intake to reduce dependence on laxatives and enemas.	
b. Encourage relaxation techniques for pain and anxiety reduction.	Involves client in self-care activities and potentially reduces dependency.
c. Encourage using energy in physical activity rather than in somatization.	Energy is used for more constructive behavior.
2. Offer client a backrub or encourage client to use a technique that promotes relaxation, such as a warm bath, a warm glass of milk, a cup of nonstimulant herbal tea, or becoming involved in an activity to distract from preoccupation with physical complaints, as a substitute for medication.	To provide alternatives to present behavior.
3. Observe and note situations that precede requests for medications.	Emotional distress or certain irrational beliefs are expressed in somatic terms. The distress or beliefs seem to be "automatic" and are not consciously attended to; however they can be brought to conscious attention by discussing events, feelings, and thoughts that precede medication requests. It is important for client to discover the connection between emotional distress or irrational beliefs and somatic symptoms. The nurse can assist the patient in this process by noting similarities in situations that precipitate medication requests.
4. Help client identify antecedent conditions to requests for medications or other treatments.	Same as #3.
5. Discuss with client potentially harmful effects of polypharmacy.	To increase client's knowledge and awareness of drug interactions. This client is notorious for consulting with many doctors and taking a variety of prescribed and over-the-counter drugs.
Emotional Dimension	
1. Assist the client in identifying affective components rather than somatic components of experience by:	To assist in separating the emotional, mood state, from the somatic aspects of experience. Often client has not learned appropriate words to express emotional feelings.
a. Learning to distinguish between a thought and a feeling.	
b. Learning to describe the bodily sensations that occur with particular thoughts.	
c. Giving a name to the feeling, using a word that has a nonphysical connotation. Affective words may be suggested initially to help client start.	
2. Give positive reinforcement for direct expression of feelings.	To increase the likelihood the behavior will be repeated. The individual whose behavior is rewarded tends to repeat that behavior.
3. Allow expression of anger.	The client can express physical complaints more easily than anger and may use physical symptoms as the medium for expression of anger.
4. Discuss physical sensations associated with anger.	To begin to discover the relationship between physical symptoms and anger.

PLANNING—cont'd

NURSING ACTIONS	RATIONALE
5. Explore with client situations that produce anger.	To recognize situations that produce anger so that the association between anger and somatic symptoms can be made.
6. Help client recognize how own behavior contributed to situation and in assuming responsibility for that behavior.	To learn to behave in a more satisfying and responsible manner and reduce reliance on secondary gain that accompanies physical illness.
7. Assist client in noticing and naming the feeling of anxiety.	Anxiety is emotional distress expressed in somatic terms. The distress seems to be "automatic" and is not consciously attended to; however it can be brought to conscious attention by discussing events, feelings, and thoughts that produce anxiety. It is important for client to discover the connection between emotional distress and somatic symptoms.
Intellectual Dimension	
1. Involve client in establishing goals for own care.	To learn to care for self and to reduce dependency on others. Goal setting is an affirmation of self, of the ability to act independently.
2. Avoid any implication that symptoms are imaginary or "in the head."	Client is sincere in the belief that symptoms are real. To discount symptoms increases anxiety and can possibly exacerbate symptoms.
3. Allow limited expression of somatic complaints.	To set limits to reduce continual expression of complaints so that undesirable behavior is not reinforced by someone listening to complaints.
4. Respond with interest and verbally or nonverbally reward client's willingness to talk about personal issues.	To provide positive reinforcement, and client is less likely to focus on somatic complaints.
5. Convey a personal interest in client rather than in physical symptoms.	To recognize client as a person of worth and to restructure the interpersonal relationship by focusing on the person rather than the complaint.
6. Encourage discussion of topics other than symptoms.	Client is self-centered and has a narrow and limited interest in the world.
7. Verbally and nonverbally reward discussion of other topics.	Same as #4.
8. Assist client in identifying relationship between exacerbation of symptoms and anxiety or stress.	Often anxiety is not felt and relief behavior, symptoms, occur automatically and become the characteristic response to anxiety or stress.
9. Be cautious in confrontations and in interpretations of symptom behavior.	Symptoms serve a purpose for client. Confrontations and interpretation may be extremely anxiety provoking. As new behaviors are learned, the necessity for maintaining symptoms will be reduced.
10. Teach assertiveness training.	To reduce dependency.
11. Reinforce assumption of responsibility in all situations.	To reduce dependency.
12. Make comments such as, "You have a remarkable capacity to persevere with such pain," rather than dismiss client's complaints.	To recognize client's experience and to reduce the need to be defensive.
13. Use minimal reassurance when discussing the bases of physical complaints; focus on affective states related to fears and complaints.	To recognize and to verbalize mood states. Beliefs about illness are fixed and difficult to change. Client will give up the beliefs as the need to maintain them is reduced.
14. Encourage client to make own decisions rather than rely on others to make decisions.	To encourage self-care and to reduce dependency.
15. Provide attention when client is not complaining.	To reinforce noncomplaining behavior.
16. Teach client to be self-nurturing (regularly getting a massage, giving self a special treat, taking a bubble bath).	To fill the need to be nurtured and to provide a more satisfying means than the secondary gain derived from the attention of others.
17. Discuss life goals with client to ascertain client's perception of achievement or failure to achieve those goals.	Client may not be or may perceive that he is not living up to his potential.
18. Teach client techniques of thought stopping.	To reduce obsessive thoughts regarding symptoms.
19. Teach client to covertly reward self for thought stopping by saying to himself, "Good, you did that well."	To provide reinforcement for desirable behavior and remind client that self-reinforcement is beneficial.

NURSING ACTIONS	RATIONALE
Social Dimension	
1. Enhance client's self-esteem (a) by helping client recognize strengths and (b) by establishing small goals that allow success.	Hypochondriasis is seen in individuals with low self-esteem.
2. Involve family in treatment plan.	Dysfunction of a family member indicates a dysfunction in the family system.
3. Develop a plan with family and client to allow client to assume more family responsibility.	A change in functioning of a family member results in a change in other family members. If the family expects responsibility, client is more likely to respond in a responsible manner.
4. Teach family to reward nonillness behavior.	To reduce illness behavior. Nonillness behavior that is reinforced is more likely to be repeated. Ignoring illness behavior will reduce repetition of that behavior.
5. Discuss with family or significant other needs that client may be meeting with behavior and plan ways for client to meet those needs more directly.	Dependency or other needs may be satisfied by client's behavior. The family can assist client in restructuring interpersonal relationships when there is an awareness of client's needs.
6. Help client focus more on others and less on self.	To learn to focus on others rather than self and physical problems.
7. Encourage expression of care and concern for others.	To decrease self-centeredness.
8. Explore ways of making friends.	To encourage involvement with others.
9. Reverse roles with client.	To discover the effect of behavior on others.
10. Teach client social skills.	To increase self-esteem, reduce feelings of social inferiority, and increase awareness of others.
11. Refrain from excusing client from participation in activities because of symptoms.	To communicate expectation of involvement in normal role responsibilities.
12. Encourage client to initiate conversations that focus on a topic other than symptoms or illness.	To shift focus from self to others. To decrease self-centeredness.
13. Act as a model for client, and by your example let client see pleasure missed in relationships with others.	To assist learning.
14. Determine if family or culture devalues emotional experience but accepts physical illness.	To determine if client's behavior may be influenced by family or cultural values.
15. Develop ways for family to allow and encourage client's expression of feelings.	To involve the family in the treatment plan. Client has difficulty in separating emotional mood state from somatic aspects of experience. Client has not learned appropriate words to express emotional feelings.
16. Encourage client's participation in community activities.	To enlarge client's social system to help change focus from self to others.
17. Involve client in group therapy.	To encourage formation of relationships.
Spiritual Dimension	
1. Accept client as is and become familiar with client's perceptions of the world before expecting change.	The therapeutic relationship is one of mutual learning and conveys caring and respect.
2. Discuss with client the meaning of making choices.	Client is primary agent in determining own behavior and makes choices even though client may not be consciously aware of those choices.
3. Discuss choices that are presently being made.	Same as #2.
4. When client makes an "I will try" statement, explain that trying is a subtle provision for an excuse. Ask him to change the statement to "I will" or "I won't."	To increase awareness and a commitment to a choice.
5. Avoid discussing past failures; stay in the present.	The past cannot be changed, but the present can be.
6. Excuses that present behavior is result of past experiences are unacceptable.	Blaming the past (experiences, people, environment, genetic makeup) is absolving oneself from responsibility and excusing present behavior.
7. Explore client's value system. Challenge irrational thoughts associated with values.	To assist in more rational thinking.
8. Convey a sense of hope that it is possible for change to occur.	If hope is present, client will continue to work on changing behavior.
9. Share personal growth experiences with client.	To help client grow to know self.

PLANNING—cont'd

NURSING ACTIONS	RATIONALE
10. Encourage creative expression (writing, painting, ceramics, music, and dance).	To lessen preoccupation with physical complaints.
11. Discuss client's values, his chosen direction, and his total orientation toward life.	Value systems provide a framework for how and why we live.
12. Encourage client to frequently restate positive values and beliefs of own life.	To divert attention to positive aspects and away from negative self-defeating behavior.
13. Encourage client to deepen and enlarge religious ideas.	To encourage client to transcend self.
14. Discuss client's perception of purpose in life.	To encourage client to discover the meaning of own life.
15. Help client formulate philosophy of life.	To encourage client to become more self-actualized.

EVALUATION

Hypochondriasis is refractory to treatment, which may be a source of frustration to caregivers. Movement toward goals may be a slow and tedious process. If outcome criteria are not met, goals may be too ambitious and beyond the capacity of individual achievement. A reevaluation of goals may require a slower change in behavior and changes in smaller increments. The following behaviors indicate that the client is making changes:

1. Reduces the frequency of somatic complaints
2. Is able to distinguish the emotional from the somatic aspect of experience and to give a name to the feeling
3. Assumes responsibility and demonstrates initiative
4. Focuses on others instead of self
5. Makes friends
6. Expresses care and concern for significant others
7. Discusses personal values and beliefs

BIBLIOGRAPHY

Barsky AJ, Geringer E, Wool CA: A cognitive-educational treatment for hypochondriasis, *Gen Hosp Psychiatry* 10(5):322, 1988.

Barsky AJ, Wyshak G: Hypochondriasis and related health attitudes, *Psychosomatics* 30(4):412, 1989.

Brodsky CM: Sociocultural and interactional influences on somatization, *Psychosomatics* 25(9):673, 1984.

Ford CV: *The somatizing disorders: illness as a way of life,* New York, 1983, Elsevier Science Publishing Co.

Holt RE, LeCann AF: Use of an integrative interview to manage somatization, *Psychosomatics* 25(9):663, 1984.

House A: Hypochondriasis and related disorders. Assessment and management of patients referred for a psychiatric opinion, *Gen Hosp Psychiatry* 11(3):156, 1989.

Katon W, Kleinman A, Rosen G: Depression of somatization: a review, Part I, *Am J Med* 72(1):127, 1982.

Katon W, Kleinman A, Rosen G: Depression and somatization: a review, Part II, *Am J Med* 72(2):241, 1982.

McCranie J: Hypochondriacal neurosis, *Psychosomatics* 20(3):11, 1979.

Pilowsky I: The concept of abnormal illness behavior, *Psychosomatics* 31(2):207, 1990.

Sifenos PE: *Short-term psychotherapy and emotional crisis,* Cambridge, Mass., 1972, Harvard University Press.

Slavney PR, Teitelbaum ML, Chase GA: Referral for medically unexplained somatic complaints: the role of histrionic traits, *Psychosomatics* 26(2):103, 1985.

Smith GR, Brown FW: Screening indexes in DSM-III-R somatization disorder, *Gen Hosp Psychiatry* 12:148, 1990.

Smith GR, Monson RA, Livingston RL: Somatization disorder in men, *Gen Hosp Psychiatry* 7(1):4, 1985.

Sullivan HS: *The interpersonal theory of psychiatry,* New York, 1953, W.W. Norton & Co.

Warwick HM: A cognitive-behavioral approach to hypochondriasis and health anxiety, *J Psychosom Res* 33(6):705, 1989.

Warwick HM, Salkovskis PM: Hypochondriasis, *Behav Res Ther* 28(2):105, 1990.

Whitney JD et al: A validation study of the nursing diagnosis "somatization", *Arch Psychiatr Nurs* 2(6):345, 1988.

Loneliness

Loneliness is a subjective phenomenon characterized by a lack of intimacy. Intimacy, a need throughout life, can be defined as a reciprocal closeness and sharing between individuals and is characterized by a sense of involvement. Lack of intimacy leads to emotional and social isolation.

Accompanying loneliness is a feeling of unexplained dread, desperation, or restlessness. Early life experiences in which remoteness, indifference, and emptiness characterize the child's relationships with others may contribute to loneliness. Peplau considers loneliness an unbearable experience that is always hidden, disguised, defended against, and expressed in other forms.

To understand loneliness, it is necessary to differentiate among the following terms; aloneness, lonesomeness, existential loneliness, and loneliness anxiety. *Aloneness,* sometimes referred to as solitude, implies being without company. To be alone is desirable when retreat, seclusion, or protected isolation is sought. The intense, encompassing feeling of being lonely is not a part of aloneness. *Lonesomeness* occurs when an individual is alone physically or psychologically and has a desire to feel closer to others. Lonesomeness may be expressed as a feeling. In *existential loneliness* the individual is fully aware of himself as an isolated and solitary individual, yet this phenomenon produces triumphant creation from long periods of desolation. In *loneliness anxiety* the individual is separated, or alienated, from himself as a feeling and knowing person.

Episodes of loneliness are likely to be preceded by precipitating events. Significant losses (of spouse, pet, or job) or the anniversary of a traumatic event in the client's life may serve as these precipitating events.

The nurse needs to recognize that loneliness is contagious. The nurse may experience personal unexplained feelings of anxiety when caring for the lonely person. The nurse's awareness can help her accept the phenomenon as a human emotion.

The original content for this section was contributed by Margaret Payne, R.N., M.N.Sc.

Related DSM-III-R disorders

Psychoactive substance-use disorders
Schizophrenia
Post-traumatic stress disorder
Somatoform pain disorder
Somatization disorder
Adjustment disorders
   With depressed mood
   With anxious mood
   With mixed disturbance of mood and conduct

Other related conditions

Social isolation
Long-term illness and confinement
Developmental crises of adolescence and aging
Grief reactions
Anniversary of a crisis situation

PRINCIPLES

▶ Physical Dimension

1. Physical mobility limitations and losses in the elderly may serve as precipitating factors for loneliness.
2. A long-term physical illness that results in confinement and isolation from significant others and groups may produce loneliness.
3. Hearing and speech deficits produce communication hindrances that foster loneliness.

▶ Emotional Dimension

1. The need for intimacy is located, in hierarchical order, just above the physiological and safety needs and just below the needs for self-esteem and self-actualization.
2. A significant loss may precipitate loneliness.
3. In adolescents, feelings of loneliness and isolation accompany the move out of childhood; an intense need for closeness, love, and understanding ensues.

193

4. Loneliness anxiety causes an individual to constantly seek the companionship of others, while avoiding the vital issues of life.
5. Loneliness anxiety consists of a complex system of defense mechanisms.
6. Loneliness is emotionally paralyzing and nonconstructive and can ultimately lead to psychosis.
7. Anniversaries of events (deaths or disasters) precipitate feelings of loneliness.
8. Loneliness is an overwhelming, persistent experience.
9. The lack of an intimate, close person, such as a spouse or lover, results in emotional loneliness.
10. The need for involvement is built into the human nervous system; thus loneliness produces pain, as well as constant, gnawing, uncomfortable feelings that commonly are manifested as anxiety, depression, and fatigue.

▶ Intellectual Dimension

1. An individual experiencing the phenomenon of loneliness does not recognize the cause. After recovery, the individual no longer wishes to recall and discuss the painful experience of loneliness.
2. The lonely individual has two streams of thought. The first stream is verbalized. The other stream is more difficult for the client to recognize and involves thoughts that are automatic and subliminal. Frequently, they do not relate to reality or follow logic. Such perceptions are referred to as cognitive distortions.

▶ Social Dimension

1. Loneliness is an absence or perceived absence of satisfying social relationships, with accompanying psychological distress related to the actual or perceived absence.
2. The roots of loneliness are in infancy. The infant enjoys being loved and admired but must wait for others to satisfy needs.
3. Loneliness anxiety is a defense to avoid dealing with issues of life and death and is manifested by the individual who constantly seeks the companionship of others.

4. Loneliness is a phenomenon of modern society that results from a decline in primary group relationships and from increases in both family and social mobility.
5. Loneliness is characterized by a lack of intimacy. Intimacy, a need throughout life, is a reciprocal closeness and sharing between individuals.
6. Social loneliness consists of a recognized lack of meaningful friendships or a sense of community with others.
7. Loneliness results when interpersonal communications lack honesty.
8. The older adult with ego integrity can tolerate losses and reduce the likelihood of loneliness.
9. The despairing older adult is susceptible to loss and responds with loneliness.
10. The lonely person can be surrounded by others and still experience loneliness.
11. For the lonely person, past relationships are for the most part forgotten and there is little hope of future relationships.
12. Poor self-concept contributes to loneliness.
13. Lack of self-esteem is also a factor in loneliness.

▶ Spiritual Dimension

1. Because they fear loneliness, most individuals feel it must be avoided at all costs.
2. If it is impossible to avoid loneliness, it is better to deny its existence than experience it.
3. Loss of meaning contributes to loneliness.
4. Lack of commitment to a personal destiny fosters a sense of purposelessness.
5. Sensory deprivation in the widowed elderly leads to hopelessness, with a perceived inability to find someone with whom to share the remainder of life.
6. Fear of dying alone and of having no one attend the funeral characterizes a situation among some institutionalized elderly who have few visitors and who retreat from interactions with staff.
7. A strong religious belief can prevent loneliness. Belief in a supreme being provides a feeling of ever-present help and fellowship and assures the individual of an ultimate destiny of eternal life after death.

ASSESSMENT

▶ Physical Dimension

I. History

A. Activities of daily living
  1. Nutrition
    a. Loss of appetite
  2. Sleep
    a. Changes in sleep patterns
  3. Previously enjoyed activities discontinued
  4. Immobility or physical limitations
  5. Sexual activity decreased

B. Habits
  1. Increased use of alcohol

  2. Medications
    a. Excessive use of over-the-counter drugs
    b. Abuse of prescribed drugs
    c. Abuse of illegal drugs
  3. Increased smoking

C. Destructive behavior
  1. Possible depression with thoughts of suicide
  2. Aggressive behavior

D. Health history
  1. Physical problems such as illnesses, injury, and long-term hospitalization

▶ Physical Examination

CLIENT DATA	ANALYSIS	NURSING DIAGNOSIS
Long-term illness and confinement	Institutionalization may result in isolation from significant others and social situations.	*Loneliness: related to confinement for long-term illness
Physically limited	May cause immobility; results in an inability to pursue previously productive activity.	Social isolation: related to physical limitations
Weight loss or gain	Depression, often associated with loneliness, may be manifested by appetite changes.	Altered nutrition: more or less than body requirements related to depression associated with loneliness
Physical complaints	Loneliness may be evidenced by physical symptoms—backache, headache.	Anxiety: somatic complaints and fears of having a disease related to loneliness
Changes in sleep patterns	Early morning awakening and insomnia are characteristic of depression, which may be complication of loneliness.	Sleep pattern disturbance: related to difficulty in falling asleep or early morning awakening

▶ Emotional Dimension

CLIENT DATA	ANALYSIS	NURSING DIAGNOSIS
Sadness, brooding	Client's predominant feelings provide clues to internal mechanisms of loneliness phenomenon.	*Sadness: brooding related to loneliness
	Loneliness may be result of past losses, present situations, or anticipated future losses.	Dysfunctional or anticipatory grieving: related to past or anticipated losses
Anger	May precede acts of violence involving client or significant others. Client may hurt or humiliate those around him.	High risk for violence: related to impaired ability to control aggression associated with loneliness.
		*Anger: related to complications of loneliness
Depression	Client may be suicidal.	High risk for violence: to self, related to feelings of hopelessness and loneliness
Anxiety	Anxiety associated with the experience of loneliness may be expressed as somatic symptoms.	Ineffective individual coping: related to altered ability to constructively manage stressors of loneliness
Feelings of helplessness	Client is emotionally paralyzed; feels unable to relieve feelings of loneliness or emptiness.	Ineffective individual coping: helplessness related to loneliness

▶ **Intellectual Dimension**

CLIENT DATA	ANALYSIS	NURSING DIAGNOSIS
Distorted perceptions	Believes life has no meaning without someone to share it. Unrealistic underlying assumptions result in distorted perceptions.	Altered thought processes: cognitive distortion, unrealistic assumption related to loneliness
Time-oriented complaints—"the days are endless"	Client claims to be waiting for an event to occur but makes no preparation for it.	Ineffective individual coping: related to inability to become involved in activity
Anticipation of future loss	Thoughts of loneliness may arise when significant other develops an illness or disability.	Anticipatory grieving: related to illness or disability of significant other
Blaming and dissatisfaction	Client blames others for dissatisfactions and problems related to loneliness.	Altered thought processes: related to cognitive distortions blaming others for dissatisfactions
Depression or symptomatic complaints on anniversary dates of traumatic event	Anniversaries may bring on symptoms even when client is unaware the anniversary is approaching.	Ineffective individual coping: depression or somatic complaints related to approaching anniversary of traumatic event and associated with loneliness
Denial	Defense mechanism to reduce anxiety; loneliness is disguised, defended against, and expressed in different forms.	Ineffective denial: related to inability to accept devastating feelings of loneliness
Talkativeness	Focus and content of conversation are superficial. Keeps others at a distance.	Social isolation: related to inability to form relationships

▶ **Social Dimension**

CLIENT DATA	ANALYSIS	NURSING DIAGNOSIS
Superficial relationships	Client may have many acquaintances on a first-name basis, about whom he knows little (barroom-type relationships).	Impaired social interaction: related to superficial relationships
Seeking contact with numerous people	Clinging, dependent behaviors are defense mechanisms used by lonely individual.	Ineffective individual coping: related to dependent behavior
Little hope of future relationships	Self-worth is affected by pain of loneliness.	Self-esteem disturbance: related to low self-worth
Usual support system unavailable	Spouse or pet may have died. Client may be geographically separated from family, church, or regular groups.	Social isolation: related to death or geographic separation from significant others
Inability to be intimate	Intimacy is a need throughout life. Knowing how to relate to others is lacking.	Impaired social interaction: related to developmental deficits
Busy, hectic home situation	Home situation precludes the privacy necessary for honest communication with significant others. Home may be physically small or there may always be others (children, friends, etc.) around.	Impaired home maintenance: management related to lack of privacy for communications with significant others
Inability to recall the quality of past relationships; thus inability to form new ones	Past relationships are for the most part forgotten, and individual is unable to derive comfort from those memories.	Impaired social interaction: related to the inability to recall past relationships

▶ **Social Dimension—cont'd**

CLIENT DATA	ANALYSIS	NURSING DIAGNOSIS
Clinging, touching behavior	Clinging, dependent behavior of client may be experienced by staff or observed with other clients. Touching and clinging to others are attention-seeking behaviors.	*Social intrusiveness: related to the need for attention
Lack of self-esteem	Individual's concept of self-worth impacts on his relatedness to others. Isolated individual does not receive affirmation of self from others.	Self-esteem disturbance: related to isolation from others

▶ **Spiritual Dimension**

CLIENT DATA	ANALYSIS	NURSING DIAGNOSIS
Powerlessness	Philosophy of life, beliefs, and values affect way client views loneliness.	*Spiritual despair: related to feelings of estrangement and remoteness between events in life and personal meaning and purpose for being
Loss of meaning in life	Lack of commitment to a destiny fosters a sense of purposelessness.	Spiritual distress: related to loss of meaning in life
Fears of dying alone and no one attending the funeral	In the later stages of life, the individual gives much thought to own death. If reminiscing is painful and life is perceived as less than desired, death is feared. Some institutionalized elderly who have few visitors and who retreat from interactions with staff have such fears.	Spiritual distress: related to fears of dying alone
Regrets about the kind of life lived	Has doubts about the life lived. Client is separated from usual source of religious comfort.	Spiritual distress: related to concerns about not living life to full extent
Hopelessness	In the widowed elderly, the perceived inability to find someone to share the remainder of life leads to hopelessness.	Spiritual distress: hopelessness related to loss and fear of spending the remainder of life alone

PLANNING

Long-Term Goal

To establish an intimate relationship with at least one other person

SHORT-TERM GOALS	OUTCOME CRITERIA
Physical Dimension	
To relate somatic complaints to precipitating event of loneliness	1. Identifies relationship between somatic complaints and loneliness
To maintain adequate nutrition	1. Relates nutritional deficiencies or excesses to the loneliness episode 2. Eats three balanced meals per day
To reestablish sleep patterns as they were before the episode of loneliness	1. Uses relaxation techniques to assist the return of satisfying sleep patterns (see Sleep disorders, p. 307)

PLANNING—cont'd

SHORT-TERM GOALS	OUTCOME CRITERIA
To reestablish recreational patterns and hobby interests	1. Relates stopping recreation and hobbies to the onset of loneliness 2. Chooses a hobby appropriate to physical limitations 3. Learns to paint, do crossword puzzles, write, or cook
To become sexually active or to find alternatives for sexual expression	1. Discusses reduction in sexual activity 2. Discusses various methods of alternative sexual activity 3. Discusses activities that produce pleasure and serve as substitutes for sexual activity
To reduce reliance on drugs or alcohol	1. Identifies the ineffective coping associated with substance abuse and the potential for addiction (see Dependence, p. 122)
To refrain from self-destructive behavior	1. Makes a contract with the nurse to refrain from self-destructive behavior for a given amount of time (see Suicidal behavior, p. 316)
To refrain from aggressive acts	1. Refrains from aggressive behavior regarding others 2. Associates aggressive urges with loneliness 3. Verbalizes constructive methods for dealing with aggression
To differentiate between warm, touching behaviors and attention-seeking behavior	1. Differentiates between touching behaviors that convey sincere warmth and those that promote dependency needs.
Emotional Dimension	
To recognize and constructively deal with feelings associated with loneliness	1. Verbalizes feelings of anger, helplessness, and sadness 2. Deals with feelings of anger appropriately 3. Identifies relationship between anger, helplessness, sadness, and loneliness
To decrease feelings of loneliness	1. Identifies feeling of loneliness 2. Discusses cause of loneliness 3. Tolerates increasing periods of aloneness 4. Uses time alone to become involved in a pleasurable activity, to sit in contemplative silence, or to experience the pain or pleasure of being alone 5. Distinguishes between aloneness and lonesomeness 6. Discusses the meaning of intimacy 7. Shares intimate feelings and thoughts with others 8. Identifies ways to relieve loneliness
To decrease feelings of helplessness	1. Recognizes the relationship between feelings of helplessness and loneliness 2. Assumes responsibility for reducing feeling of loneliness
Intellectual Dimension	
To discover adequate substitutes for times when human company is unavailable	1. Identifies times of day when human company is unlikely. 2. Becomes involved in substitute activities.
To deal realistically with potential future losses	1. Approaches the potential of future losses with problem solving and considers alternatives, including the worst things that could happen
To identify and deal with anniversaries of painful events in client's past	1. Verbalizes relationship between anniversary dates of traumatic events and own feelings and behaviors 2. Verbalizes acceptance of feelings and sadness associated with anniversary dates

SHORT-TERM GOALS	OUTCOME CRITERIA
To reduce cognitive distortions associated with feelings of loneliness	1. Identifies distortions in beliefs that increase feelings of loneliness 2. Identifies relationship between cognition and feelings of loneliness 3. Identifies situations in which others have been blamed for his loneliness
Social Dimension To determine the difference between superficial relationships and intimate ones	1. Identifies the responsibilities of an individual to maintain an intimate relationship 2. Communicates with others at both a feeling level and an intellectual level 3. Upholds the commitment for confidentiality and reciprocal sharing in a relationship
To renew previously enjoyed relationships	1. Recalls satisfying relationships before the onset of loneliness 2. Initiates actions to renew previously enjoyed relationships (phone calls, attending church, attending club meetings, doing volunteer work)
To overcome the loss of a significant other	1. Seeks to cultivate a support system to replace the loss of a significant other 2. Contacts friends and becomes involved in singles groups, senior citizen groups, special interest groups
To increase self-esteem	1. Makes positive statements about self 2. Identifies strengths, skills, assets
Spiritual Dimension To relate beliefs and values to the loneliness episode	1. Identifies values and beliefs that increase loneliness 2. Identifies values and beliefs that decrease loneliness
To increase client's sense of meaning in life	1. Identifies values and activities in which client finds meaning 2. Discusses meaning and meaninglessness of life
To appreciate self as an individual who makes choices and enjoys being alone	1. Chooses to spend time alone. 2. Statements indicate comfortableness with alone time.
To decrease the fear of dying alone	1. Explores the possibility of significant others being with him at the time of death 2. Discusses fears associated with dying alone 3. Discusses the meaning of death
To decrease discomfort felt about this life lived	1. Identifies the "good" things done in life 2. Identifies unrealistic expectations of self 3. Identifies sources of guilt-producing feelings caused by religion 4. Seeks ways to participate in religious experiences 5. Forgives self

Discharge Planning

The following client behaviors demonstrate readiness for discharge:
1. Initiates and maintains a satisfying intimate relationship
2. Substitutes activities for times when human company is not available
3. Deals with feelings (anger, depression, and anxiety) associated with loneliness
4. Associates with groups that are satisfying to client

IMPLEMENTATION

NURSING ACTIONS	RATIONALE
Physical Dimension	
1. Assist client in identifying the relationship between somatic complaints and loneliness.	To learn the cause (loneliness) and effect (somatic complaints) relationship.
2. Encourage client to correct eating habits through psychotherapeutic techniques: behavior modification, cognitive restructuring, and goal setting for weight loss or gain.	Weight loss or weight gain can be a manifestation of loneliness.
3. Assist client with relaxation exercises and preparation for sleep.	To reestablish previous sleep patterns. Sleep pattern disturbances that are characteristic of depression can be a complication of loneliness.
4. Encourage client to accept physical limitations.	Acceptance can lead to development of alternative behaviors that decrease loneliness.
5. Encourage client to discuss reduction in sexual activity. a. Explore feelings related to reduction in sexual activity. b. Discuss alternative methods of sexual expression. c. Discuss activities that produce pleasure and serve as substitutes for sexual activity.	Physical limitations may interfere with usual modes of sexual expression. Sexual activity may change after loss of a partner through death or divorce.
6. Encourage client to develop appropriate behaviors for dealing with long-term confinement resulting in social isolation. a. Encourage learning a new hobby. b. Encourage making friends with staff and others who are confined. c. Engage in pursuing some long-desired reading. d. Help in learning new self-help mechanisms.	Client learns self-support by becoming involved in activities that can reduce loneliness.
7. Assist client in differentiating between touching behaviors that convey genuine warmth and those that fulfill dependency needs. a. Assess feelings at the time of the touching behaviors. b. Touch or hug client frequently when client is not engaged in attention-seeking behavior. c. Model appropriate touching behavior. d. Be aware that the elderly may experience little contact. e. Use touch as a method of sensory stimulation for the elderly.	The lonely client may touch excessively as a way of getting attention.
8. Encourage warm soapy baths or massages.	This can be a method of caring for self to relieve loneliness.
9. Encourage and provide opportunity for strenuous exercise appropriate to client's physical condition. Include exercise plans for the bedridden.	Exercise increases physical fitness and can increase interpersonal contact. It also uses energy that may have been used to maintain feelings of loneliness.
Emotional Dimension	
1. Assist client in identifying and labeling the experience of loneliness.	Feelings of loneliness may be dissociated; naming or labeling the experience indicates recognition of the feeling.
2. Encourage client to recognize and deal with feelings of loneliness.	Recognition of the feeling of loneliness provides opportunity for adaptive coping.
3. Encourage constructive expression of anger. a. Engage in physical exercise. b. Pound a pillow. c. Talk in a therapy session.	Anger may be a complication of loneliness.
4. Assist client in determining the relationship between feelings of depression and loneliness.	To learn the relationship between cause and effect.
5. Allow or give client permission to cry.	Crying may be seen as a sign of weakness. Encourage expression of feelings.
6. Respond empathetically to expressions of feelings and provide feedback.	Empathy is an important factor in bringing about learning and change.
7. Discuss situations that produce feelings of loneliness.	Provides a basis for interventions.

NURSING ACTIONS	RATIONALE
8. Help client recognize aggressive urges and impulses.	Anger may be a more acceptable feeling than the pain of loneliness.
9. Discuss constructive methods for dealing with aggression.	Aggression may be a complication of loneliness.

Intellectual Dimension

NURSING ACTIONS	RATIONALE
1. Assist client in identifying the precipitating event for loneliness.	Recognizing the precipitating event provides the means for adaptive coping.
2. Support client as he shares the loneliness episode and its associated feelings.	It is a painful experience and having a supportive person may reduce some of the pain.
3. Assist client in identifying substitute activities (pets, television, radio, hobbies, exercise) for times when human company is unlikely.	To learn alternative behaviors.

4. Assist client in a cognitive exercise of reacting to potential future losses.
  a. List alternatives following the potential loss.
  b. Include the worst things that could happen.
  c. Make decisions about how to handle these consequences if they occurred.
  d. Recall how often the worst possible thing one can imagine happens.
	To learn anticipatory coping and to reduce hopelessness.

5. Encourage client to identify times when he blames another person for problems that he himself caused.
  a. Encourage realistic appraisal of the situation to reduce blaming.
  b. Assist client in recognizing his reaction to problems of this nature.
  c. Assist client in taking responsibility for his own actions.
	To teach client to use logic when analyzing a situation.

6. Explore with client the painful feelings associated with the anniversary of a traumatic event.
  a. Encourage client to get in touch with and experience the feelings associated with the traumatic event.
  b. Encourage client to reminisce about the positive happenings associated with the individual or pet related to the traumatic event.
	Depression or somatic complaints may be precipitated by the anniversary of a traumatic event.

7. Encourage initiation of activities and trying new things.	To encourage self-care and reduce dependency on others.
8. Use humor when interacting with client.	It is constructive coping behavior.
9. Teach the value of humor and laughter.	Same as #8.

10. Teach client techniques of active listening and responding empathetically in conversation. Model good listening.
  a. Give complete attention to content of message.
  b. Restate content.
  c. Reflect feelings that are conveyed.
  d. Make good eye contact.
  e. Use nonverbal gestures such as nodding head or smiling.
To teach cause-and-effect relationship.
	To learn to focus on others and to increase social competence.
	11. Assist client in determining effects of withdrawal.

12. Model warmth and friendliness.	Learning occurs through observation and imitation.
13. Be aware of own feelings of loneliness.	Loneliness is contagious and anxiety can be reduced by recognition of the phenomenon.
14. Use self-disclosure regarding own feelings of loneliness.	To convey genuineness, honesty, and empathy.
15. Encourage mutual self-disclosure with a trustworthy friend.	It invites interpersonal intimacy.

16. Assist client in overcoming sadness and anxiety of being alone.
  a. List benefits of being alone.
  b. List activities that provide satisfaction while alone.
  c. Assist client in recognizing anxiety when alone.
	To teach self-support and to increase independence.

IMPLEMENTATION—cont'd

NURSING ACTIONS	RATIONALE
17. Help client identify cognitive distortions associated with loneliness, depression, or anger.	To help client discover the irrational thoughts that contribute to these feelings.
18. Help client substitute rational thoughts for irrational thoughts related to loneliness, depression, or anger.	Cognitive distortions are changed by rational thinking.
19. Encourage client to make a scrapbook of pictures of events, family, friends, or pets.	To teach client constructive coping.

20. Encourage client to find someone he can help.
    a. Do volunteer work (blood bank, thrift shops, food or clothing distribution centers, senior citizen centers).
    b. Coach little league teams or be a boy or girl scout leader.
    c. Become a foster grandparent.
	Focusing on another person or activity lessens loneliness.

21. Assist client in recognizing positive attributes. a. Make a list of positive qualities (include such things as health, material needs met, children, education, skills or ability to work, hobbies, pets, and friends).	To increase self-esteem and emphasize skills and abilities.
22. Assist client in recalling previous coping skills a. Keep a list of these behaviors and identify current situations in which these coping skills would be useful.	To promote positive thinking; at some time in life he coped adaptively and can again.

23. Encourage client to be honest with self about substance (alcohol, drug) intake.
    a. Explore reasons for substance abuse.
    b. Teach long-term effects of substance abuse.
    c. Explore substitute activities that are more productive for the individual.
	To reduce denial and confront behavior.

24. Teach client the responsibilities of an intimate relationship.
    a. Communicate at both a feeling and an intellectual level.
    b. Show warmth when interacting with others.
    c. Make a commitment for confidentiality in relationships.
    d. Make a commitment for reciprocal sharing in relationship.
	To teach client ways to develop interpersonal intimacy.

Social Dimension
1. Assist clients in recognizing the difference between a superficial relationship and an intimate one.
2. Encourage client to renew previously enjoyed relationships.
    a. Role-play the first encounter with an individual he has not contacted in a while.
    b. Prepare for both anticipated and unanticipated reactions.
3. Assist client in identifying dependent behavior. Encourage substitution for dependent behavior.
4. Help and encourage client to overcome loss of a significant other.
    a. Foster idea that "life goes on."
    b. Help client to restructure his support system.
    c. Explore the cultivating of others and of substitute activities.
    d. Share the feeling that the void of a significant other may be filled, but the person, pet, or object cannot be replaced.
5. Assist client in exploring the home situation for opportunities for private, honest communication with significant others.
	Lack of intimate satisfying relationships contributes to loneliness.
	Role playing is a way of learning and rehearsal of behavior can reduce the anxiety of the encounter.
	
	Dependent behaviors are methods used by lonely client in an attempt to draw others closer to him.
	To promote resolution of grief process.

NURSING ACTIONS	RATIONALE
a. Explore own schedules and those of others. b. Explore physical layout of home to provide space for private communication. c. Encourage client to develop plans to schedule time with significant other to discuss important private matters.	Environmental factors may create isolation and contribute to loneliness.
6. Use nurse-client relationship as a beginning interaction for lonely client. a. Point out positive and negative aspects of relationship. b. Offer feedback as client expresses feelings regarding the therapeutic relationship. c. Assist client in recognizing aspects of self-esteem and self-worth in the nurse-client relationship.	Nurse-patient relationship is a learning process used to bring about behavioral changes in client.
7. Encourage client to initiate contact with one person (ask to share lunch, discuss a book, admire a pet).	To promote social interaction, to learn to become involved with another person, to learn to assume responsibility in maintaining a relationship, and to increase self-esteem.
8. Give positive feedback for paticipating in a relationship.	Behavior that is rewarded is likely to be repeated.
9. Help client move toward goals of group relatedness.	To facilitate involvement with others.
10. Involve client in group therapy.	Groups can provide support and assist client in understanding own behavior, as well as helping client learn new behaviors.
11. Involve client in family therapy.	To improve communication, to allow constructive expression of feelings, and to demonstrate affection.
12. When appropriate, sit quietly in silence with client.	Silence can be intimate communication.
13. Reinforce client's attempts to initiate caring, intimate relationships with others.	Same as #8.
14. Help client form networks where others with similar interests would congregate. (Groups may already be established, as in the case of church groups, political interest groups, exercise groups, or singles' groups.)	Groups provide social support and reduce feelings of isolation.
15. Encourage client to accept physical limitations. Help client accept an altered body image.	Acceptance can lead to development of alternative behaviors.
Spiritual Dimension 1. Help client identify own beliefs and values.	Client's philosophy of life can change loneliness to a positive creative experience.
2. Relate beliefs and values to present situation of loneliness.	Same as #1.
3. Encourage client to identify activities in which he finds meaning.	To reduce sense of purposelessness and to encourage client to discover own purpose in life.
4. Help client identify situations when he may feel like a meaningless number.	To encourage client's awareness of feelings of isolation and provide basis for intervention.
5. Assist client who has fears of dying alone to explore the possibility of a significant other being with him at the time of death. Enlist the aid of significant others to confirm that they will be personally present when he dies.	A plan will provide solace and comfort by reducing the anxiety of dying alone.
6. Encourage client who has had previously satisfying religious experiences to resume religious activities. a. Arrange a visit from a chaplain or clergyman. b. Arrange for client to attend church services, engage in church activities, or receive communion in the institution or home situation.	Religious activities can provide comfort and focus on others rather than on self.
7. Help client identify feelings produced by not meeting ideals a. Help client to confront these feelings, experience them, and resolve guilt.	To provide a means of relieving guilt and to allow client to form meaningful relationships.

IMPLEMENTATION—cont'd

NURSING ACTIONS	RATIONALE

b. Help client understand that guilt feelings pervade his being and interfere with relationships and intimacy with others.
8. Explore fear that client will spend the remainder of life alone.
  a. Help client discuss the worst possible consequences of spending remainder of life alone.
  b. Help client determine possible alternatives to living alone (moving to senior citizen complex, living with children, making a residential agreement with another person.)
9. Encourage client to spend alone times in prayer or meditation.
	Client can confront fears of loneliness and can find constructive methods to deal with it.
	
	Restorative benefits can be gained from prayer or meditation.

EVALUATION

Evaluation of the lonely client consists of an ongoing observation of the quality of the relationships in which the client is participating. The client and the nurse maintain a close, trusting relationship to foster openness regarding problems the client may be having in relationships with others. The following behaviors indicate that the client is making changes in the desired direction:

1. Eats adequate amounts of nutritional foods
2. Reestablishes sleep pattern
3. Has fewer physical complaints
4. Becomes involved with a pet or hobby
5. Recognizes and constructively deals with feelings associated with loneliness
6. Assumes responsibility for reducing loneliness

BIBLIOGRAPHY

Austin AG: Becoming immune to loneliness: helping the elderly fill a void, *J Gerontol Nurs* 15(8):16, 1989.

Beck AT: *Cognitive therapy and the emotional disorders,* New York, 1976, International University Press.

Beck C et al: Predictors of loneliness in older men and women, *J Women Aging* 2(1):3, 1990.

Booth R: Toward an understanding of loneliness, *Soc Work* 28(2):116, 1983.

Calvert MM: Human pet interaction and loneliness: a test of concepts from Roy's adaptation model, *Nurs Sci Q* 2(4):194, 1989.

Cohen N: On loneliness and the aging process, *Int J Psychoanal* 63(pt. 2):149, 1982.

Copel LC: Loneliness, *J Psychosoc Nurs* 26(1):14, 1988.

Davis, BD: Loneliness in children and adolescents, *Issues Compr Pediatr Nurs* 13(1):59, 1990.

Derlaga VJ, Marguli ST: Why loneliness occurs: the interrelationship of social-psychological and privacy concepts. In Perlman D, Peplau, L, editors: *Loneliness: a sourcebook of current theory, research and therapy,* New York, 1982, John Wiley and Sons.

Foxal MJ, Ekberg JY: Loneliness of chronically ill adults and their spouses, *Issues Ment Health Nurs* 10(2):149, 1989.

Francis GM: Loneliness: the syndrome, *Issues Ment Health Nurs* 3:1, 1981.

Jones WH: Loneliness and social contact, *J Soc Psychol* 113:295, 1981.

Labun E: Spiritual care: an element in nursing care planning, *J Adv Nurs* 13:314, 1988.

Mahon NE: Developmental changes and loneliness during adolescence, *Topics Clin Nurs* 5(1):66, 1983.

Miller J: Assessment of loneliness and spiritual well-being in chronically ill and healthy adults, *J Professional Nurs* 1(2):79, 1985.

Moustakas C: *Loneliness and love,* Englewood Cliffs, N.J., 1972, Prentice-Hall.

Okoneski D: Gay grief: issues of love, loss and loneliness, *Occup Ther Health Care* 7(2/3/4):213, 1990.

Peplau H: Loneliness, *Am J Nurs* 55:1476, 1955.

Perry GR: Loneliness and coping among tertiary-level adult cancer patients in the home, *Cancer Nurs* 13(5):293, 1990.

Ribeiro V: The forgotten generation: elderly women and loneliness, *Rec Adv Nurs* (25):20, 1989.

Russell D, Peplau LA, Ferguson M: Developing a measure of loneliness, *J Pers Assess* 42(3):290, 1978.

Walton CG et al: Psychological correlates of loneliness in the older adult, *Arch Psychiatr Nurs* 5(3):165, 1991.

Weiss R: *Loneliness: the experience of emotional and social isolation,* Cambridge, Mass., 1973, MIT Press.

Young Y: Loneliness, depression, and cognitive therapy: theory and application. In Perlman D, Peplau L, editors: *Loneliness: a sourcebook of current theory, research and therapy,* New York, 1982, John Wiley and Sons.

Malingering

Malingering is the deliberate feigning of some mental or physical defect for a consciously desired end. The individual is aware of the gain for self from displaying the defect.

Malingering may be chosen to avoid a situation perceived as unpleasant. An example of such a situation is the military service. Physical defects such as poor eyesight, severe low back pain, or paralysis of hand or arm may be faked. Mental or behavioral faking is also used, including feigning a mental illness or claiming to be a homosexual, which excludes a person from military service. Undesirable job situations, jury duty, or standing trial may also be avoided by malingering if the individual cannot or will not directly confront the situation. Malingering affects family, friends, and authority persons in that one cannot "blame" an individual who is ill or mentally incapable.

Related DSM-III-R disorders

Factitious disorders
Antisocial personality disorders
Münchausen's syndrome

PRINCIPLES

▶ Physical Dimension

1. The individual consciously chooses to fake a physical defect.
2. Physical symptoms appear authentic.
3. Malingering is a symptom, not a disease.
4. Malingering is found in situations that offer probable benefits for the presence of disease.

▶ Emotional Dimension

1. Malingering is a conscious act; therefore it originates from the ego.
2. The superego is not adequately developed, and the id is able to gain gratification by faking a mental or physical defect.
3. Severe anxiety results over conflicts and attempts to solve problems.
4. The person who malingers fears being caught in the deception.

▶ Intellectual Dimension

1. Malingering is an attempt to achieve a desired goal.
2. It is a conscious act for which the person receives a desired reward.
3. Malingering is an accusation rather than a diagnosis.
4. Malingering may be deliberate deception involving the description of nonexistent symptoms or their production in the absence of actual disease.
5. Malingering may be a conscious and voluntary exaggeration of symptoms of a real disease.
6. Malingering may involve attribution of an actual disability to an injury or accident that did not cause it.
7. The act of malingering causes less anxiety than the object being avoided.
   a. The behavior must be reinforced if it is to continue.
   b. To change the behavior the person must consider the punishment less desirable than the reward.

▶ Social Dimension

1. If inadequate standards have been set within the personality of the person, he looks only at self-gain.
2. The resultant value system narrows personal action to what is least likely to create anxiety.
3. The person in the sick role is released from the normal and usual social obligations of society, such as going to work or attending school.
4. The person in the sick role is absolved from blame for own condition.
5. The person in the sick role is expected to want to get well, to seek help, and to cooperate with the treatment.

The original content for this section was contributed by Mary Flo Bruce, R.N. Ph.D.

6. To be sick is to be different, to have deviant status.
7. Falsely enacting the sick role is malingering.
8. The malingerer claims an identity he does not have, which forces other people to play correlative and meaningless roles.
9. The malingerer consciously takes the sick role with full awareness of the consequences.
10. The sick role may be used to rationalize personal failures or inadequacies.

▶ **Spiritual Dimension**

1. Malingering is an act freely chosen by the individual.
2. It is an attempt by the person to confront existential anxiety.
3. The behavior can be understood by knowing the individual's subjective experiences.
4. Malingering causes intrapersonal conflict and this conflict further increases the existential anxiety the person is trying to avoid.

ASSESSMENT

▶ **Physical Dimension**

I. **History**
   A. Habits
      1. Medications and drugs
         a. Use of medications to fake symptoms
         b. Toxic substances or medications detected in drug screens
   B. Destructive behavior
      1. Methods used to fake symptoms possibly injurious to health
         a. Uses anticoagulants to promote blood in urine
         b. Self-dislocates shoulder
         c. Fakes hearing loss
   C. Health history
      1. Injuries appear self-inflicted

   2. Numerous hospitalizations, clinic visits, and emergency room visits for fake symptoms
   D. Review of systems—any body system may be affected, depending on the client's choice of illness

II. **Physical examination**
   A. Affected area examined
   B. Results not in support of complaint

III. **Diagnostic tests**
   A. Perform appropriate tests according to symptoms
   B. Drug screens
   C. Minnesota Multiphasic Personality Inventory (MMPI)

▶ **Emotional Dimension**

CLIENT DATA	ANALYSIS	NURSING DIAGNOSIS
Anxiety	Attempts to solve problem or meet needs. Experiences conflict over conscious decision to malinger. Experiences anxiety over attempts at deception.	Ineffective individual coping: malingering related to inability to appropriately meet needs Anxiety: related to conflict over making a decision to malinger
Fearfulness	Fears being caught in deception. Fears being unable to attain conscious goal. Fears having insufficient knowledge to carry out deception.	Fear: related to being caught in deception, to possible inability to attain goal associated with malingering, or to possible lack of sufficient knowledge to deceive others
Distrustfulness	Is unable to trust caregiver, since caregiver may discover deception and client's inability to discuss actual condition.	Anxiety: related to distrust of caregiver
Feelings of inferiority	Has low self-esteem, contributing to overly confident and self-assertive act.	Self-esteem disturbance: feelings of inferiority related to malingering

▶ **Intellectual Dimension**

CLIENT DATA	ANALYSIS	NURSING DIAGNOSIS
Distorted perception	Attempts to manipulate environment by lies and deception.	Altered thought processes: distorted perception related to malingering
Denial	Perceives others as incapable of recognizing fake behavior.	Ineffective individual coping: denial related to malingering
Unusual lack of comprehension	Is overly evasive and vague because of fear of giving incorrect or invalid information.	Altered thought processes: vague and evasive responses related to malingering
Impaired judgment	Makes decisions, which may or may not be valid, with intent of attaining goal. Focuses on present payoff without thought for how malingering may affect future. Is unable to generalize goals.	*Altered judgment: related to malingering
Lack of insight	Realizes consequences of behavior but believes that environment can be manipulated.	Altered thought processes: impaired insight related to malingering
Avoidance	Does not accept reality-oriented approach to solving problems.	Altered thought processes: use of avoidance related to malingering
Inappropriate use of rationalization	Uses rationalization to reach goal.	Defensive coping: related to malingering
Rigid thinking	Uses rigid manner to solve problems. Promotes a more secure feeling.	Altered thought processes: rigid thinking related to malingering

▶ **Social Dimension**

CLIENT DATA	ANALYSIS	NURSING DIAGNOSIS
Low self-esteem	Does not live up to own expectations of self.	Self-esteem disturbance: related to malingering
Dependence on others	Shows maladaptive dependence. Chooses role of deception with belief that caregivers and others can be bluffed. Receives secondary gains.	Ineffective individual coping: dependence related to malingering
Lack of support system	Attempts to manipulate others by lies and deception; deception makes it impossible to relate well or trust anyone.	Impaired social interaction: inadequate support system related to deception
Impaired role functioning	Has reduced ability to function in social and occupational roles because of anxiety associated with deception.	Altered role performance: impaired role functioning related to malingering

▶ **Spiritual Dimension**

CLIENT DATA	ANALYSIS	NURSING DIAGNOSIS
Conflict with inner self	Experiences conflict within personality.	Spiritual distress: inner conflict related to malingering.
Lack of faith in achieving goals authentically	Fails to have sufficient belief in solving problem or meeting needs without deception.	Spiritual distress: inadequate faith in self related to malingering
Disturbed or distorted faith	Experiences a distortion in faith because must either rationalize deception or consciously decide to not be truthful.	Spiritual distress: distorted faith related to malingering

PLANNING

Long-Term Goal

To develop an effective way of dealing with anxiety that does not require malingering
(feigning mental or physical defect)

SHORT-TERM GOALS	OUTCOME CRITERIA
Physical Dimension To identify situations that lead to malingering behavior	1. Describes sequence of events leading to malingering behavior 2. Identifies goals achieved by behavior
Emotional Dimension To identify feelings involved in decision to malinger	1. Verbalizes feelings involved in decision to malinger 2. Examines other methods of coping with stress and anxiety caused by not attaining goal 3. Examines other ways to manage feelings 4. Identifies needs that are unmet 5. Communicates needs in direct manner
Intellectual Dimension To identify an effective method of problem solving	1. States goal he wishes to attain 2. Identifies problems in attaining goal 3. Verbalizes thoughts and feelings about problem 4. Lists possible methods of attaining goal 5. Discusses consequences of each method 6. Chooses an option 7. Tests option 8. Evaluates results
To identify needs	1. Explores needs 2. Differentiates needs from wants 3. Directly asks for what he needs and wants
Social Dimension To identify effects of malingering on significant others	1. Identifies significant others 2. States how significant others view the act of malingering 3. States ways goals can be met without malingering
To identify ramifications of malingering on broader social life	1. States how community (job, school, church) views malingering 2. Examines effect on own life if malingering act is discovered 3. Investigates the meaning behind malingering
Spiritual Dimension To examine beliefs and values in regard to deception	1. Explores beliefs and values that are being violated 2. Verbalizes how this behavior affects value system 3. Examines rationalization used to attempt deception 4. Acknowledges responsibility for own behavior 5. Accepts consequences of own behavior 6. Acknowledges that goal attainment by deception is not being true to self

Discharge Planning

The following client behaviors demonstrate readiness for discharge:
1. Identifies steps that lead to the decision to malinger
2. Identifies use of rationalization
3. Uses a support system that accepts and rewards positive problem solving
4. Has a realistic perception of the consequences of malingering
5. Outlines method of problem solving to attain goal
6. Works with social worker or others to resolve problems with occupation or education
7. Confronts self with responsibility and accountability for own behavior
8. Increases self-esteem and self-awareness

IMPLEMENTATION

NURSING ACTIONS	RATIONALE
Physical Dimension	
1. Be consistent in follow-up of physician's information to client.	To clearly convey the message that deception is counterproductive and reduces manipulation.
2. Reaffirm diagnostic findings by confronting client directly in regard to any manipulation attempted concerning illness or defect.	Same as #1.
3. Encourage client to continue activities of daily living to the same degree as client was capable of before attempting deception.	To increase self-esteem and reinforce client's ability to solve problems realistically.
Emotional Dimension	
1. Work with client to explore feelings that led to decision to malinger.	To associate feelings with behavior provides a basis for developing more appropriate behavior.
2. Assist client in verbalizing anxiety and guilt associated with the decision by listening actively and clarifying.	To help client to recognize the feelings and consequences of own choices.
3. Develop a therapeutic relationship with client.	The therapeutic relationship is one of mutual trust. Trust in the nurse is an important factor in facilitating change in behavior.
4. Assist client in dealing with underlying feelings concerning the possibility of not attaining desired goal by increasing self-awareness.	To promote self-awareness and a basis for changing behavior.
Intellectual Dimension	
1. Have client confront and acknowledge accountability for behavior by making observations about his behavior.	When client accepts responsibility for behavior, he can recognize that he can choose to change that behavior.
2. Discuss client's attempts to manipulate the environment by deception.	To confront client's self-defeating and unacceptable behavior.
3. Discuss sources of client's fears and anxiety.	Awareness of fears and anxiety provides a means for identifying potential coping mechanisms.
4. Explore guilt-producing situation in which client has placed self.	To help client become aware of consequences of own behavior.
5. Help client identify needs in an open manner.	Awareness of needs and an honest expression of those needs provide a means for realistically meeting them.
6. Identify steps client used in reaching decision to malinger.	To assist client in gaining insight into own behavior.
7. Explore other methods of problem solving that use positive ways to attain goal.	To help client discover other ways to successfully meet needs.
8. Explore consequences of client's behavior.	To establish the cause-and-effect relationship between behavior and undesirable consequence.
9. Give feedback about how others view client's behavior.	To promote self-awareness.
10. Explore use of rationalization to justify deception.	To point out how client is deceiving self while deceiving others.
11. Assist client in using direct methods to attain goal instead of avoidance by use of effective communication skills.	To help client learn other more effective ways of behaving.

IMPLEMENTATION—cont'd

NURSING ACTIONS	RATIONALE
Social Dimension	
1. Assist client in identifying a support system that encourages use of positive methods of attaining goal.	Support from others reinforces positive behavior and increases the likelihood that it will be repeated.
2. Refer to social worker if client has encountered difficulty with occupation or education because of malingering.	Social worker can provide occupational or educational guidance.
3. Maintain positive attitude toward client but not his behavior.	Indicates acceptance of client but not of his behavior.
4. Explore methods of attaining interdependence in relationships.	To encourage client to be more self-reliant and to increase confidence in his own ability.
5. Discuss environmental factors that produce and lead to malingering such as dissatisfaction at work.	To help client associate malingering with stress. When client accepts responsibility for his behavior, he recognizes that he can choose to change that behavior.
6. Provide group therapy.	Groups are supportive and can assist in understanding behavior and in learning new behaviors.
7. Encourage sharing of feelings regarding malingering.	To learn to share feelings with others, which is a part of establishing a trusting relationship.
8. Promote self-esteem.	To increase self-esteem. Client does not live up to own expectation of self.
Spiritual Dimension	
1. Assist client in clarifying conflict between personal goals and values with individual and group therapy.	To establish the relationship between the violation of values and the attempt to achieve a desired goal.
2. Promote client's self-awareness without making a judgment.	To accept client.
3. Assist client in developing faith that problem can be solved without deception.	To promote hope and instill belief that behavior can be changed.
4. Encourage client to use creative energy in developing positive ways to attain goal.	To promote a more satisfying life.

EVALUATION

Evaluation is based on measurable goals and outcome criteria that provide the data needed to assess the client's ability to attain a desired goal without malingering. Development of a therapeutic relationship with the nurse enables the client to set goals and determine outcome criteria by which progress can be evaluated. As the client progresses in his ability to solve problems by facing the problem and working toward attaining his goal, evaluation is positive. Other positive indications include:

1. Discusses feelings associated with the decision to malinger
2. Discloses difficulties in attaining desired goals
3. Uses other methods of problem solving
4. Becomes more assertive in stating needs
5. Identifies the effect of malingering on self and others
6. Acknowledges the discrepancy between values and behaviors

The nurse identifies and controls anger at the client that frequently emerges when treatment efforts are frustrated by malingering. She also realizes that she does not have to prove a client is malingering. A simple statement that no explanation exists for the disease process is sufficient.

BIBLIOGRAPHY

Cassem E: When symptoms seem groundless, *Emerg Med* 19(12):62, 1987.

Collins M: The dreaded Mrs. Scott . . . never "assume" a patient was malingering, *AD Nurse* 2(3):18, 1987.

Cosgrove R, Fawley R: Could it be Ganser's syndrome? *Arch Psychiatr Nurs* 3(4):241, 1989.

Goebel R: Detection of faking on the Halstead-Reitan neuropsychological test battery, *J Clin Psychol* 39:731, 1983.

Gold S: Speech discrimination scores at low sensation levels as possible index to malingering, *Audit Res* 21:137, 1981.

Gorman W: Defining malingering, *J Forensic Sci* 27(2):401, 1982.

Gorman W: Malingering: detection and reporting, *Ariz Med* 41(3):179, 1984.

Headley B: Delayed recovery: taking another look, *J Rehabil* 55(3):61, 1989.

Hesterbert R et al: A review of ocular malingering and hysteria for the flight surgeon, *Aviat Space Environ Med* 54:934, 1983.

Little N: The body electric short-circuits: the hysterical or malingering patient, *Emerg Med* 16(1):187, 1984.

Lyssitt D: Back rehabilitation programs speed recovery of injured worker, *Occup Health Saf* 53:5, 1984.

Niebuhr B, Marion R: Detecting sincerity of effort when measuring grip strength, *Am J Phys Med Rehabil* 66(1):16, 1987.

Niebuhr B, Marion R: Voluntary control of submaximal grip strength, *Am J Phys Med Rehabil* 69(2):96, 1990.

Rappaport M et al: Neuropsychiatric assessment of a spinal cord injury patient with sudden recovery, *Arch Phys Med Rehabil* 69(6):455, 1988.

Spanos N et al: Disorganized recall, hypnotic amnesia and subjective faking: more disconfirmatory evidence, *Psychol Rep* 50(2):383, 1984.

Suvanich S: Pepper grains as artifactual urinary calculi, *N Engl J Med* 310:129, 1984.

Szasz TS: Malingering: diagnosis or social condemnation? *Arch Neurol Psychiatry* 76:432, 1956.

Manic Behavior

Manic behavior is a mood (affective) disturbance found in clients diagnosed as having bipolar disorder. In this instance, *mood* refers to a prolonged emotion that colors the psychic life; it generally involves elation or depression in those with bipolar disorders. The manic and depressive syndromes each consist of characteristic symptoms that tend to follow each other in cycles. Occasionally the manic and depressive symptoms intermingle, occurring at the same time. They may alternate rapidly, that is, within a few days, or alternate cyclically, with periods of highs and lows lasting from several weeks to several months (see Depression, p. 133).

The manic episode is characterized by a predominately elated mood associated with symptoms of hyperactivity, pressure of speech, flight of ideas, inflated self-esteem, decreased need for sleep, distractibility, irritability, and excessive involvement in activities that may have painful consequences. Because clients with manic behavior may go for days without adequate nutrition and sleep, the situation may become life-threatening. Skillful nursing interventions are essential to provide comfort and relief for the client and the client's family.

Related DSM-III-R disorders

Bipolar disorder
Attention-deficit hyperactivity disorder (ADHD)
Anxiety disorders
Psychoactive substance use disorders

Other related conditions

Hypomania
Brain damage

PRINCIPLES

▶ Physical Dimension

1. There is a high incidence of manic behavior in families with a history of bipolar disorder.
2. Changes in mood reflect both physiological and psychological processes.
3. Changes in biogenic amines, including increased levels of norepinephrine and catecholamines, may lead to manic behavior.
4. Predisposing factors include mental retardation, epilepsy, cerebral palsy, neurological disorders, and endocrine disorders.
5. Heredity may increase the potential for mood disorders, biological factors may trigger them, and environmental factors may influence how symptoms are exhibited.
6. Neurotransmitter imbalances are related to manic episodes.
7. Mood disorders are related to the ebb and flow of hormonal factors—cortisol, human growth hormone (HGH), and thyroid-stimulating hormone.
8. Disturbances in electrolyte metabolism play an important role in mood disorders.
9. Mood disorders are associated with toxic pharmacological agents and physical disease.
10. Any condition that impairs functioning of the central nervous system (CNS) may produce manic behavior.
11. Euphoric reaction has been associated with right-sided brain damage.
12. Mania is characterized by greater left-sided hemispheric activation in electroencephalographic asymmetry.

▶ Emotional Dimension

1. The struggle between the ego and the id, in which the id is stronger, determines manic behavior.

2. Mania is a defense against depression.
3. Feelings of insecurity and inadequacy are disguised by manic behavior.
4. Feelings of aggression lurk beneath the manic episode.
5. A distinct period of abnormally and persistently elevated, expansive, or irritable mood is present.

▶ Intellectual Dimension

1. Predisposing personality characteristics of manic behavior include egocentricity, ambivalence, and envy.
2. Disappointments in later life may lead to regression to earlier forms of relating and may result in manic behavior.
3. Mania is a defense-oriented strategy for dealing with stress; it is a means of escape.

▶ Social Dimension

1. Manic behavior is seen as a return to acting out infantile freedom.
2. Individuals are highly dependent on esteem and approval from others.
3. Inconsistent parental discipline with punishment at times for behavior that at other times brought no punishment leads to hyperactivity (manic behavior).
4. Environmental stimuli (colors, sounds, and activities) affect manic behavior.

▶ Spiritual Dimension

1. Mania provides a pathological "high" that the individual is unable to experience in everyday life.
2. An exaggerated sense of well-being and value is seen in clients with manic behavior.

ASSESSMENT

▶ Physical Dimension

I. History
  A. Activities of daily living
   1. Nutrition
    a. Does not take time to eat meals; becomes malnourished
    b. Lack of concern about nutrition
    c. Weight loss
    d. Inadequate eating patterns
    e. Inadequate fluid intake
    f. May eat voraciously
   2. Sleep
    a. Inability to sleep
    b. Decreased need for sleep without fatigue
   3. Recreation, hobbies, and interests
    a. Pursues many activities but is too distractible to complete them
    b. Is disorganized
   4. Physical activities and limitations
    a. Increased physical activity
    b. Participation in ceaseless, wild, disruptive activities
    c. Boundless energy
   5. Sexual activity
    a. Sexual activity not usual for the individual
    b. Sexual indiscretions
  B. Habits
   1. Alcohol
    a. Abuse, misuse, and excessive consumption
   2. Smoking
    a. Excessive
   3. Medications and drugs
    a. Noncompliance with medication regimen
   4. Caffeine
    a. Excessive intake of coffee, tea, and colas
  C. Destructive behavior
   1. Life-threatening when client does not eat, drink, or sleep adequately
   2. Pays little attention to health needs
   3. Ignores bruises, fever, and injuries
   4. Impulsive actions
   5. Reckless driving
   6. Aggressive activity
  D. Health history—previous hospitalizations for similar symptoms
  E. Genetic factors
   1. Family history of bipolar disorder
  F. Review of systems
   1. General
    a. Change in weight
    b. Change in appetite
    c. Change in sleep habits
   2. Neurological
    a. Mood changes
     (1) Elation and euphoria
     (2) Mood swings

II. Diagnostic tests
  A. EEG
  B. CAT scan
  C. Differential blood count; blood culture
  D. Basal metabolic rate; Chem 20
  E. Blood levels
  F. T_7, T_3, and T_4

▶ **Physical Examination**

CLIENT DATA	ANALYSIS	NURSING DIAGNOSIS
Restless, ceaseless activity	Accelerated motor activity, impulsive actions.	High risk for injury: related to accelerated motor activity
Inappropriate dress for weather or situation	Judgment impaired.	Dressing/grooming self-care deficit: Inappropriate dress related to impaired judgment associated with manic behavior
Unusual dress—flamboyant, bizarre, or eccentric	Judgment impaired, mood of elation, euphoria.	Dressing/grooming self-care deficit: unusual or eccentric dress: related to impaired judgment associated with manic behavior
Disheveled and unkempt	Unable to take time for self-care.	Dressing/grooming self-care deficit: unkempt appearance related to manic behavior
Neglected personal hygiene	Unable to take time for self-care.	Bathing/hygiene self-care deficit: neglects personal hygiene related to manic behavior
Accelerated speech with flight of ideas	Thoughts speeded up, causing rapid speech and flight of ideas.	Impaired verbal communication: flight of ideas related to accelerated thinking

▶ **Emotional Dimension**

CLIENT DATA	ANALYSIS	NURSING DIAGNOSIS
Euphoria, elation, cheerfulness, "high," and playfulness	Elated, expansive mood, an exaggerated sense of well-being to cover up feelings of inadequacy or inferiority.	Ineffective individual coping: related to elated, expansive mood
Irritability, anger and rage	Emotional lability when immediate needs are not met.	High risk for violence directed at others: related to anger or rage
Infectious quality to elated mood	Cheerful good-naturedness that affects others.	Ineffective individual coping: excessively cheerful, good-natured, related to elevated mood
Unceasing and unselective enthusiasm	Elevated, expansive mood; hyperactivity.	Ineffective individual coping: unceasing, unselective enthusiasm related to elevated mood
Unwarranted optimism	Elevated mood.	Ineffective individual coping: unwarranted optimism related to elevated mood
Grandiosity	Inflated self-esteem.	Altered thought processes: grandiosity related to elevated mood
Emotional lability	Unstable moods; moves from cheerfulness to irritation easily, with little provocation.	Ineffective individual coping: related to emotional lability associated with manic behavior

▶ **Intellectual Dimension**

CLIENT DATA	ANALYSIS	NURSING DIAGNOSIS
Grandiosity and delusional thinking	Defense against anxiety, an escape from reality.	Altered thought processes: related to delusional thinking
Belief that he is well-known political, religious, or entertainment leader	Grandiose delusions.	Altered thought processes: related to delusions of grandeur

▶ **Intellectual Dimension—cont'd**

CLIENT DATA	ANALYSIS	NURSING DIAGNOSIS
Expansive; thinks he can write novels, run hospitals or the United Nations, compose music, write poetry, or is being sought for political office or some impractical invention	Inflated, expansive thinking.	Altered thought processes: related to expansive thinking
Lack of judgment	Impaired judgment leading to buying sprees or inappropriate business deals.	*Altered judgment: related to expansive thinking
Lack of insight	Unaware of intrusiveness or domineering, demanding nature of his behavior.	Altered thought processes: lack of insight related to expansive thinking
Excessive planning for participation in activities (social, sexual, occupational, political, or religious)	Accelerated thinking.	Altered thought processes: related to accelerated thinking
Short attention span; difficulty concentrating	Easily distracted.	Altered thought processes: decreased attention span and difficulty concentrating related to accelerated thinking
Hostile comments, complaints, and angry tirades	When thwarted and needs are unmet, is emotionally labile.	High risk for violence directed at others: related to hostile, angry behavior
Obscenities; uninhibited sexual interest	Judgment impaired; sexual indiscretions.	Altered thought processes: related to obscenities and uninhibited sexual indiscretions associated with manic behavior
Denies illness and problems of any nature	A defense against depression and/or aggression.	Defensive coping: denial of illness and problems related to manic behavior
Uses jokes, puns, plays on words, rhymes, and amusing irrelevancies	Creative, expansive thinking; id influences.	Altered thought processes: creative, expansive verbal activity related to euphoria
Theatrical or dramatic mannerisms (singing)	Inflated self-esteem.	Ineffective individual coping: related to theatrical, dramatic mannerisms associated with manic behavior
Clanging	Sounds, rather than meanings, form conceptual relationships, govern word choice.	Altered thought processes: clanging speech related to euphoria
Flight of ideas	Continuous flow of accelerated speech, skipping from topic to topic with minimal associations.	Altered thought processes: flight of ideas related to accelerated thinking
Distractibility	Rapid changes in speech and activity as a result of responding to various, irrelevant external stimuli.	Altered thought processes: related to high level of distractibility
Overresponsive to stimuli	Easily distractible.	Sensory-perceptual alterations: related to easy distractibility, overresponsiveness to stimuli
Pressured speech	Accelerated thinking; highly responsive to environmental stimuli, accompanying flight of ideas.	Impaired verbal communication: related to pressured speech

▶ **Social Dimension**

CLIENT DATA	ANALYSIS	NURSING DIAGNOSIS
Unrealistic perception of self	Sees self as well-known figure (athlete, political or religious leader, one of God's anointed), delusional.	Self-esteem disturbance: related to unrealistic perception of self associated with manic behavior
Self-esteem unrealistically inflated; self-indulgent	Euphoric mood to defend against insecurity and inferiority.	Self-esteem disturbance: unrealistically elevated self-esteem related to manic behavior
Open to anyone, everyone; extreme gregariousness; increased social interactions with others; excessive participation with others; uninvitingly intimate and unwelcomely personal; renewing old acquaintances (calls at all hours of night); helping self to others' possessions; pilfers from others	Unconcerned with trust, is friendly, and initiates interactions with others excessively with little sensitivity to others' interests.	Impaired social interaction: related to elated and expansive mood
Impaired social functioning	Inflated perception of self and increased activity alienates others.	Impaired social interaction: related to manic behavior
Constantly seeking involvement with the environment	Overinvolvement and overreactivity to external environmental stimuli.	Sensory-perceptual alterations: overinvolvement and overreactivity to environmental factors related to manic behavior

▶ **Spiritual Dimension**

CLIENT DATA	ANALYSIS	NURSING DIAGNOSIS
Life values and beliefs change rapidly	Responses to environmental stimulation or interactions with others.	Spiritual distress: related to rapid value changes associated with manic behavior
"Everything is great" attitude toward life	Euphoria, exaggerated sense of well-being.	Spiritual distress: related to euphoria
Prefers "high" of illness to pain of reality	Elevated, euphoric mood relieves pain in real life; elation and overinvolvement as defense against despair. Is alienated from self.	Spiritual distress: preference of euphoric mood with "highs" related to inability to deal with pain in life
Identifies with a religious leader	Esteem is low with delusions of grandeur.	Spiritual distress: related to delusions of grandeur associated with manic behavior
Increase in creative activities	Writes, paints, and sings even though lacks talent; perceives self with unrealistic abilities.	Spiritual distress: related to unrealistic creative abilities associated with manic behavior

PLANNING

Long-Term goals

To resume effective functioning without manic episodes
To know signs and symptoms of an approaching manic episode in order to seek
  help early

SHORT-TERM GOALS	OUTCOME CRITERIA
Physical Dimension	
To control motor activity	1. Sits in chair for increasing periods of time without getting up and disturbing others

SHORT-TERM GOALS	OUTCOME CRITERIA
	2. Works at a task or activity until completion 3. Identifies times when restless and agitated and needs to move about
To perform self-care	1. Attends to personal hygiene and grooming: cares for hair and teeth, showers, launders clothes, and uses appropriate make-up 2. Verbalizes sense of pride in self-care
To meet basic physical needs	1. Takes short naps 2. Uses quiet time for self 3. Sleeps 5 to 7 hours at night without interruption 4. Engages in moderate amounts of exercise and activities 5. Establishes elimination regularity with proper diet 6. Sits down to eat a balanced diet regularly each day 7. Drinks adequate fluids without being asked 8. Verbalizes satisfaction from being able to meet own needs adequately
To comply with medication regimen	1. Takes medications as directed 2. Verbalizes reasons for taking medications 3. States side effects of medications 4. Verbalizes importance of taking medications, perhaps for rest of life 5. Verbalizes importance of having blood levels taken regularly while on medication (lithium) 6. Develops a plan for interventions when signs and symptoms are increasing
To have outlets for tension and energy	1. Engages in physical activities, such as jogging, swimming, sweeping, raking leaves, and cutting grass 2. Engages in solitary activities 3. Identifies activities that can be performed successfully 4. Avoids competitive activities 5. Extends attention span while engaged in activities 6. Completes activities started 7. Participates in activities without being disruptive 8. States feelings of pleasure associated with various activities
Emotional Dimension To identify painful feelings—sadness, anger, guilt, or anxiety—beneath the euphoria	1. Verbalizes painful feelings 2. Able to differentiate between feelings of anger, sadness, guilt, and anxiety 3. Identifies situations, events, and people associated with painful feelings 4. Verbalizes feelings of anxiety and of being overwhelmed 5. Develops a plan of self-care when feeling anxious and overwhelmed 6. Statements indicate it is OK to have painful feelings 7. Verbalizes relief felt by discussing painful feelings with another person 8. States other ways to express painful feelings
Intellectual Dimension To control verbal activity	1. Focuses on one topic for discussion 2. Allows others to interrupt stream of conversation 3. Limits own verbal activity 4. States effect of verbal activity on others
To express realistic ideas	1. Expresses no grandiose ideas 2. Expresses no exaggerated ideas of self-importance 3. Identifies ideas that are grandiose, unrealistic, or fictional 4. Expresses needs and wants clearly and directly

PLANNING—cont'd

SHORT-TERM GOALS	OUTCOME CRITERIA

Social Dimension
To enhance self-concept
	1. Identifies the relationship between grandiosity and own self-worth
	2. Realistically appraises self
	  a. Identifies strengths and weaknesses
	  b. Accepts weaknesses
	3. Differentiates between idealized self and perceived self

Spiritual Dimension To gain satisfaction from a less adventuresome life-style	1. Receives pleasure from reading, ball games, swimming, and other activities 2. Identifies activities that provide satisfaction without producing stress 3. Verbalizes satisfaction with life when not "high" 4. Does not have to be center of attention and can listen to others 5. States that "high" periods interfere with health and safety and lead to problems, such as overspending, poor health, and hospitalization

Discharge Planning

The following client behaviors demonstrate readiness for discharge:
1. Complies with medication regimen, including periodical blood tests
2. States purpose, side effects of medications, and consequences of not taking medications
3. States signs and symptoms of an approaching manic episode
4. Knows who to contact when early symptoms appear
5. Has a supportive person to express feelings and thoughts with and receive support from during stressful times

IMPLEMENTATION

NURSING ACTIONS	RATIONALE
Physical Dimension	
1. Provide genetic counseling if client has family history of bipolar disorder.	Hereditary factors are involved in mood disorders.
2. Monitor sleep patterns.	The client is susceptible to exhaustion because he is too busy to eat, drink, or sleep.
3. Provide rest and quiet time.	To promote physical health.
4. Use comfort measures to promote sleep; decrease stimuli, provide darkness, limit interactions at night.	To prevent exhaustion.
5. Monitor eating, drinking, and elimination.	To ensure adequate nutrition, elimination.
6. Provide finger foods and nutritious drinks if client is unable to sit down for meals.	To maintain nutrition.
7. Encourage large motor activities (jogging, sweeping, raking leaves) as outlets for energy.	Provides a means of decreasing overactive behavior, uses energy in effective manner, and reduces anxiety.
8. Promote solitary activities to limit distractions.	Client is overstimulated and responds to any stimuli in the environment.
9. Provide simple activities within client's abilities to perform.	Client may move from one task to another and have difficulty completing a task that is too complex.
10. Urge client to avoid competitive activities.	Competitive activities escalate manic behavior.
11. Assist client in completing activities.	The manic client has difficulty in task completion and may initially need assistance.

NURSING ACTIONS	RATIONALE
12. Help client learn adaptive ways to channel energy without being disruptive through use of large motor skills; sweeping, raking, vacuuming.	To prevent or reduce acting-out behavior seen in the manic client. Excessive energy results in impulsive behavior.
13. Present an attitude of positive expectation that client will take medications.	To ensure cooperation with pharmacotherapy.
14. Discuss consequences of not taking medications.	Medication compliance may be problematic because client enjoys the feeling of elation.
15. Explain action of medications and side effects to client and significant others.	An understanding of the purpose and side effects of medications increases medication compliance by client and encourages significant others to become involved in treatment plan. Certain precautions need to be observed with lithium therapy.
16. Assist with personal hygiene and appropriate dress and grooming.	Hyperactive client is too busy to care for self and dresses inappropriately.
17. Provide positive reinforcement for appropriate dress and grooming.	To increase the likelihood that appropriate dress and grooming will be continued.
18. Limit hoarding of items (e.g., newspaper or gum wrappers).	Excesses are a hallmark of manic behavior and setting limits increases feelings of security.
19. Observe for infections, bruises, and injuries.	Pays little attention to health needs and may be unaware of illness or self-harm resulting from manic behavior.
20. Observe for escalating activity.	Early intervention prevents behavior from getting out of control.
21. Observe for signs of depression.	Depression is seen in conjunction with mania, and the potential for suicide becomes serious.
22. Substitute purposeful activity for disorganized action.	To assist client in regaining control of behavior.
23. Limit caffeine intake and smoking.	These drugs are often abused and may increase manic behavior.
24. Assist client to identify inappropriate sexual behaviors.	To protect client from being sexually indiscreet or making sexual references that may become a source of embarrassment following recovery.
25. Protect client from going on spending sprees or participating in unwise business ventures.	Judgment is impaired.
26. Monitor lithium level.	High levels of lithium are toxic.
27. Monitor fluid and electrolyte balance.	Inattention to eating and drinking, excessive sweating, and the gastrointestinal effects of lithium can result in a fluid and electrolyte imbalance.
28. Monitor dietary salt intake.	Lithium is a salt, and reduced sodium intake can accelerate lithium retention with subsequent toxicity; consequently, salt is included in the diet.

Emotional Dimension

1. Help client identify painful feelings (sadness, anger, guilt, and anxiety) with feedback and positive reinforcement.	Manic behavior may disguise painful feelings, and conscious awareness provides a means for dealing with them effectively.
2. Help client express painful feelings.	To promote self-awareness of feelings.
3. Assist client in staying with the painful feeling and experiencing it.	Helps client identify and name feeling.
4. Discuss other ways client can express painful feelings (e.g., writing or painting).	To increase coping skills.
5. Help client learn to enjoy simple pleasures.	To learn that satisfaction can be gained from a less adventuresome life-style.
6. Help client learn to live with a state of mind that is less than euphoric; that it is OK to be sad and disappointed at times.	Euphoria is self-rewarding, and client may be reluctant to give it up.
7. By listening actively and reflecting, help client identify feelings of being overwhelmed.	To decrease anxiety.
8. Listen to client's "feeling tone" rather than the content of client's words.	Painful feelings are not a part of client's awareness and are implied rather than verbalized.
9. Provide materials to write or draw on.	To provide an alternative to verbal expression of feelings.
10. Encourage client to assume responsibility for own health care with positive reinforcement.	To increase self-control and self-esteem.

IMPLEMENTATION—cont'd

NURSING ACTIONS	RATIONALE
Intellectual Dimension	
1. Present reality to client when ideas are unrealistic.	Reality testing is impaired.
2. Limit excessive verbal activity by focusing on one topic at a time.	To encourage self-control.
3. Interrupt when necessary to slow down stream of conversation.	To increase client's awareness of behavior.
4. Help client stay with subject being discussed.	To set limits, increase attention span.
5. Provide paper to write or draw on as a way to express thoughts.	Since logical speech is disturbed, provides an alternative to verbal expression of thoughts.
6. Ignore or distract from grandiose ideas.	To encourage a more realistic view of self.
7. Limit flight of ideas by clarifying and validating meaning of message.	To focus on logical thought processes and speech.
8. Help client become aware of effects of intrusive, domineering, and demanding behavior on others using feedback from self and others.	To reduce alienation and rejection by others.
9. Listen to hostile comments, obscenities, angry tirades, and arguments nonjudgmentally and without punitive reactions, yet set appropriate limits.	To convey acceptance of client, reduce alienation, and provide a sense of security.
10. Provide regularly scheduled activities.	To promote effective use of energy and time and reduce impulsive behavior.
11. Refrain from encouraging theatrical performing or being the center of attention.	Paying attention will escalate behavior.
12. Refrain from encouraging jokes, puns, and amusing anecdotes.	Same as #11.
13. Provide short-term activities.	Client's attention span is short; client is easily distracted and is unable to concentrate.
14. Have client explore consequences of manic behavior.	To encourage reality testing; behavior interferes with health and safety and causes client to overspend and make unwise business investments.
15. Be persuasive and authoritative in approaching client.	To prevent resistance or attempts to manipulate.
16. Assist client in developing a plan of self-care for when client is anxious or overwhelmed.	To convey the expectation that client can control own behavior.
17. Promote clients's motivation and willingness to participate in treatment by: a. Educating client and significant others about the illness. b. Teaching client and family importance of taking medications as prescribed, symptoms of side effects, and need for follow-up checks. c. Discussing thoughts and feelings associated with the possible necessity of staying on lithium for the rest of client's life.	To encourage client to assume control of behavior.
Social Dimension	
1. Provide flexible routine based on client's needs.	Attention span and concentration are decreased and client may not be able to focus on one activity for a concentrated period of time.
2. Identify environmental limits, controls, and unit regulations clearly and specifically (use of phone or visitors).	To establish limits and to provide structure.
3. Protect from overstimulation by monitoring activities.	Highly responsive to environmental and external stimuli.
4. Decrease environmental stimulation (colors, pictures, noise, furniture, people) when possible.	Same as #3
5. Limit participation in group activities and interactions.	To prevent dominating, overinvolvement.
6. Discourage others from encouraging inappropriate behavior.	Paying attention to jokes and witticisms increases the behavior to extreme levels.
7. Protect client from group's response to disruptive behavior by staying with client or moving client to another area.	Client's behavior may precipitate anger or rejection by others.

NURSING ACTIONS	RATIONALE
8. Confront discrepancies in client's perceived self and real self once relationship has been established.	To promote a more realistic self-concept.
9. Have client return articles pilfered from others.	Behaves impulsively with little regard for others; tends to take those articles that appeal to him.
10. Provide group or family therapy when activity level is decreased.	To improve functioning in family or with others.
11. Avoid being taken in by client's playful, entertaining ways.	To discourage behavior, which if encouraged will rapidly become inappropriate.
12. Limit number of staff who come in contact with client.	To decrease stimulation.
13. Refer to manic-depressive self-help groups.	To provide social support.
14. Involve family in treatment regimen.	To increase the likelihood of client cooperation with treatment plan.
Spiritual Dimension	
1. Help client accept his illness as one for which medication can relieve symptoms.	There may be a reluctance to accept lithium therapy as a lifetime need. Acceptance can release energy for more creative and productive efforts. To encourage self-actualization, to prevent future hospitalization.
2. Discuss with client ability to live a less disruptive and more satisfying life as long as client takes his medications.	Same as #1.
3. Discuss with client the fact that the "high" he experiences provides only a temporary release from the pain of reality and the fact that real life can offer "highs" with less disruption to life.	Same as #1.

EVALUATION

Measurable goals and outcome criteria provide the data for evaluating the client with manic behavior. Initial focus is on meeting the client's basic needs for health and safety. As therapeutic levels of medication are reached and behavior becomes more stabilized, observations made by the nurse, other health professionals, family members, and significant persons in the client's life contribute to an evaluation of client's readiness to learn about and understand the disease process. The following behaviors indicate that the client is making satisfactory progress:

1. Knowledgeably discusses factors contributing to behavior
2. Verbalizes the need for and cooperates with medication regimen
3. Is able to control own behavior
4. Identifies painful feelings and the way in which they affect own behavior
5. Makes realistic self-appraisals
6. Participates in less stimulating activities that provide satisfaction

BIBLIOGRAPHY

Alprazolam linked to manic behavior: *Nurses' Drug Alert* 10(1):3, 1986.

Brenners D, Harris B, Weston P: Managing manic behavior, Am *J Nurs* 87(5):620, 1987.

Fieve R: *Moodswings*, New York, 1975, Bantam Books.

Hunn S: Nursing care of patients on lithium, *Perspect Psychiatr Care* 18:214, 1980.

Keltner N: Drugs for treatment of depression and mania. In Shlafer M, Marieb E, editors: *The nurse, pharmacology, and drug therapy*, Redwood City, 1989, Addison-Wesley.

Kuyler P: Rapid cycling bipolar 1 illness in three closely related individuals, *Am J Psychiatry* 145:114, 1988.

McEnany G: Psychobiological indices of bipolar mood disorder: future trends in nursing care, *Arch Psychiatr Nurs* 4(1):29, 1990.

Pollack L: Improving relationships: groups for inpatients with bipolar disorder, *J Psychiatr Nurs* 28(5):17, 1990.

Ryan L, Montgomery A, Meyers S: Impact of circadian rhythm research on approaches to affective illness, *Arch Psychiatr Nurs* 1(4):236, 1987.

Secunda S: Diagnosis and treatment of mixed mania, *Am J Psychiatry* 144:96, 1987.

Simmons-Alling S: Genetic implications for major affective disorders, *Arch Psychiatr Nurs* 4(1):67, 1990.

Spence G: Lithium therapy: a group approach to patient education, *Can Nurse* 78(9):33, 1982.

Tirrell C, DeForest D: Neuroendocrine factors in affective disorders, *Arch Psychiatr Nurs* 1(4):225, 1987.

Young M: Establishing diagnostic criteria for mania, *J Nerv Ment Dis* 171(11):676, 1983.

Manipulation

Manipulation is controlling behavior used as a protection against failure or frustration and as a means to gain power over another person. Through manipulative behavior an individual uses others to meet his needs or achieve his goals. Either passive behavior or aggressive behavior may be directed toward or against others. The manipulator is frequently charming, full of fun, and entertaining on a superficial social level. He rarely sees himself as having difficulty and usually does not seek help voluntarily. He demonstrates little motivation for change because his behavior has inherent rewards—he accomplishes his goals. He is self-oriented, yet gives the impression of involvement with others. Other characteristics include attempts to influence others, deception, insincerity, feeling of "having put something over on another," rationalization, procrastination, and extreme compliance.

Manipulation may be subtly used by children and adolescents. Children learn to manipulate parents at an early age. Adolescents manipulate parents and teachers indirectly and directly. Manipulating behaviors test the limits of both parents and teachers.

A more serious form of manipulation is seen in the individual diagnosed as having an antisocial personality. Disrupted relationships over a period of time (or a lifetime) are characteristic of persons with an antisocial personality.

Manipulative behavior tends to evoke strong negative feelings within the individual being manipulated. Feelings include dislike, rejection, retaliation, and punishment. Such responses reinforce the manipulative individual's dependency, increase his anxiety, and foster the continued use of manipulation.

Related DSM-III-R disorders

Psychoactive substance use disorders
Antisocial personality
Conduct disorders

Other related conditions

Antisocial behavior

PRINCIPLES

▶ Physical Dimension

1. A family history of antisocial personality disorder may indicate a possible genetic basis.

▶ Emotional Dimension

1. Satisfaction of needs is the primary goal of the person who manipulates.
2. Unmet needs in infancy result in anxiety and early feelings of insecurity, with a corresponding need to manipulate.
3. Manipulation may result from parental love with "strings attached"; that is, the parents withhold love or shower the child with love as a way of coercing the child to comply with parental wishes or requests.
4. Dependence on others causes anger about being in this frustrating position and precipitates subsequent manipulation.
5. The child represses his angry feelings, fearing he will be punished for expressing them, and reveals them in his manipulation.

▶ Intellectual Dimension

1. Manipulative behavior is both consciously and unconsciously motivated.
2. Unconscious impulses and needs, usually hostile and aggressive, are communicated verbally and nonverbally and influence the behavior of the manipulator.
3. Verbal and nonverbal communication tends to be coercive, illogical, or skillfully deceptive to others.
4. If conscious needs in the person being manipulated are in conflict with those of the manipulator, the person being manipulated may respond with anger or withdrawal.
5. A power struggle may result when the unconscious needs of both the manipulator and the person being manipulated are in conflict.
6. Sporadic or inconsistent love and guidance may cause a child confusion and insecurity about himself and

about parental feelings toward him; thus manipulative behavior is adopted as a way to obtain the love and direction necessary to resolve the confusion.

▶ Social Dimension

1. Difficulty in relating to others, rejection, and punishment result in an increased need to manipulate.
2. Manipulative behavior is promoted when an individual feels incapable of meeting his own needs, does not trust himself to act, and becomes hurt when he tries; he then attempts to influence others to act for him.
3. Intense needs the individual cannot meet using his own strengths prompt the use of others.
4. The person who manipulates skillfully influences others to behave in ways intended to satisfy his own social needs.

5. When a repertoire of learned responses involves the use of others to meet personal needs, the automatic behavior that emerges is destructive manipulation.
6. The person who manipulates fails to accept responsibility for his own behavior.

▶ Spiritual Dimension

1. Lack of self-respect and self-esteem coupled with a strong need to manipulate leaves the person with little or no capacity to care about others.
2. Failure to experience comfort and protection from a parent or caretaker may lead to the development of possible identification with negative, devaluing, nongiving aspects.
3. Manipulation prevents the individual from valuing himself and achieving a sense of self-worth.

ASSESSMENT

▶ Physical Dimension

I. History
- A. Activities of daily living
  - 1. Physical activities and limitations
    - a. Exercises actively
    - b. Dawdles and is slow to move
  - 2. Sexual activity
    - a. Disturbed
    - b. Inappropriate
- B. Habits
  - 1. Alcohol
    - a. Excessive use
  - 2. Medications and drugs
    - a. Uses over-the-counter, prescribed, and illegal medications or drugs

- C. Destructive behavior
  - 1. Acts impulsively; possibly is assaultive
  - 2. Takes risks
    - a. Speeding
    - b. Drug abuse
    - c. Alcohol abuse
    - d. Legal violations
  - 3. Suicide attempts
- D. Health history
  - 1. Hospitalizations
    - a. Numerous previous admissions associated with manipulative behavior (for example, threat of suicide)
    - b. Incarceration in jail before hospital admission

▶ Emotional Dimension

CLIENT DATA	ANALYSIS	NURSING DIAGNOSIS
Depression	A response to failure in having needs met.	Ineffective individual coping: depression related to unfulfilled needs.
Abrupt mood swings	Has difficulty delaying gratification of needs. Moods change abruptly depending on whether needs are met.	Ineffective individual coping: related to abrupt mood swings
Low tolerance for frustration	Easily frustrated when obstacles interfere with meeting needs.	Ineffective individual coping: related to low tolerance for frustration
Lack of control of anger— inappropriate or exaggerated responses	Easily angered when needs are not met; dependence on others causes resentment and anger.	Ineffective individual coping: related to inappropriate anger
Lack of emotional responses, no remorse or guilt	Has difficulty knowing right from wrong; lacks social norms, a socialized conscience.	Ineffective individual coping: related to inappropriate emotional responses, no remorse or guilt

▶ **Emotional Dimension—cont'd**

CLIENT DATA	ANALYSIS	NURSING DIAGNOSIS
Lack of empathy	Caring about and understanding others demonstrated in terms of getting own needs met.	Ineffective individual coping: related to lack of empathy
Inability to tolerate boredom	Lacks ability to accept responsibility for own actions; may antagonize or intimidate others to ease boredom.	Ineffective individual coping: related to antagonizing behavior

▶ **Intellectual Dimension**

CLIENT DATA	ANALYSIS	NURSING DIAGNOSIS
Poor judgment	Thinks and acts impulsively; personality dominated by desire for pleasure. Satisfaction of needs is primary goal.	Altered thought processes: impaired judgment related to impulsivity
Lack of insight	Aspects of client's behavior seen as acceptable and consistent with client's total personality (ego syntonic); lacks understanding about why others do not comply with requests and demands.	Altered thought processes: lack of insight related to inability to see behavior as unacceptable
Preoccupation with own interests	Self-centered and narcissistic; lacks self-respect and esteem, leaving person with little capacity to care about others.	Altered thought processes: inability to show genuine interest in others related to manipulation
Impaired problem-solving abilities	Lacks insight about problem; thinks there is not one.	Altered thought processes: impaired problem-solving abilities related to lack of insight
Use of stipulations and threats	Response to anxiety and insecurity.	Ineffective individual coping: threats and stipulations related to manipulation
Intimidation of others	To make self feel better and to cover up own insecurity (compensation).	Ineffective individual coping: intimidation of others related to manipulation
Lying	To meet own needs; has difficulty knowing right from wrong; primary goal to have own needs met.	Ineffective individual coping: tells lies related to manipulation
Projection	Blames others; unable to accept responsibility for own behavior; protects self from anxiety.	Altered thought processes; use of projection related to manipulation
Denial	Denies allegations and thus reduces anxiety.	Defensive coping: use of denial related to manipulation
Rationalization	Justifies own behavior and thus reduces anxiety.	Altered thought processes: use of rationalization related to manipulation
Multiple demands or requests; presses issue or person	Attempts to get others to meet needs; communication tends to be coercive, illogical, and deceptive.	Altered thought processes: multiple demands related to manipulation
Requests special privileges	To have needs met.	Altered thought processes: requests special privileges related to manipulation
Pits personnel against each other	To get what he wants.	Altered thought processes: pits personnel against each other related to manipulation
Betrays confidences	To better serve self.	Altered thought processes: betrayal of confidences related to manipulation

▶ **Social Dimension**

CLIENT DATA	ANALYSIS	NURSING DIAGNOSIS
Feelings of inadequacy	Covers up inadequacies with feelings of power and control; feels incapable of meeting own needs.	Self-esteem disturbance: feelings of inadequacy related to manipulation
Boasting about self and achievements	To cover up feelings of inadequacy.	Self-esteem disturbance: boasts about self and achievements related to manipulation
Lack of self-respect: reprimanding self, derogating self, self-pity	A way to get others to meet needs; primary goal is to satisfy own needs.	Self-esteem disturbance: lack of self-respect related to manipulation
Overly friendly and solicitous	An approach to get own needs met by others; a repertoire of learned responses that uses others to meet needs.	Ineffective individual coping: is overly friendly and solicitous related to manipulation
Charming, flattering, seductive, or ingratiating	A way to get others to do what he want them to do; when needs are intense and he cannot meet them through use of own strengths, he seeks to satisfy them through others.	Ineffective individual coping: charming, flattering, seductive, ingratiating behavior related to manipulation
Calculating and demanding	An approach to have others meet needs.	Ineffective individual coping: calculating and demanding behavior related to manipulation
Mistrust of self	Unable to trust self without being hurt so feels safe influencing others to act for him; unmet needs in infancy result in anxiety and insecurity.	Self-esteem disturbance: inability to trust self related to manipulation
Immature, transient, and superficial in relationships	Unable to develop meaningful relationships with others.	Impaired social interaction: related to manipulation
Inability to invest in or depend on others	Mistrust of others.	Impaired social interaction: related to manipulation
Seeks others' admiration and approval	To compensate for inadequacy.	Self-esteem disturbance: seeking approval and admiration related to manipulation
Impaired ability to sustain close, warm, lasting, responsible relationships with family, friends, and sex partner	Use of others impairs ability to sustain relationships with others; parental love with "strings attached" provides client with inconsistent model.	Impaired social interaction: inability to sustain relationships related to manipulation
History of family member diagnosed as antisocial personality disorder	Possible genetic basis to client's behavior, a learned behavior.	Ineffective individual coping: manipulation related to family history of antisocial personality
Lifelong pattern of maladaptive relationships: in school, on the job, and in the community	Inability to be successful in school, at work, or in the community.	Altered role performance: impaired social functioning related to manipulation
Frequent job changes	Maladaptive relationships on the job.	Altered role performance: impaired job functioning related to manipulation
Conflicts with the law	Violates laws, fails to accept responsibility for own behavior.	Ineffective individual coping: violations of the law related to manipulation

▶ **Spiritual Dimension**

CLIENT DATA	ANALYSIS	NURSING DIAGNOSIS
Lack of socially accepted values	Inadequately socialized; accepts values as they meet needs; has difficulty clarifying values; poorly developed conscience.	Ineffective individual coping: lack of socially accepted values related to manipulation
Perception of self functioning well in life	Thinks the trouble is with others; lacks insight.	Ineffective individual coping: related to denial of problems
Use of sick role to meet own needs and avoidance of jail sentence	An approach to have needs met by others.	Ineffective individual coping: use of sick role related to manipulation
Inability to learn and grow from life experiences	Lifelong pattern of maladaptive behavior prevents growth.	Spiritual distress: inability to learn from experiences related to manipulation
Use of religion as it meets needs	Usually lacks a religious background but uses it to meet needs.	Ineffective individual coping: use of religion related to manipulation
Political, economic, or military success	Own needs met through successful use of others.	Self-esteem disturbance: ability to achieve success related to manipulation of others

PLANNING

Long-Term Goal

To express needs and wants in a clear, direct manner that does no harm to others ✓ and demonstrates responsibility for own actions

SHORT-TERM GOALS	OUTCOME CRITERIA
Physical Dimension	
To refrain from inappropriate sexual activity	1. Does not engage in inappropriate sexual activity 2. States ways to satisfy sexual needs without manipulating partner
To demonstrate habits that promote general health	1. Stops smoking 2. Refrains from excessive use of alcohol, drugs
To decrease inpulsive acts	1. Thinks through consequences of actions 2. Demonstrates self-control
Emotional Dimension	
To express feelings of frustration, powerlessness, and inadequacy	1. Expresses feelings of frustration, powerlessness, and inadequacy appropriately
Intellectual Dimension	
To identify manipulative behavior	1. Discusses events or situations that evoke manipulation 2. States behaviors that indicate manipulation
To identify own wants and needs	1. Asks for what he wants or needs directly 2. States when he cannot meet needs himself 3. Asks for help to meet need 4. Verbalizes that it is OK to ask for help
To limit manipulating behavior	1. Identifies behaviors that are manipulative 2. Limits self from using the identified manipulation 3. States alternative ways to meet needs 4. Demonstrates other ways to meet needs
To gain insight on effects of manipulative behavior on himself and others	1. States ways behavior affects himself 2. States ways behavior affects others 3. Verbalizes responsibility for own behavior 4. Verbalizes anxieties and feelings of inadequacy 5. Demonstrates willingness to participate in own treatment planning

SHORT-TERM GOALS	OUTCOME CRITERIA
To learn to delay immediate gratification of needs and wants	1. Distinguishes between needs and wants 2. Able to wait willingly for requests to be fulfilled 3. Decreases number of requests and demands 4. Attempts to be responsible for fulfilling requests himself
Social Dimension To accept responsibility for own actions	1. States he is responsible for own actions 2. Does not blame others or intimidate others 3. Does not tell lies 4. Does not rationalize or justify behavior
Spiritual Dimension To respect and value self as an adequate person who can meet needs without manipulating others	1. Makes realistic positive statements about self 2. Believes it is OK to ask directly for wants and needs 3. Asks for what he wants clearly 4. States satisfactions with independence and autonomy

Discharge Planning

The following client behaviors demonstrate readiness for discharge:
1. Identifies manipulative patterns
2. Controls impulses to achieve immediate need gratification
3. Decreases attempts to manipulate others
4. States wants and needs openly, directly

IMPLEMENTATION

NURSING ACTIONS	RATIONALE
Physical Dimension 1. Provide sex counseling.	To assist client in understanding disturbances in sexual activity.
2. Help client to lessen smoking, alcohol consumption, and indiscriminate use of drugs.	To promote general health.
3. Encourage activities that bring pleasure with fewer risks.	To enhance self-respect.
4. Direct attention to client's behavior (actions).	Focuses on behavior of others rather than on own behavior (less threatening).
5. Avoid client's attempts to focus on others' behavior (actions).	Client needs to examine own behavior.
6. Help client control impulsive actions.	To teach client how to control own behavior.
Emotional Dimension 1. Facilitate expression of angry, frustrated, or hostile feelings in a socially acceptable manner using feedback, role modeling.	Self-control is improved when energy used for acting out is converted into acceptable behavior.
2. Encourage expression of feelings of inadequacy by empathy.	To increase conscious awareness of feelings of inadequacy.
3. Promote acceptance of feelings of inadequacy in specific situations, that is, help client understand that others feel inadequate at times, that it is a normal feeling.	Client who feels inadequate is unable to provide self-support and attempts to get others to provide it. When client recognizes own feelings of inadequacy, client can begin to develop own source of self-support.
4. Promote increased frustration tolerance using stress-reducing techniques.	To teach client how to control own behavior.
5. Provide outlets for frustration.	To prevent acting-out behavior.
6. Avoid rejecting and retaliating behavior.	Manipulative client will create nurse discomfort as a way of meeting needs, and client's behavior invites rejection, retaliation, or both.

IMPLEMENTATION—cont'd

NURSING ACTIONS	RATIONALE
7. Assist client in identifying situations that produce anger, frustration, and hostile feelings.	Impulsive behavior of client requires helping him identify ways to control it.
Intellectual Dimension	
1. Explore with client consequences of behavior (threats, demands, and questions).	Client is present-oriented and has little anxiety about consequences in the future.
2. Mobilize anxiety when appropriate.	Client whose life-style is manipulative or impulsive is insensitive to anxiety. Anxiety and fear are warning signals of danger. Activating anxiety or fear is a way for client to learn to anticipate danger, to consider the consequences of actions, and to control impulsive behavior.
3. Refrain from responding to behavior such as self-pity, teasing, flattery, or use of vulgar language and risqué jokes.	Negative reinforcement of undesirable behavior decreases the likelihood of it being repeated.
4. Give feedback regarding any type of manipulative behavior.	Consistent feedback is required to increase client's awareness of own behavior.
5. Confront lies.	Increases client's awareness of behavior.
6. Accept testing of interpersonal limits.	To help client learn to control own behavior. Client will maneuver to establish interpersonal patterns that satisfy his immediate needs.
7. Help client clarify what he wants.	To discover what needs client is trying to fill through manipulation.
8. Be nonjudgmental as client examines his manipulative behavior.	Being judgmental or resentful will interfere with the therapeutic process.
9. Clarify reasons for setting limits and consequences for breaking limits.	To model open, direct communication.
10. Ensure documentation of behavior among members of health care team.	To foster among the health care team a coordinated and consistent effort to deal with manipulative behavior.
11. Be consistent in following specified limits.	Inconsistency in follow-up encourages manipulative behavior.
12. Demonstrate willingness to admit own mistakes.	Client is quick to recognize mistakes and will use them in an effort to gain control of an interpersonal situation.
13. Assist client in identifying when his needs are met and the interactions in which he was given respect and consideration.	To establish the cause-and-effect relationship between getting needs met and maintaining respect and consideration of others.
14. Use a kind, firm, matter-of-fact attitude.	To convey acceptance and consistency.
15. Continuously direct attention to client's behavior.	Same as #4.
16. Convey expectations in a clear, direct manner and request clarification from client.	So that client cannot use the excuse of misunderstanding as a way to manipulate.
17. Help client develop an ability to delay need gratification.	To help client learn by informing client of consequences of specific behaviors before behavior occurs.
18. Teach client problem-solving techniques.	To teach client effective ways of meeting needs.
19. Use modeling.	To teach client how to modify socially unacceptable behavior.
20. Foster client's motivation and willingness to participate in treatment planning with positive reinforcement.	To increase self-esteem and self-respect.
21. Promote a realistic perception of self by identifying discrepancies.	Behavior is immature and client is unaware of immature responses.
Social Dimension	
1. Explore problems in relationships.	To help client gain awareness of behavior. Has difficulty learning from experience.
2. Help client meet needs for self-respect.	To increase self-esteem.
3. Discuss alternative ways of relating to others (without seduction, or intimidating).	To teach client other modes of behavior.
4. Spend time with client when client is not demanding to be noticed.	To teach client that interpersonal needs can be met through socially acceptable behavior.

NURSING ACTIONS	RATIONALE
5. Provide a confrontation group for client to have interactions with others who manipulate.	Same as #1.
6. Include family in plans for helping client.	To teach family ways to intervene in client's manipulations and to promote cooperation with treatment plan.
7. Refer to social worker for job counseling.	Client has a history of job losses.
8. Discuss conflicts with law and consequences of violations.	Same as #1.
9. Use behavior modification.	To reinforce socially acceptable behavior.
10. Use role playing and psychodrama.	To promote awareness of behavior.
11. Positively reinforce behaviors that indicate sensitivity toward others.	Behavior that is positively reinforced is likely to be repeated.
12. Promote mature behavior and feelings of adequacy with positive feedback.	To encourage personal growth and increase feelings of self-worth.
Spiritual Dimension	
1. Help client clarify personal values and beliefs.	Client does not have a clear sense of direction in life; tends to feel carried along by events.
2. Decrease denial of problems by discussing in a nonthreatening manner the client's behavior in relation to life as a whole rather than in relation to specific hospital policies, except to examine how client's behavior on the unit reflects general behavior pattern in life.	Focuses on process rather than content.
3. Assist client in learning and growing from experiences by replacing destructive behavior with realistic, self-directed behavior that builds and maintains respect, security, and independence.	Client has difficulty in learning from past experience.
4. Promote self-awareness.	To experience a sense of self-respect and adequacy.
5. Encourage responsibility for choices by suggesting options.	To reduce dependency on others for needs satisfaction and to teach client to be self-supportive rather than relying on others for support.

EVALUATION

Measurable goals and outcome criteria provide the data for evaluating the progress in intervening with a client's manipulative behavior. Because the client may be unable to see the problem realistically, confirmation is obtained by observations of those who come in contact with client, from sources (e.g., family) that provide a developmental and social sketch of the client, and with validation from discussions with others.

Interventions are aimed at helping the client gain some insight into the effect of own behavior on self and others. The potential for meeting goals is variable and depends on the client's motivation to change behavior and capacity to learn from experience.

The following behaviors are indicators of successful intervention:

1. Recognizes and verbalizes manipulative behaviors
2. Asks directly for what he wants or needs
3. Demonstrates alternative ways to meet needs
4. Demonstrates that he is learning from past experiences

Successful intervention promotes satisfying relationships and decreases the need to manipulate.

Evaluation also involves looking at staff behavior. An effect of manipulation is parallel manipulation by staff. Staff members may react to the client by assuming that client's behavior and verbal expressions are a personal attack. Consequently, client is seen as a troublemaker, complainer, a noncooperative person, or an inappropriate admission, which results in sabotage of the treatment and disinterest in treatment outcomes.

BIBLIOGRAPHY

Bursten B: *The manipulator: a psychoanalytic view*, New Haven, Conn., 1973, Yale University Press.

Chitty K, Maynard C: Managing manipulation, *J Psychosoc Nurs Ment Health Serv* 24(6):8, 1986.

Davidhizer R: Handling manipulation, *Health Care Superv* 8(3):37, 1990.

Hirst S: The difficult patient, *Nurs Manage* 14(2):68, 1983.

Hughes J: Manipulation: a negative element in care, *J Add Nurs* 5:21, 1980.

Johnson G, Werstlein P: Reframing: a strategy to improve care of manipulative patients, *Issues Ment Health Nurs* 11(3):237, 1990.

McMurrow M: The manipulative patient, *Am J Nurs* 8(6):1188, 1981.

McMurrow M: The manipulators: how to help them and yourself, *Crit Care Update* 10(7):35, 1983.

Pelletier L, Kane J: Strategies for handling manipulative patients, *Nurs* 19(5):82, 1989.

Reid W: *The psychopath: a comprehensive study of antisocial disorders and behaviors*, New York, 1978, Brunner/Mazel.

Richardson J: The manipulative patient spells trouble, *Nurs* 11:48, 1981.

Schlemmer J, Barnett P: Management of manipulative behavior of anorexia nervosa patients, *J Psychiatr Nurs* 15(11):35, 1977.

Shahady E: Uncovering the real problems of "crocks" and "gomers," *Consultant* 24(4):33, 1984.

Shostrom E: *Man, the manipulator*, New York, 1967, Abbington Press.

Wiley P: Manipulation. In Zderad L, Belcher H: *Developing behavioral concepts in nursing*, Atlanta, 1968, Southern Regional Educational Board.

Negative Self-Concept

Self-concept consists of all the ideas, feelings, and attitudes that a person has about his own identity, worth, capabilities, and limitations. Such factors as values and opinions of others, especially in the formative years of early childhood, play an important part in the development of a person's self-concept. The nature of an individual's self-concept is a vital aspect of his overall personality. Problems with self-concept are seen in individuals having difficulty functioning in social and work situations. In addition, many emotional and mental disorders are characterized by a negative self-concept.

Negative self-concept is a composite of negative ideas an individual develops about himself. This conception of self is based on a set of values that tend to develop on perceived failures to perform adequately, in general, and on belittling responses from other individuals, particularly those deemed significant. Body image, self-esteem and self-worth, personal identity, and roles are associated with a person's self-concept. *Body image* is an individual's concept of his physical appearance and functioning. A negative body image reflects a negative perception of a person's appearance and functioning. *Self-esteem* and *self-worth* are additional components of the self-concept, reflecting the incorporation of goals and/or ideals. Negative self-esteem or self-worth reflects an individual's sense of failure to achieve at a level of performance consistent with his own expectations or ideals or those of others. *Personal identity* is the awareness of a sense of being oneself, which is derived from self-observation and judgment. It implies consciousness of oneself as an individual with a definite place in the scheme of life. Behavior that conforms with the self-concept is viewed as behavior that preserves a person's sense of identity. The roles that an individual occupies and the value that society places on those roles influence self-concept. *Roles* are sets of socially expected behaviors and influence an individual's function in various social groups. Roles may be ascribed or assumed. Ascribed roles are those over which the individual has no control, such as age and sex. Assumed roles include occupational and marital or family roles.

Each individual responds uniquely to life experiences. Therefore it is important that the nurse determine a person's usual responses to experiences before attempting intervention for persons with a negative self-concept.

Related DSM-III-R disorders

Anxiety disorders
Personality disorders
Mood disorders
Psychoactive substance-use disorders
Schizophrenia
Delusional (paranoid) disorders
Anorexia nervosa
Bulimia nervosa

Other related conditions

Obesity
Victims of abuse
Losses (body parts, body function, job, or status)
Separation or divorce
Pregnancy
Social and/or economic oppression

PRINCIPLES

▶ Physical Dimension

1. The image of one's body is central to the concept of self.
2. Body image is the mental idea a person has about his body.
3. Body image is constantly changing.
4. The quality of early life experiences with others determines how secure a child learns to feel about his body.
5. Body image gradually evolves as a component of self-concept.

The original content for this section was contributed by Elizabeth Brophy, R.N., Ph.D.

6. School experiences reinforce or weaken a child's perceptions of body and self.
7. The body is a channel through which rejection or acceptance occurs.
8. Disturbances of the body influence self-concept.
9. Body type and size influence personality development.
10. Illness causes changes in body image.
11. Physical changes in adolescence and aging may alter body image.
12. Body image is based on biological factors and experiences.
13. Intrusive procedures threaten a person's sense of wholeness.

▶ Emotional Dimension

1. Fear of rejection is inherent in those with a negative self-concept.
2. Persons with a negative view of self have feelings of inferiority, failure, incompetence, and inadequacy.
3. Suicidal feelings, the ultimate in self-hate, may be seen in persons with a negative self-concept.

▶ Intellectual Dimension

1. The ability to use conceptual systems such as language helps the individual differentiate himself from the environment.
2. The self is capable of changing.
3. Irrational assumptions about self lead to self-defeating behaviors.
4. Therapy promotes an awareness of irrational beliefs about self.
5. Parental overprotection and domination lead to feelings of helplessness and diminished curiosity.
6. Parental lack of control leads to unrealistic and frightening feelings of being all powerful.
7. Identity is a component of self-concept.
8. The individual with low self-esteem views himself, others, and the world negatively.
9. Opinions of significant others are important to the development of self-concept.

▶ Social Dimension

1. Self-esteem is an individual's personal judgment of his own worth and a component of his self-concept.
2. The frequency with which goals are achieved directly affects the development of high self-esteem.
3. Persons with high anxiety tend to have low self-esteem.
4. Persons with a lack of confidence in themselves are characterized by low self-esteem.
5. Self-esteem is derived from self and others.

6. Self-esteem is lowered when one fails to receive approval from others.
7. Self-esteem originates in childhood and is based on acceptance, praise, and respect.
8. Self-esteem is threatened whenever role changes occur.
9. Self-esteem is most threatened during adolescence.
10. Self-esteem is threatened in the aged by the challenges of retirement, menopause, loss of spouse, and physical disabilities.
11. When stressed, an individual with low self-esteem becomes anxious and responds with defenses.
12. The person with low self-esteem has difficulty meeting intimacy needs.
13. Many individuals with low self-esteem are passive dependent.
14. The self system develops in infancy and is a means of avoiding anxiety.
15. The self develops as a means to win the mothering figure's love.
16. Self-perceptions are selective and based on interpersonal feedback.
17. A positive self-concept is correlated with effective group functioning and acceptance of others.
18. Persons with negative self-perceptions tend to have ineffective communication patterns and social maladjustment.
19. Persons behave in terms of their perceptions of themselves.
20. The self-concept is learned and can be unlearned and relearned.
21. Significant others in the environment influence self-concept.
22. The primary dynamic in shaping a person's concept of self is developed from feelings of approval or disapproval in interactions with others.
23. Confirmation and validation of self by another are basic to identity formation.
24. Self-concept is influenced by social and sex roles.
25. Interactions with others in a social world determine one's concept of self.
26. During self-concept development significant others are those who provide rewards and punishments.
27. The self-concept is the self at all times and in all situations, and once established, it usually has a degree of stability.
28. Self-concept is also seen as constantly evolving and directing behavior.
29. The aspect of self in which we perceive ourselves as others see us is the social self or the "looking-glass" self.
30. Behaviors labeled good or bad influence the self-concept.
31. People tend to live up to the expectations that significant others have of them.

32. The family has a powerful influence on the child's sense of adequacy or inadequacy.
33. Cultural patterns such as social class and ascribed roles influence an individual's self-concept.
34. Individuals with positive self-concepts function effectively because they view themselves and the world positively.

▶ Spiritual Dimension

1. The self is characterized by freedom of choice.
2. The self focuses on the moment, not the past.

3. Self-concept is a system of beliefs, feelings, and attitudes a person has about himself and is predominately outside of awareness.
4. Being able to be close to another or share love is based on a person's self-concept.
5. Self-concept includes feelings of existing in one's own right and of being worthwhile as a person.
6. An individual with low self-esteem can learn to love others best after he learns to love himself.
7. An individual's tendency is toward self-actualization; those with a negative self-concept have difficulty achieving self-actualization.

ASSESSMENT

▶ Physical Dimension

I. History
  A. Activities of daily living
    1. Nutrition
      a. Overeating (obesity)
      b. Undereating (anorexia nervosa)
    2. Little or no participation in physical activities
    3. Sexual activity
      a. Excessive
      b. Inappropriate
      c. Diminished
  B. Habits
    1. Alcohol abuse
    2. Medication and drug abuse
  C. Destructive behavior
    1. Accident proneness
    2. Suicide
  D. Health history
    1. Illnesses

    a. Eating disorders
      (1) Anorexia nervosa
      (2) Bulimia nervosa
    2. Injuries—any trauma may affect self-image
    3. Surgeries—any disfiguring surgery may affect self-image
  E. Family health history
    1. Depression
    2. Suicide
    3. Substance abuse
    4. Psychoses
  F. Review of systems
    1. General
      a. Increased or decreased food intake
      b. Weight gain or loss
    2. Psychiatric—anxious, tense, and nervous

II. Diagnostic tests
  A. Electrolyte analysis (anorexia nervosa)

▶ Physical Examination

CLIENT DATA	ANALYSIS	NURSING DIAGNOSIS
Unkempt, neglects personal hygiene	Manifestation of negative self-image.	Bathing/hygiene self-care deficit: unkempt with neglect of personal hygiene related to negative self-image
Overalertness and restlessness	Low self-esteem and insecurity contribute to symptoms of anxiety.	Anxiety: overalertness and restlessness related to negative self-image
Diminished eye contact	Lessened in persons with low self-esteem; possibly a cultural norm.	Self-esteem disturbance: diminished eye contact related to negative self-image
Low, soft voice	Manifestation of negative self-image.	Self-esteem disturbance: low, soft voice related to negative self-image
Slouched posture	Manifestation of negative self-image.	Self-esteem disturbance: slouched posture related to negative self-image

▶ **Emotional Dimension**

CLIENT DATA	ANALYSIS	NURSING DIAGNOSIS
Fear of rejection	Need for approval from others; the opinions of significant others affect the development of self-concept. Rejection of self results in the expectation of rejection by others.	Self-esteem disturbance: related to fears of rejection
Feelings of inferiority	Failure to receive approval, praise from others. Reality is what the individual perceives it to be. Lacks confirmation and validation of self by another.	Self-esteem disturbance: related to feelings of inferiority
Fear of losing control	Perceived powerlessness. Experiences not consistent with the self-concept produce anxiety. Parental overprotection leads to feelings of helplessness.	Self-esteem disturbance: related to fear of losing control
Sense of self-diminution; feelings of failure, incompetency, worthlessness, inadequacy, and unimportance	Painful personal experience; responses of inadequacy from others and/or unrealistic standards contribute to inability to accept personal assets and exaggerated personal weaknesses. Irrational assumptions lead to self-defeating behaviors.	Self-esteem disturbance: related to self-diminution and feelings of failure
Lack of self-confidence; shyness and timidity	Fearfulness resulting from sense of inadequacy; difficulty with intimacy.	Self-esteem disturbance: shyness and timidity related to sense of inadequacy
Self-hate; suicidal feelings	Self-punishment and depression; persons behave in terms of their self-perception.	Self-esteem disturbance: related to self-hate and suicidal feelings

▶ **Intellectual Dimension**

CLIENT DATA	ANALYSIS	NURSING DIAGNOSIS
Poor academic performance	Insecurity and anxiety, negative perception of intellectual abilities, test anxiety. Individual labeled a failure behaves as a failure.	Self-esteem disturbance: related to poor academic performance
Inability to make decisions	Insecurity and inadequacy.	Self-esteem disturbance: related to inability to make decisions
Impaired judgment	Inability to trust self-perceptions and interpretations. Negative view of self influences view of others and world.	Self-esteem disturbance: related to impaired judgment
Preoccupation with physical symptoms	Negative perceptions of self-worth; focus on physical symptoms.	Self-esteem disturbance: related to preoccupation with physical symptoms
Sensitivity to criticism	Validates sense of inferiority.	Self-esteem disturbance: related to sensitivity to criticism
Lacking in assertiveness	Parental overprotection leading to feelings of helplessness and inadequacy.	Self-esteem disturbance: related to lack of assertiveness
Negative statements about physical appearance	Manifestation of negative self-image.	Self-esteem disturbance: related to negative self-image
Self-criticism	Manifestation of negative self-concept; self-rejection.	Self-esteem disturbance: related to self-criticism
Procrastination	Related to anxiety. Difficulty with decision making.	Self-esteem disturbance: related to anxiety over making decisions

▶ Intellectual Dimension—cont'd

CLIENT DATA	ANALYSIS	NURSING DIAGNOSIS
Denial; blaming others	Defense mechanism; reduces anxiety; self-system develops as a means to avoid anxiety.	Ineffective individual coping: related to use of defense mechanisms
Worrying	Preoccupation with inability to succeed.	Self-esteem disturbance: related to worrying
Denial of deformity, body change, and loss of function	Inability to accept body change or loss of function.	Ineffective individual coping: denial related to body changes
Grandiose thinking, boasting, and delusions	Compensation using exaggerated positive perceptions of self.	Self-esteem disturbance: exaggerated sense of self-importance related to feelings of inadequacy and inferiority

▶ Social Dimension

CLIENT DATA	ANALYSIS	NURSING DIAGNOSIS
Feelings of discomfort at social events	Lack of confidence in self; inability to fulfill self-expectations, which are unrealistic.	Self-esteem disturbance: related to unrealistic ideals and standards
Refusal to compete	Taking risks is threatening; sense of habitual failure; social maladjustment.	Self-esteem disturbance: related to perceived inadequency in competitive activities
Dependence on others	Sense of powerlessness, helplessness, and passiveness.	Self-esteem disturbance: related to dependence on others
Responsiveness to flattery	Relief of painful feelings of incompetence; need for approval from others.	Self-esteem disturbance: related to need for approval
Withdrawal from others	Belief that self is unacceptable to others.	Self-esteem disturbance: withdrawal from others related to perceived unacceptability to others
Impaired role functioning	Lack of confidence in self and abilities contributing to perceived sense of inadequacy in roles.	Altered role performance: related to inability to perceive self as capable of functioning in a given role
Lack of participation in group activities	Fearfulness caused by perceived inadequacies; fear of rejection.	Self-esteem disturbance: related to fear of inadequacies and of rejection

▶ Spiritual Dimension

CLIENT DATA	ANALYSIS	NURSING DIAGNOSIS
Perceived worthlessness and inability to succeed	Sense of inadequacy based on family and cultural influences.	Spiritual distress: related to perceived worthlessness and inability to succeed
Belief that fate controls life	Insecurity about personal values; external locus of control.	Spiritual distress: related to lack of ability to control own destiny
Negative feelings of self-worth; devaluation of self	Negative self-concept contributing to sense of worthlessness.	Spiritual distress: related to feelings of negative self-worth
Lack of clarity about personal values	Inability to clarify values because of unrealistic self-perceptions.	Spiritual distress: related to lack of clarity of values
Avoidance of responsibility for own behavior	Insecurity and fear about consequences.	Spiritual distress: related to avoidance of responsibilities
Focus on past failures	Preoccupation with past failures.	Spiritual distress: related to preoccupation with past failures
Experience of the present as "passing time"	Life without energy or excitement; sense of self dulled, and awareness of joy of living diminished or absent.	Spiritual distress: related to diminished or absent joy in living

PLANNING

Long-Term Goals

To cope adequately with threats to the self and maintain a realistic perception
   of self

To establish a positive self-concept

SHORT-TERM GOALS	OUTCOME CRITERIA
Physical Dimension	
To accept and like own body	1. Makes positive statements about body 2. Uses humor when discussing less well-liked parts of body 3. Emphasizes well-liked parts 4. Identifies distortions in beliefs regarding body image 5. Verbalizes acceptance of imperfections, disfigurements, and losses 6. Identifies the relationship between negative self-concept and body image
Emotional Dimension	
To have positive feelings about self	1. Makes positive statements about self 2. Makes positive statements about others 3. Experiences success in activities and tasks 4. Identifies strengths, skills, and assets 5. Loses (or gains) weight 6. Makes own decisions 7. Accepts compliments
To reduce anxiety	1. Identifies threats to self 2. Uses anxiety-reducing techniques (see Anxiety, p. 48)
Intellectual Dimension	
To identify the causes of negative self-concept	1. Explores sources of threats 2. Discusses negative self-concept related to family and cultural norms 3. Discusses negative self-concept related to religious beliefs 4. Discusses negative self-concept related to past personal failures 5. Discusses negative self-concept related to perceptions of inadequately performed role functions
To alter ineffective coping mechanisms related to a negative self-concept	1. Identifies commonly used coping mechanisms pertaining to a negative self-concept 2. Discusses the degree of effectiveness achieved by the use of previously employed coping mechanisms 3. Explores pros and cons of alternative coping mechanisms related to perceptions of self 4. Selects and begins to use alternate coping mechanisms 5. Gives self positive affirmations for new coping mechanisms 6. Involves family and significant others for support with new coping behaviors
To identify negative thoughts about self	1. Describes perception of self 2. States differences in idealized self and perceived self 3. Recognizes self as being what one is and not what one wishes to be 4. Stops blaming, criticizing, and devaluing himself

SHORT-TERM GOALS	OUTCOME CRITERIA
Social Dimension	
To assume responsibility for enhancing own self-concept	1. Acknowledges influence of previous experience in the formation of own self-concept
	2. Identifies chosen modes of behavior based on a rational exploration and evaluation of own behavior
	3. Is aware of alternate modes of responses to given situations
	4. Acknowledges behavior that enhances self-concept
Spiritual Dimension	
To identify values and beliefs that create negative thoughts about self	1. Explores values and beliefs related to self
	2. Clarifies personal values and beliefs
To be able to love self and others	1. Responds spontaneously in presence of others
	2. Verbalizes the components of love, for example, respect, sensitivity, and responsibility
	3. Verbalizes acceptance of self and others

Discharge Planning

The following client behaviors demonstrate readiness for discharge:
1. Identifies common manifestations of a negative self-concept
2. Uses effective coping mechanisms in threatening situations that do not devalue self
3. Perceives self realistically

IMPLEMENTATION

NURSING ACTIONS	RATIONALE
Physical Dimension	
1. Work with client toward acceptance of physical deformities, disfigurings, and/or loss of function by identifying areas of concern and suggesting options for thinking and feeling about them.	Disturbances of the body influence self-concept.
2. Explore with client ways he can maximize his physical potential.	Body image is a component of self-concept; a positive change in body image will have positive effects on self-concept.
3. Help client identify physical strengths and assets.	Body image is a component of self-concept. Improving the body image will have beneficial effects on the self-concept.
4. Help client learn to like his body despite imperfections.	To accept self.
5. Assist client in improving personal hygiene and grooming.	To promote self-esteem.
6. Help client gain (or lose) weight.	Same as #5.
7. Help client learn to speak in a loud, clear voice.	To promote confidence in self.
8. Help client improve posture.	Same as #6.
9. Encourage client to become involved in activities in which he can be successful.	To improve self-concept.
10. Discuss contemporary or historical persons who succeeded despite handicaps or limitations.	To provide a model, to provide inspiration, and to motivate the client.
11. Help client identify inappropriate emphasis on physical symptoms.	Negative perceptions of self-worth are manifested by preoccupation with physical symptoms.

IMPLEMENTATION—cont'd

NURSING ACTIONS	RATIONALE
Emotional Dimension	
1. Examine with client specific feelings regarding self.	Client's view of self is a vital aspect of his personality.
2. Encourage client to express emotions, fears, feelings of inferiority, sadness, and grief about body changes by listening actively, reflecting, and clarifying.	To provide catharsis.
3. Reduce anxiety with stress-reduction methods.	To experience more security and more confidence in self.
4. Help client accept body changes and losses in functioning and feel good about body by discussing changes and considering other ways to view them.	To improve body image, which will have beneficial effects on self-concept. Body image is a component of self-concept.
5. Help client focus on what he feels rather than why he feels.	To increase awareness of dissociated feelings. Emphasizes wholeness of human experience.
6. Have client identify an emotion and then explore manifestations of that emotion.	To increase awareness of emotions and their physiological effects.
7. Discuss relationship between feelings of worthlessness and failure with negative thoughts about self.	To teach the relationship between thoughts and feelings.
Intellectual Dimension	
1. Explore client's underlying negative assumptions about self.	To identify causes of negative self-concept.
2. Focus on current behaviors and experiences.	To reduce self-criticism of past behaviors and to reduce blaming past events for present behavior.
3. Reward behaviors based on new insights.	Behavior that is rewarded is likely to be repeated.
4. Teach problem-solving techniques.	Learning to solve problems helps in decision making and increases self-esteem.
5. Provide opportunities to make decisions.	Has difficulty making decisions because of anxiety.
6. Encourage client's responsibility for own behavior.	To teach client that he has choices and to reinforce ability to be supportive to self.
7. Explore jointly client's previously used coping mechanisms and their usefulness.	To determine and alter ineffective coping mechanisms that perpetuate a negative self-concept.
8. Discuss the pros and cons of alternate coping mechanisms.	To help client learn he has choices.
9. Help client affirm and strengthen identity by exploring feelings about self and focusing on positive attributes, skills, talents.	To improve self-concept.
10. Explore with client realistic perception of self.	Irrational assumptions about self lead to self-defeating behaviors.
11. Explore client's negative perception of self, focusing on reasons for it, where it comes from, who else agrees with it, what purpose it serves.	To increase reality testing.
12. Teach client positive affirmations about self.	To focus on the positive rather than on the negative. Promotes self-care.
13. Limit client's self-criticism.	To interrupt preoccupation with self-blame.
14. Limit worry time to 10 to 15 minutes per day.	To reduce preoccupation and to teach client that there are alternatives to worrying.
15. Be aware that grandiose thinking is compensation for low self-esteem.	The nurse's awareness of psychodynamics increases the effectiveness of interventions.
16. Have client list positive assets.	To increase reality testing.
17. Teach client to change negative statements about self to positive ones.	To change negative irrational beliefs about self to rational positive beliefs.
18. Teach techniques to stop self-defeating thoughts.	To promote new coping mechanisms.
19. Teach stress management.	To reduce anxiety.
20. Assist client in recognizing that feeling worthless, like a failure, inadequate, and incompetent do not mean that he is any of these.	To increase reality testing.
21. Assist client in recognizing that thoughts of failure and inadequacy may result in feelings of failure and inadequacy.	To establish cause-and-effect relationship.
22. Teach client to become aware of negative self-statements and their emotional and physical effects.	Same as #21.

NURSING ACTIONS	RATIONALE
23. Teach client to give and receive compliments.	To increase self-confidence and social skills.
24. Teach client to focus on others, as well as on self.	To lessen preoccupation with negative thoughts about self.
25. Involve client in assertiveness training.	Same as #23.
26. Reinforce positive self-statements.	Behavior that is reinforced is likely to be repeated.
27. Explore negative stereotypes associated with sexual identity and social roles.	Self-concept is influenced by social and sex roles.
28. Discuss ways client avoids reality or excuses behavior.	To promote insight.
29. Discuss client's beliefs about success and failure and realistic or unrealistic aspects of each.	To increase reality testing.
30. Discuss fears about taking risks in relationships.	To increase assertive behavior. To lessen helplessness.
31. When client excuses self with "I tried," remind that trying affords an excuse and ask to change the statement to "I will."	To interrupt self-defeating behavior and encourage responsibility.
32. Assist client in recognizing that worrying about the future will not change it.	To teach constructive coping.

Social Dimension

1. Encourage participation in group interactions.	To increase social skills and self-confidence.
2. Identify and discuss past behaviors that were functional and those that were dysfunctional in group interaction.	To encourage awareness of own behavior.
3. Identify and discuss self-expectations in group setting.	To encourage reality testing.
4. Practice alternate behaviors through role playing.	To increase client's understanding of own and others' behavior.
5. Encourage interaction with allied professionals, for example, vocational counselors.	To improve role functioning.
6. Involve family and/or significant others in therapy.	To increase cooperation with treatment plan.
7. Explore the meaning of dependence, independence, and interdependence and discuss how these concepts apply to client's life.	To clarify the meaning of dependence, independence, and interdependence. Client feels powerless and helpless; depends on others and has difficulty acting independently.
8. Provide social group activities and interactions in which client can feel successful.	To increase self-confidence.
9. Help client learn to trust self by building self-confidence.	To increase confidence in self.
10. Help client improve social skills.	Same as #9.
11. Promote independence in relationships; be aware that flattery meets client's needs for approval and acceptance, and that he can be easily manipulated by those who flatter him.	To prevent manipulation by flattery.
12. Have client initiate new friendships.	Confirmation and validation of self by another is essential for a positive self-concept.
13. Explore with client how negative self-concept affects relationship.	To establish a cause-and-effect relationship.
14. Refer client for vocational guidance if needed.	Lack of confidence in self and abilities may have interfered with career goals.

Spiritual Dimension

1. Identify values and beliefs related to client's negative self-concept.	To determine rational and irrational aspects of client's beliefs.
2. Explore client's beliefs and those of any organized religious group of which he is a member that may contribute to his negative self-concept.	Client lacks clarity about personal values and may be unable to make a realistic appraisal of the religious group's beliefs.
3. Examine unrealistic moral principles regarding self.	To determine rational and irrational aspects of client's beliefs.
4. Help client objectively review perceived past inadequacies.	To promote reality testing.

IMPLEMENTATION—cont'd

NURSING ACTIONS	RATIONALE
5. Promote feelings of worth and uniqueness as an individual through caring and empathy.	To increase self-esteem.
6. Help client gain sense of inner control so that he feels more in control of own destiny.	To increase feelings of adequacy and of control of own destiny.
7. Play games with client.	To encourage spontaneous, pleasurable responses.
8. Help client see humor in situations and laugh.	To reduce despair and to provide a different perspective.
9. Promote self-awareness through use of all senses and an appreciation of things seen, smelled, heard, touched, and tasted.	To encourage movement toward self-actualization.

EVALUATION

Evaluation of nursing interventions is essential because of the dynamic, changing character of human behavior. Measurable goals and outcome criteria form the basis for measuring a client's progress in achieving a positive self-concept. The following behaviors indicate a positive evaluation:

1. Accepts self as a person with unique characteristics, flaws, and imperfections
2. Experiences success in activities and tasks
3. Makes positive statements about self and others
4. Becomes successful in work, school, or home performance and in interactions with others

BIBLIOGRAPHY

Akhtar S: The syndrome of identity diffusion, *Am J Psychiatry* 141(11):1381, 1984.

Austin J, Champian V, Tzeng O: Cross-cultural relationships between self-concept and body image in high school boys, *Arch Psychiatr Nurs* 3(4):234, 1989.

Brundage D, Broadwell DC: Altered body image. In Phipps W et al, editors: *Medical-surgical nursing: concepts and clinical practice*, ed 4, St Louis, 1991, Mosby—Year Book.

Campbell J: A test of two explanatory models of women's responses to battering, *Nurs Res* 38(1):18, 1989.

Coopersmith S: *The antecedents of self-esteem*, San Francisco, 1967, WH Freeman.

Crouch M, Straub V: Enhancement of self-esteem in adults, *Fam Commun Health* 6(2):65, 1983.

Erikson E: *Childhood and society*, New York, 1963, WW Norton.

Stanwyck D: Self-esteem through the life span, *Fam Commun Health* 6:11, 1983.

Steffenhagen R, Burns J: *The social dynamics of self-esteem,* New York, 1987, Praeger.

Suls J: *Psychological perspectives on the self,* vol 1, Hillsdale, NJ, 1982, Lawrence Erlbaum Associates.

Taft L: Self-esteem in later life: a nursing perspective, *Adv Nurs Science* 8(1):77, 1985.

Negativism

Negativism is behavior characterized by marked resistance to a stimulus in which an individual actively or passively opposes conformation with the stimulus. Resistance and opposition are behaviors commonly displayed by individuals experiencing negativistic feelings. Resistance is exhibited as sullen, contrary, unaccommodating, antagonistic, and pessimistic verbal and nonverbal behaviors toward an object, person, or situation. Opposition is the refusal to do something that is expected or requested, or doing exactly what one is not expected or requested to do. These behaviors are characteristic of everyone during specific developmental levels and at various times, but what distinguishes the negativistic personality are the erratic and vacillating frequency and intensity with which these behaviors are displayed. The negativistic individual perceives his negative behavior as based on reality and is unaware of avoiding reality. He views his negativistic behavior as a demonstration of his strength, but the negativism actually arises from feelings of immaturity, inadequacy, and ambivalence.

Related DSM-III-R disorders

Anxiety disorders
Disorders of impulse control not elsewhere classified
Mood disorders
Delusional (paranoid) disorders
Personality disorders
Schizophrenia
Psychoactive substance-use disorders
Conduct disorders
Oppositional defiant disorders

Other related conditions

Chronically physically ill
Spinal cord injuries
Cerebrovascular accidents
Grief reactions

The original content for this section was contributed by Jo Cox Hasley, R.N., M.N.Sc.

PRINCIPLES

▶ Physical Dimension

1. The erratic and vacillatory behaviors displayed by the negativistic individual may arise in the limbic system.
2. Negativistic individuals may possess an intrinsic irritability or hyperreactivity to stimulation.

▶ Emotional Dimension

1. Negativistic behaviors of resistance and opposition normally occur around the second year of life when the child is developing a superego and internalizing a system of control.
2. Adolescents display negativistic behaviors during their quest for independence and separation from parental control.
3. Some individuals, when threatened by external controls, persist in exhibiting resistance and opposition, and thus negativistic behaviors become a personality trait.
4. Negativistic individuals react immaturely, that is, with little control and few other defense mechanisms. They behave erratically and vacillate in their response to persons, events, and situations.
5. Negativism, as a psychological defense reaction, may be carried to great extremes.
6. Extreme negative behavior may be expressed as mutism and refusal of food or care.

▶ Intellectual Dimension

1. Illogical thought patterns of being flawed, inadequate, worthless, or unsuccessful generate negativistic perceptions by the individual about himself.
2. Assigning excessive significance to events or situations involving loss or failure as well as to obstacles hindering successes perpetuates negativistic thought patterns.
3. Expectations of gloom and doom regarding future events or situations result in a negativistic outlook.

▶ **Social Dimension**

1. Children learn by observing behavior displayed by their parents or caregivers and then enact the same behaviors in similar situations.
   a. The negativistic adult may have developed a resistant and oppositional personality as a product of childhood exposure to parents in frequent conflict.
   b. A child's ambivalent behavior occurs when he is told by his parents that he should think, behave, or feel one way and then observes contradictory modeling by his parents.
2. Sibling rivalry results in negativism when an elder child feels replaced by a younger sister or brother.
3. The feeling of intense loss of a parent's love or attention can bring about negative thoughts of never regaining what was lost.
4. The loss of security may result in a lifelong negative feeling that nothing good or secure is lasting.
5. A child exposed to contradictory parental communications, that is, verbal praising and nonverbal criticizing, becomes caught in the bind of not knowing how to correctly interpret the message.
6. Intrafamilial communication transmits simultaneous messages that incompatibly convey acceptance and rejection.
7. Reinforcement of negativistic behaviors occurs when people with whom the negativistic individual interacts either continue trying to keep the negative person content and appeased or stop trying because of the futility of such efforts.
8. The elderly individual with organic brain syndrome who desires another's attention may display childlike negativistic behaviors as a manifestation of regression.

▶ **Spiritual Dimension**

1. When an individual feels bad about the future, negativistic behaviors may occur.
2. An individual who believes there is no real purpose to life has a negativistic outlook.
3. Negativistic behaviors occur when an individual is without a sense of well-being about the direction of life.
4. When an individual does not perceive strength and support from God or a supreme power, a negativistic outlook may occur.
5. An individual who believes a supreme being is not interested in his life may develop negativistic personality traits.
6. Judeo-Christian-Islamic beliefs view the individual as being loved and valued by God, an important factor for alleviating negativism.
7. The Hindu and Buddhist belief that humans are the victims of ignorance of their true identity and will continue to suffer as long as they remain in unenlightened ignorance may be used to encourage the negativistic person to examine his response to life.

ASSESSMENT

▶ **Physical Dimension**

I. History
   A. Activities of daily living
      1. Nutrition
         a. Appetite
            (1) Absent or poor
         b. Eating patterns
            (1) Rejects food
            (2) Undereats
         c. Weight changes
            (1) Loss
      2. Sleep
         a. Insomnia
         b. Refusal to get out of bed
      3. Recreation, hobbies, and interests
         a. Initially engrossed
         b. Quickly disenchanted
      4. Physical activities and limitations
         a. Little or no involvement in activities
         b. Muscular rigidity when touched by others
      5. Sexual activity
         a. Abstinence
         b. Aclimactic sexual behavior
   B. Health history
      1. Drug and alcohol abuse
      2. Smoking
   C. Review of systems
      1. Gastrointestinal
         a. Refusal to swallow
         b. Vomiting
         c. Constipation
      2. Genitourinary
         a. Urine retention

▶ **Physical Examination**

CLIENT DATA	ANALYSIS	NURSING DIAGNOSIS
Untended, unkempt, with disheveled clothing	Lack of concern for personal appearance because of poor self-concept and negative outlook.	Bathing/hygiene self-care deficit: related to decreased interest in body, inability to make decisions, and feelings of worthlessness
Weight loss	Diminished appetite and reduced eating resulting from feelings of personal worthlessness and future hopelessness.	Altered nutrition. less than body requirements related to refusal to eat
Muscular rigidity	Possible response to external stressors; usually seen in catatonic schizophrenia; extreme resistance.	*Altered motor behavior: related to feelings of loss of control, fear of others, or avoidance
Reduced physical activity	Possible response to external stressors.	*Altered motor behavior: related to feelings of loss of control, fear of others, or avoidance
Insomnia	Preoccupation with dismal thoughts may diminish ability to achieve peaceful rest.	Sleep pattern disturbance: related to decreased activity level and interest in life activities
Refusal to swallow; vomiting	Feelings of poor self-concept and hopelessness for the future may precipitate lost or diminished appetite; usually seen in schizophrenics, and then only rarely.	Altered nutrition: less than body requirements related to ineffective individual coping
Constipation	Feelings of loss of control and fear of others or altered life-style may slow gastrointestinal processes.	Colonic constipation: related to self-induced resistance, inadequate diet, or inadequate exercise
Failure to void	May stem from feelings of fear of others or loss of control; usually seen in schizophrenics, and then only rarely.	Altered patterns of urinary elimination: urine retention related to self-induced resistance or inadequate fluid intake
Sexual abstinence, aclimactic sexual behavior	Feelings of poor self-concept or pessimistic attitude toward relationship or future.	Sexual dysfunction: related to decreased sex drive, loss of interest and pleasure, secondary to altered self-concept

▶ **Emotional Dimension**

CLIENT DATA	ANALYSIS	NURSING DIAGNOSIS
Sullen	Upset at course of events, person, or situation; dissatisfied; frequency of sullenness a distinguishing characteristic.	Ineffective individual coping: related to habitual resistance
Antagonism	Antagonism toward whatever is encountered.	Ineffective individual coping: related to antagonistic behavior
Contrariness	Stubborn resistance to cooperation; inflexibility.	Ineffective individual coping: related to contrariness
Discontent	Never satisfied; vacillates from one thing to another.	Ineffective individual coping: discontent; inability to find satisfaction in events, situations, self, or others related to negativism
Lability	Displays a rapid succession of moods; emotions are "worn on their sleeves"; excitable and impulsive; may burst into tears or anger.	Ineffective individual coping: marked mood shifts related to negativistic behavior
Easily angered	Quick tempered; easily provoked by minor events or insignificant behaviors on the part of others.	*Anger: related to irritations with minor events or behaviors of others
Guilt	Result of anger and resentment and is used to curtail those emotions.	*Guilt: related to anger and resentment

▶ Intellectual Dimension

CLIENT DATA	ANALYSIS	NURSING DIAGNOSIS
Distorted perceptions, preoccupation with negative thoughts, belief that all relationships are doomed, excessive thoughts of failure	Discrepancies with reality; attaches exaggerated significance to irrational thoughts of unworthiness and unreal expectations.	Altered thought processes: cognitive distortions related to negative cognitive set
Marked ambivalence	Vacillates between dogmatically held views; feelings of insecurity in capabilities and lack of confidence in choices and self.	*Altered decision making: ambivalence related to lack of confidence in choices and in self
Indecisiveness	Unable to make a commitment to anything.	*Altered decision making: related to inability to make commitments
Expecting difficulties	Perceives and anticipates difficulties where none exist.	Altered thought processes: cognitive distortions related to negative expectations
Projection	Defense mechanism to relieve anxiety; blames others for causing feelings of anger.	Ineffective individual coping: projection related to inability to accept own angry, negative feelings
Impulsiveness	Every new situation seems to elicit a separate and different emotion; no consistency and no predictability to reactions.	*Altered impulse processes: related to unpredictability and inconsistencies of emotional responses to new situations
Inflexibility	Perceives different events as if they were the same.	Altered thought processes: related to inflexible perception of events related to negativism

▶ Social Dimension

CLIENT DATA	ANALYSIS	NURSING DIAGNOSIS
Worthlessness	Belief that one has little or no value as a person; disregard of successes and emphasis of failings possibly stem from low self-esteem; belief that one is destined to fail.	Self-esteem disturbance: chronic low self-esteem related to feelings of worthlessness and failure
Pushes others to the limit; antagonizes others	Efforts directed at testing relationships; expedites failure of relationships through the other's display of perceived disloyalty.	Impaired social interaction: related to inability to maintain enduring attachments
Explodes unpredictably	Easily exasperated and angered.	Impaired social interactions: related to alienation of others by unpredictable explosive behavior
Expects difficulties in relationships	Believes that good things do not last and protectively disengages when things are going well.	Impaired social interactions: related to expectations of difficulties; inability to maintain enduring attachments
Does the opposite of what is normally expected	Exposed to incompatible messages, which convey acceptance and rejection.	Impaired social interactions: related to effects of negative behavior on forming and maintaining relationships

▶ **Spiritual Dimension**

CLIENT DATA	ANALYSIS	NURSING DIAGNOSIS
Pessimistic	Taking the gloomiest outlook for future; forlorn; irrational feelings of low self-concept and hopelessness for future.	Hopelessness: related to negative beliefs about self-worth and abilities
Purposelessness	Lacking a worthwhile direction in which to channel life.	Spiritual distress: related to negative beliefs about purpose in life
Godforsaken	Belief that God or any supreme being is neither interested in nor supportive of client.	Spiritual distress: related to alienation from a higher power

PLANNING

Long-Term Goal

To identify and explore negative thoughts and learn ways of reducing negativism

SHORT-TERM GOALS	OUTCOME CRITERIA
Physical Dimension	
To identify physical sensations precipitated by negative thoughts and feelings	1. Verbalizes awareness of physical changes related to negative thoughts and feelings 2. Verbalizes identification of specific alterations in specific physical sensation occurring with negative thoughts and feelings
Emotional Dimension	
To recognize the feeling of anger	1. Verbalizes description of angry feelings 2. Acknowledges nonverbal cues that communicate anger 3. Verbalizes a name for angry feelings 4. Discusses discomfort of experiencing anger
To recognize the feeling of irritation	1. Verbalizes description of the feeling of irritation 2. Acknowledges nonverbal cues that communicate irritation 3. Verbalizes a name for feelings of irritation 4. Discusses discomfort of experiencing irritation
To recognize the feeling of resentment	1. Verbalizes description of feelings of resentment 2. Acknowledges nonverbal cues that communicate resentment 3. Verbalizes a name for feelings of resentment 4. Discusses discomfort of experiencing resentment
To recognize the relationship between feelings of anger, irritation, resentment, and negativism	1. Discusses relationship between feelings of anger, irritation, and resentment 2. Acknowledges similarities in anger, irritation, and resentment 3. Acknowledges differences in anger, irritation, and resentment
Intellectual Dimension	
To identify thoughts that precipitate negative feelings	1. Verbalizes how thoughts are related to negative feelings 2. Discusses how past feelings are related to beliefs and values 3. Discusses how feelings of failure and unworthiness are related to unrealistic expectations
To identify situations that precipitate negative thoughts	1. Discusses details of situations that precipitate negative thoughts
To explore past experiences and interactions that resulted in negative beliefs and values	1. Verbalizes awareness of prior life events and relationships that affect current values and beliefs

PLANNING—cont'd

SHORT-TERM GOALS	OUTCOME CRITERIA
To examine negative thought-provoking situations and contrast to positive thought-provoking situations	1. Verbalizes that different situations produce different results; not all situations are negative, and not all situations are positive. Balance can be achieved.
To alter irrational beliefs and values	1. Verbalizes irrational aspects of beliefs and values
To identify and explore alternative constructive behaviors	1. States how future behavior can facilitate an increase in positive thought-provoking situations
Social Dimension	
To identify aspects of behavior that contribute to negative outcomes in interactions and relationships	1. Discusses behavior and those aspects that produce failures and unsatisfactory relationships 2. Discusses behavior and its role in producing successful outcomes and satisfying interpersonal relationships 3. Verbalizes behaviors that, in probability, will contribute toward positive experiences and successes
To examine effect of past failures, successes, and satisfactory and unsatisfactory experiences and relationships on current situations and relationships	1. Discusses impact of past behavior and experiences on current value and belief system
To elevate self-esteem	1. Acknowledges own worthiness and personal value 2. Verbalizes realistic self-expectations 3. Discusses positive attributes 4. Verbalizes method of reinforcing self for positive thought-producing behaviors 5. Verbalizes positive self-concept and belief in ability to positively direct life 6. Verbalizes acceptance for responsibility of changing from negative thought and behavior patterns to positive thought and behavior patterns
Spiritual Dimension	
To pursue successes and positive outcomes in life experiences and relationships	1. Verbalizes optimistic prediction for present and future successes in situations and relationships and for satisfying experiences
To examine and clarify values and beliefs about the meaningfulness of life	1. Acknowledges value in performing creative and enjoyable work 2. Acknowledges freedom to choose attitude in any given situation 3. Acknowledges the right to dignity in any given situation
To clarify beliefs and resolve conflicts about God or a supreme being	1. Verbalizes value as a human being 2. Verbalizes worthiness of respect as a human being 3. Acknowledges freedom of choice to direct life experiences

Discharge Planning

The following client behaviors demonstrate readiness for discharge:
1. Identifies situations that evoke negative behavior or feelings
2. Identifies thoughts, emotions, and behaviors that reduce negativism and increase positive and successful outcomes
3. Has positive methods of coping with negative behaviors
4. Positively reinforces self for positive or success-oriented behaviors and outcomes

IMPLEMENTATION

NURSING ACTIONS	RATIONALE
Physical Dimension	
1. Encourage attendance to early physical messages associated with behaviors that precipitate negative outcomes, thoughts, and emotions.	To promote awareness of how negative emotions and thoughts elicit identifiable physical sensations.
Emotional Dimension	
1. Encourage client to examine negative emotion–evoking thoughts, behaviors, and experiences.	To promote awareness of negative behavior and its impact on client and others.
2. Verbally praise client for positive efforts resulting in successful outcomes.	To reinforce positive behavior.
3. Assist client in identifying feelings of anger, irritation, and resentment.	To promote awareness of feelings associated with negative behavior.
4. Observe for nonverbal cues that indicate anger, irritation, and resentment.	To help client acknowledge feelings of anger, irritation, or resentment.
5. Encourage client to discuss uncomfortable feelings of hurt, irritation, or anger.	To promote awareness of uncomfortable feelings and consider options for handling them.
6. Discuss relationship between feelings of anger, irritation, or resentment and behavior.	To help client link feelings to behavior and gain an understanding of his behavior.
7. Convey to client that irritation, resentment, and anger are normal responses.	To assist client in accepting feelings and understanding that it is the way he handles them that may be troublesome.
8. Be aware that client places responsibility on others for his negativism.	To identify use of defense mechanism, projection.
9. Assist client in experiencing situations that result in laughter, fun, and spontaneous expression of positive feelings.	Experiencing positive feelings leads to pleasure and optimism and tends to reduce negativism.
Intellectual Dimension	
1. Encourage identification of past experiences that produced negative expectations.	To help client consider causes of negative behavior and reevaluate conclusions.
2. Assist client in exploring and verbalizing thoughts about situations surrounding negative experiences.	To consider other ways of viewing situations.
3. Encourage identification of irrational aspects of negative beliefs about situations.	To promote realistic thinking.
4. Encourage identification of success behaviors with positive outcome.	To provide experiences that result in positive attitudes.
5. Encourage identification of realistic goals and objectives.	To prevent failure and increased negativism.
6. Encourage realistic expectations of self, others, and situations.	To lessen possibility of failure with accompanying negativism.
7. Encourage identification of behaviors used to express negativism.	To increase awareness of behaviors needing to be changed.
8. Identify strength or value of reinforcers.	To determine which will offer significant rewards for behavior change.
9. Contract with client for behavioral changes that are mutually agreed on. Include a list of required daily activities and behavioral changes with rewards and punishments for, respectively, fulfilling or defaulting on agreed changes.	To clarify and delineate for client the staff's expectations.
10. Make available to client and all involved staff a copy of the contract to remind them of contract terms and goals.	To involve staff in a unified and consistent effort.
11. Assist client in exploring and verbalizing detailed thoughts about past successes.	To foster positive attitudes regarding current endeavors, situations, and relationships.
12. Teach client self-affirmation and positive self-talk (e.g., "I did a good job.").	To reinforce positive thinking.
13. Teach client thought stopping for negative and self-devaluating statements.	To reinforce positive thinking.

IMPLEMENTATION—cont'd

NURSING ACTIONS	RATIONALE
14. Positively reinforce client's positive self-statements.	To give feedback for positive attitudes and behavior.
15. Fully involve client in the plan of care.	To prevent increased negativism. Participation in planning promotes cooperation and positive attitudes by helping client feel in control of health care.
16. Assist client in focusing attention on one thing or event.	To help client sort out thoughts about a particular event and prevent him from being overwhelmed by many situations with negative outcomes.
17. Explore with client the effects of negative expectations.	To promote awareness of the self-fulfilling prophecy of negative expectations.
18. Discuss meaning of self-fulfilling prophecy.	To help client understand effects of negative expectations.
19. Ask client to keep a daily journal listing situation, emotion experienced, and negative thought.	To create awareness of negative behavior.
20. Assist client in identifying a rational alternative thought for the negative thought and then identify the emotional outcome associated with the rational thought.	To promote problem solving that results in changing negative thoughts to positive ones.
21. Encourage client to assume responsibility for this technique as client's skill level improves.	To motivate client to actively participate in behavioral change.
22. Teach problem-solving techniques that can be substituted for expressions of negativism.	To teach client a skill that may result in less negative behavior.
23. Teach client to ask for and to demonstrate affection for appropriate others.	To help client experience positive effects of warmth and affection.
24. Teach client to reduce impulsivity by saying to himself, "Stop for a minute and consider the situation before I act."	To help client reduce negative effects of impulsive behavior.
25. Teach client decision making and abiding by the decision to reduce vacillatory and contradictory behaviors.	To give client skill and confidence in his ability to change his behavior.

Social Dimension

NURSING ACTIONS	RATIONALE
1. Reduce opportunities for negative choices, outcomes, and failures.	To discourage negative behavior.
2. Promote awareness of behaviors and choices that facilitate successful relationships and interactions.	To gain insight about behaviors that result in establishing relationships.
3. Incorporate support for client from staff, other clients, and significant others.	To increase their understanding and acceptance of client and his treatment and to interrupt negative cycle.
4. Refrain from imposing demands on client that are unrealistic and premature.	To reduce probability of negative outcomes and failures.
5. Consistently verbalize positive behaviors and encourage client to consciously become aware of successful outcomes and positive responses during interactions with others. Have client count and review the positive experiences at day's end.	To promote self-motivation for changing behavior.
6. Encourage participation in pleasurable activities shared with significant others that result in positive interpersonal interactions.	To increase number of positive experiences and lessen number of negative ones.
7. Encourage role playing and role reversal.	To assist client in determining effects of negative behavior on others.
8. Avoid arguing with client regardless of provocation. Refrain from displaying anger or dissension.	To maintain therapeutic relationship and prevent client from viewing relationship as one doomed to failure.
9. Involve client in group therapy.	To promote confrontation with negative behavior.
10. Discuss client's unrealistic expectations of others, testing in relationships, and contributions to failure of a relationship.	To help client connect negative behavior to failure in relationships.
11. Discuss effects of pessimistic anticipations on relationships.	To help client understand effects of pessimistic attitudes.
12. Enhance self-concept through reduction of contradictory appraisals (see Negative Self-Concept, p. 231).	To help client reduce contradictory appraisals of self.

NURSING ACTIONS	RATIONALE
Spiritual Dimension	
1. Examine moral beliefs and values that facilitate successful living and identify those to be avoided, those which foster negative outcomes.	To promote positive experiences in living and enhance optimism about life.
2. Encourage increases in belief of worthiness, value, and successfulness.	To reduce negative value of self.
3. Promote realistic, yet optimistic, setting of appropriate goals and objectives by encouraging identification of reality, client's potential, and clarification of values and beliefs.	To foster a sense of realistic optimism about self, others, and client's potential.
4. Explore outlook for the future.	To determine client's potential.
5. Refer for appropriate religious consultation.	To increase religious faith.
6. Encourage habitual meditation or prayer.	To promote relaxation and anxiety reduction and enhance problem solving.
7. Encourage goals that lead to self-actualization.	To motivate client to enrich own life and lives of others.
8. Assist client in identifying personal attributes associated with successful living.	To encourage behavioral changes that are compatible with own value system.
9. Encourage setting of new and meaningful goals after each success.	To promote motivation toward future accomplishments.
10. Encourage activities in which something is creatively produced in an environment where others are sharing similar experience.	Being creative leads to self-actualization that generates a sense of optimism. Sharing the experience with others enhances the positive value.

EVALUATION

Measurable goals and outcome criteria provide the data for evaluating the client's negative behavior. Client self-reports, nurse observations, and family reports provide additional data for evaluation. The following behaviors indicate a positive evaluation:

1. Identifies situations that evoke negative behavior
2. Demonstrates a positive attitude toward self and others
3. Relates successfully to others
4. Uses problem-solving and decision-making skills to reduce negativism
5. Is optimistic about current life situation and future

BIBLIOGRAPHY

Bloom R: Therapy and chronicity, *New Dir Ment Health Serv* 46(Summer):29, 1990.

Coleman R, Beck A: Cognitive therapy for depression. In Clarkin J, Glazer H, editors: *Depression, behavior and directive intervention strategies,* New York, 1981, Garland STPM Press.

Decker RL: On the devalued self: implications for transtheoretical psychotherapy, *J Contemp Psychother* 19(3):221, 1989.

Earnshaw AR, Amundson NE, Borgen WA: The experience of job insecurity for professional women, *J Employ Couns* 27(1):2, 1990.

Ericson K: Further thoughts on preventing mental illness, *J Humanist Psych* 30(1):107, 1990.

Fischer R, Juni S: The anal personality: self-disclosure, negativism, self-esteem, and superego severity, *J Pers Assess* 46(1):50, 1982.

Grainger RD: Dealing with feelings: the use and abuse of negative thinking, *Am J Nurs* 91(8):13, 1991.

Hall C: *A primer of Freudian psychology,* New York, 1981, Octagon Books.

Harper R: *Psychoanalysis and psychotherapy, 36 systems,* Englewood Cliffs, N.J., 1959, Prentice-Hall.

Levy ST: Negativism and countertransference, *J Am Psychoanal Assoc* 37(1):1989.

Lorr M, Wunderlich RA: Self-esteem and negative affect, *J Clin Psychol* 44(1):36, 1988.

Pearson M: *Strecker's fundamentals of psychiatry,* ed 6, Philadelphia, 1963, J.B. Lippincott.

Ribble M: Infantile experience in relation to personality development. In Hunt J, editor: *Personality and the behavior disorders,* vol 11, New York, 1944, Ronald Press.

Ruehlman LS, Karoly P: With a little flak from my friends: development and preliminary validation of the Test of Negative Social Exchange, *Psychol Assess* 3(1):97, 1991.

Schachar R, Wachsmuth R: Oppositional disorder in children: a validation study comparing conduct disorder, oppositional disorder and normal control children, *J Child Psychol Psychiatry* 31(7):1089, 1990.

Scharfman M: The toddler. In Simons R, Pardes H, editors: *Understanding human behavior in health and illness,* ed 2, Baltimore, 1981, Williams & Wilkins.

Smith C: An atypical session: resistance and the negativistic patient, *Psychother Theory Res Pract* 8(4):276, 1971.

Smith H: *Personality development,* New York, 1968, McGraw-Hill.

Storch RS, Lane RC: Resistance in mandated psychotherapy: its function and management, *J Contemp Psychother* 19(1):25, 1989.

Suls J, Marco CA: Relationship between JAS- and FTAS-Type A behavior and non-CHD illness: a prospective study controlling for negative affectivity, *Health Psychol* 9(4):479, 1990.

Volkmar FR, Hoder EL, Cohen DJ: Compliance, "negativism," and the effects of treatment structure in autism: a naturalistic, behavioral study, *J Child Psychol Psychiatry* 26(6):865, 1985.

Watson D, Chank LA: Negative affectivity: the disposition to experience aversive emotional status, *Psychol Bull* 6(3):465, 1984.

Noncompliance

Noncompliance is personal behavior that deviates from health-related advice given by health care professionals. The client may not adhere or only partially adhere to a prescribed therapeutic or disease prevention regimen.

Noncompliance to a treatment plan is a major problem in the nursing care of clients. Suspicious clients may not take their medications. Other clients stop taking their medications because they feel better. Other reasons that clients fail to adhere to their therapeutic regimen include failure to see the condition as serious enough to require treatment, denial of the condition, side effects from the medication, fear of dependency on the medications, lack of knowledge about the disease process, excessively high or low anxiety levels, lack of family support, negative relationship with the caregiver, inability to afford the treatments or medications, and embarrassment about taking medications.

Drug reluctance is seen in psychiatric clients, and readmissions are commonly precipitated by clients, particularly those diagnosed as having schizophrenia, who lack insight into the fact that they are sick and who, as they relapse, cease taking their medications at a time when they need them most. This neglect is referred to as the "revolving door" syndrome and is seen in clients with repeated admissions and discharges from the hospital.

Related DSM-III-R disorders

Noncompliance with medical treatment
Schizophrenia
Delusional (paranoid) disorders
Bipolar disorders

Other related conditions

Conditions or diseases that clients deny (for example, diabetes or emphysema)

PRINCIPLES

▶ Physical Dimension

1. Compliance is better when there is some incentive to comply other than, or in addition to, health—for example, job incentive or prevention of a jail term.
2. Taking medications may be perceived as a stigma and influences compliance.
3. Older persons may have difficulty with compliance because of memory deficits.
4. Isolated persons comply less than those less isolated.

▶ Emotional Dimension

1. Understanding how the client feels about decisions affecting his health improves compliance.
2. Emotional factors, for example, anger, depression, and anxiety, influence compliance.
3. Clients who are overly noncompliant may be hostile and use the hospital as a focal point for further hostility and aggressive impulses.
4. High levels of anxiety promote noncompliance.
5. Persons suffering from emotional illness comply less than others.

▶ Intellectual Dimension

1. The probability that advice will be followed is a function of the client's perception of his susceptibility to the disease and of the benefits or risks likely to be derived as a result of the recommended action.
2. Denial of a condition contributes to noncompliance.
3. Enhancing client knowledge about the disease process and treatment contributes to compliance.
4. Clients with insight into their illness comply better than those without it.
5. Determining the client's preferences and using this information to modify treatment regimens promotes compliance.
6. There is a questionable area between noncompliance and making an informed decision not to adhere to health-related advice.

▶ Social Dimension

1. Satisfaction with the relationship with the caregiver is more likely to result in compliance with treatment.
2. Client attitudes contribute to decisions to cooperate with treatment regimens.
3. Client preferences contribute to decisions to cooperate with treatment regimens.
4. Effective social networks and family supervision improve compliance.
5. Noncompliance does not absolve the caregiver of further responsibility to the client.
6. Responsibility for compliance is mutually shared between the caregiver and client.
7. Environmental factors such as transportation influence compliance.
8. Cultural factors such as a belief in faith healing influence compliance.
9. Persons in lower socioeconomic groups comply less than others.
10. An individual's response to a treatment regimen depends on the expectation that the outcome will yield a positive consequence.
11. Compliance can be learned through modeling.
12. The capacity to prevent future consequences acts as a motivator of behavior and promotes compliance.
13. The sick role has deviant status in society, implies stigma, and may result in noncompliance.
14. Self-attributed behavioral changes promote compliance to a greater extent than behavioral changes attributed to an external agent or force.

▶ Spiritual Dimension

1. Client beliefs contribute to decisions to cooperate with treatment regimens.
2. Failure to behave consistently with one's beliefs is a factor in noncompliance.
3. Noncompliance is highly subjective, and caregivers are cautioned to avoid value judgments and seek causes and contributing factors for noncompliance.
4. Individuals act toward treatment regimens on the basis of the meaning the treatment regimen has for them.
5. Social interaction provides the basis for the derivation of such meanings and determines whether or not the client complies.
6. Noncompliance promotes distress when personal beliefs conflict with the treatment regimen.

ASSESSMENT

▶ Physical Dimension

I. History
  A. Habits
    1. Medications and drugs
      a. Allergic reaction
      b. Side effects
      c. Extensive medication therapy
      d. Expense
      e. Controversies regarding medications
      f. Failure to consider client preferences
      g. Inconvenience
      h. Lack of transportation to obtain medications
      i. Lack of continuity of care
  B. Destructive behavior
    1. Failure to take life-sustaining medications may result in death
    2. Procrastination or postponement of treatments
  C. Health history
    1. Illnesses
      a. Schizophrenia
      b. Bipolar disorders
      c. Delusional (paranoid) disorders
  D. Review of systems
    1. Assess each body system affected by noncompliance for
      a. Increased disease-related symptoms despite adherence to regimen
      b. Persistence of symptoms
      c. Progression of illness
      d. Severity of illness
      e. Decrease in or absence of symptoms

II. Physical examination
  A. Perform an examination on areas of body affected by noncompliance

III. Diagnostic tests
  A. Urine screens
  B. Lithium levels
  C. Breath tests

▶ Emotional Dimension

CLIENT DATA	ANALYSIS	NURSING DIAGNOSIS
High anxiety	Response to threat to health or well-being; high levels promote noncompliance; anxiety not acknowledged.	Noncompliance: related to high anxiety over threat to health
Low anxiety	Lack of motivation and/or incentives to comply; sick role has deviant social status.	Noncompliance: related to lack of motivation and/or incentives
Distrust	Unable to trust caregivers or results of laboratory tests because of suspiciousness or paranoia.	Noncompliance: related to lack of trust in caregiver
Anger and frustration	Responses to stress over health needs; may be angry at self for being ill.	Noncompliance: related to anger or frustration with health needs
Fear	Response to threat: fears diagnosis, treatment methods, setting, outcome, dependency on medications, and becoming immune to effects; sick role may require new behaviors and giving up familiar behavior.	Noncompliance: related to fears about diagnosis, treatment, setting, outcome, dependency on medications, or becoming immune to effects
Powerlessness	Nonparticipant in decisions affecting health.	Noncompliance: related to lack of participation in decisions about health
Guilt	For taking medications (prescribed or illegal); medication is perceived as a stigma.	Noncompliance: related to guilt over taking medications
Lack of feeling a personal susceptibility to future episodes of illness or condition	Denying vulnerability to possible future susceptibility; the probability that advice will be followed depends on client perception of susceptibility to disease.	Noncompliance: related to denial of susceptibility to future illness

▶ Intellectual Dimension

CLIENT DATA	ANALYSIS	NURSING DIAGNOSIS
Perceives illness as overly severe or not severe, or accepts erroneous information	Possible responses to anxiety about health needs. High levels of anxiety contribute to misperception of events and situations; low levels of anxiety prevent involvement in treatment regimen.	Noncompliance: related to distorted perception of health needs
Misinterprets facts	Anxiety affects a person's ability to hear the facts.	Noncompliance: related to misinterpretation of facts associated with anxiety
Forgets appointments, to take medications, to do treatments, or information about medications and treatments	Possible responses to high levels of anxiety, denial of condition, or aging.	Noncompliance: related to forgetfulness
Does not comprehend health needs	Lacks an understanding of treatment possibly because technical and/or clinical terms are used in explanations.	Noncompliance: related to lack of understanding of treatment
Lacks insight about health needs	Needs knowledge about disease.	Noncompliance: related to lack of insight
Refuses to take medications or treatment suggested	Participates in the decision-making process, making an informed decision not to adhere to medical advice.	Noncompliance: related to rational decision to refuse treatment

▶ **Intellectual Dimension—cont'd**

CLIENT DATA	ANALYSIS	NURSING DIAGNOSIS
Lacks motivation to learn about disease and treatment	Little or no anxiety about health needs. The inability to visualize future consequences decreases motivation.	Noncompliance: related to lack of motivation
Is immature	May lack developmental skills necessary to understand significance of taking medications.	Noncompliance: related to immaturity
Questions need for further treatment	Unable to accept health problem. Client attitudes contribute to decision to cooperate with treatment regimen; sick role has a stigma.	Noncompliance: related to perceived need for no further treatment
Is confused	Lacks knowledge about treatment; increased knowledge about disease process contributes to compliance.	Knowledge deficit: related to noncompliance with prescribed treatment regimen
Has irrational thoughts about treatment	Lacks accurate information or is unable to accept accurate information because of irrational thinking.	Noncompliance: related to irrational thoughts about health needs
Pays undue attention to negative outcomes on medication package inserts (e.g., risks and side effects)	Focuses on warnings and risk factors to support noncompliance.	Noncompliance: related to selective attention to risk factors of medication
Denies health problem	Response to anxiety; unable to accept health problem; denial contributes to noncompliance.	Noncompliance: related to denial of illness
Engages in rigid thinking	High levels of anxiety contribute to feelings of insecurity and difficulty in being open to new ideas/options.	Noncompliance: unable to consider options related to severe anxiety
Does not accept diagnosis or illness	Denying diagnosis or illness contributes to noncompliance.	Noncompliance: related to denial of diagnosis or illness

▶ **Social Dimension**

CLIENT DATA	ANALYSIS	NURSING DIAGNOSIS
Has lowered self-esteem	Sees taking medication as a sign of weakness, a handicap, an embarrassment, less than a normal person; unrealistic perception of self; stigma associated with sick role.	Noncompliance: related to low self-esteem
Lacks a feeling of value and importance	Negativism and indifference toward health needs.	Noncompliance: related to negativism and indifference toward health needs
Has negative attitude toward caregiver	Lacks a trusting, caring relationship; satisfaction with relationship with caregiver promotes compliance.	Noncompliance: related to a negative attitude toward caregiver
Negative attitude of family members or significant persons	Lacks a supportive family relationship; an effective support system improves cooperation with treatment regimen.	Noncompliance: related to negative attitude of family members
Impersonal aspects of health care setting; long waits, hurried atmosphere, lack of privacy, and uncomfortable facilities	Promotes feelings of devaluation; environmental factors influence compliance.	Noncompliance: related to impersonal aspects of health care setting

▶ **Social Dimension—cont'd**

CLIENT DATA	ANALYSIS	NURSING DIAGNOSIS
Lacks autonomy	Dependent relationships; expects others to care for him.	Noncompliance: related to lack of autonomy
Receives secondary gains from symptoms	Receives benefits and satisfaction from noncompliance.	Noncompliance: related to receiving secondary gains from symptoms
Maternalism in nurse-client relationship	Perceived as incapable by caregiver; responsibility for compliance is mutually shared between caregiver and client.	Noncompliance: related to maternalistic relationship with caregiver
Change required in life-style and habits	Pain and discomfort with change in life-style and habits; sick role may require new behaviors.	Noncompliance: related to change in life-style and habits
Dissatisfied	Relationship with caregiver is negative; client's attitudes contribute to decision to cooperate with treatment regimen.	Noncompliance: related to negative relationship with caregiver
Feels stigmatized	Sees self as having incurable illness; sick role implies stigma.	Noncompliance: related to stigma of illness
Preferences for treatment not respected	Failure to consider client preferences contributes to noncompliance.	Noncompliance: related to client's perceived lack of respect for preferences for treatment of health needs
Is isolated	Lacks support from others through isolation (living alone); no one to encourage compliance.	Noncompliance: related to isolation from others
Is elderly	Possible memory deficits of aging contribute to noncompliance.	Noncompliance: forgetfulness related to aging
Is in low socioeconomic group	Lacks finances to purchase medications or pay for treatment.	Noncompliance: related to lack of finances
Unable to get off work to get health care	Loss of a day's pay prevents compliance.	Noncompliance: related to inability to get off work
Inclement weather	Inclement weather prevents transportation to health care facility.	Noncompliance: related to lack of transportation
Relies on folk methods of treatment	Compliance influenced by cultural attitudes/beliefs.	Noncompliance: related to cultural influences on treatment

▶ **Spiritual Dimension**

CLIENT DATA	ANALYSIS	NURSING DIAGNOSIS
Lacks clarity regarding beliefs about illness	Misinterpretation and erroneous health beliefs contribute to noncompliance.	Noncompliance: related to lack of clarity regarding beliefs about illness
Lacks understanding of meaning of illness	Failure to comprehend the meaning of the illness to the individual promotes noncompliance.	Spiritual distress: inability to find meaning in the experience of illness related to noncompliance
Caretaker insensitive to client's feelings	Failure to be sensitive to client's feelings about health needs promotes noncompliance.	Noncompliance: related to insensitivity to health needs
Loss of hope and readiness to die	Feels hopeless; refuses to comply with treatment regimen.	Spiritual distress: loss of hope related to noncompliance
Religious conflicts	Prevent complying with specific treatments (blood transfusions, abortions); client beliefs influence compliance.	Noncompliance: related to religious beliefs
Attitude that God will take care of client or it is Allah's or other supreme power's will	Sees no need for treatment because of strong belief in religious leader.	Noncompliance: related to belief in God, Allah, or other religious leader

PLANNING

▶ **Long-Term Goal**

To comply with health care treatment regimen in an informed, responsible manner

SHORT-TERM GOALS	OUTCOME CRITERIA
Physical Dimension To discuss causes of noncompliance	1. Describes situations and experiences that cause client to alter prescribed treatment regimen 2. States lack of participation in making decisions about treatment causes noncompliance 3. States having no further symptoms 4. Verbalizes erroneous information about treatment 5. States lack of family support 6. Verbalizes a lack of incentive to follow treatment plans 7. Verbalizes pain in changing life-style 8. Verbalizes stigma attached to treatment 9. States uncomfortable side effects cause noncompliance 10. States treatment is not acceptable culturally
Emotional Dimension To express feelings about treatment regimen	1. Expresses feelings of fear of dependence on medication, anger about treatment regimen, embarrassment about illness, dissatisfaction with the caregiver, guilt about illness, and confusion about illness and treatment regimen
Intellectual Dimension To be informed about treatment regimen, benefits, and risks	1. States correct information about diagnosis, disease process, and treatment plans 2. Discusses benefits of treatment 3. Discusses risks of treatment 4. States preferences for treatment 5. Discusses thoughts about treatment 6. Shares feelings about treatment 7. Reads literature on treatment 8. Asks questions about treatment
To participate in making decisions about treatment	1. Discusses meaning of illness 2. Discusses beliefs about illness 3. Discusses risks and benefits about treatment regimen 4. Makes decision to comply or not to comply
Social Dimension To reestablish a trusting, supportive relationship with caregiver	1. States that he feels important to caregiver 2. Verbalizes that he is waiting less time and feels less hurried through treatments 3. Verbalizes satisfaction with amount of time spent with caregiver 4. Has an improved attitude toward caregiver 5. Verbalizes caring from caregiver 6. States incentives to comply through discussion of information with caregiver
Spiritual Dimension To discover meaning of illness as a way to restore value in self	1. Discusses impact of illness on own life 2. Verbalizes conflicting values that interfere with compliance

Discharge Planning

The following client behaviors demonstrate readiness for discharge:
1. Explains reasons for and effects of treatments
2. Describes consequences of noncompliance with prescribed treatment regimen
3. Expresses thoughts and feelings about treatment regimen
4. Develops a therapeutic relationship with caregiver

IMPLEMENTATION

NURSING ACTIONS	RATIONALE
Physical Dimension	
1. Discuss side effects of medications.	To give client accurate information, to determine if side effects are the cause of noncompliance.
2. Relieve side effects of medications with appropriate nursing measures.	To promote comfort, to demonstrate caring, and to promote compliance with medication regimen.
3. Prevent undue waiting for treatments.	To avoid giving client impression that treatment is not important.
4. Give adequate time for client in an unhurried manner.	To allow client time to ask questions.
5. Supervise treatment regularly.	To promote continuity of care.
6. Plan treatment at client's convenience when possible.	To accommodate treatment to client's schedule.
7. Consider expense of treatment.	To show sensitivity to client's financial status.
8. Assist in planning transportation for treatment.	To aid client in complying with treatment regimen.
9. Schedule individual appointments rather than a "first come, first served" basis.	To give individualized care and prevent long waits for treatment.
Emotional Dimension	
1. Facilitate expression of feelings about treatment with active listening, reflecting, and clarifying.	To determine client's feelings about treatment and plan interventions.
2. Reduce feelings of anxiety, fear, anger, guilt, powerlessness, or mistrust about treatment by helping client identify and express feelings.	To promote compliance as an understanding of client's feelings about treatment is obtained.
3. Promote comfortable, accepting attitude toward expressing feelings about treatment with positive feedback.	To help client feel safe expressing negative feelings about treatment.
4. Give feedback when feelings are expressed.	To reinforce client's expression of feelings about treatment.
Intellectual Dimension	
1. Promote realistic perception of client's illness.	To prevent reinforcing denial or minimizing the illness or disability.
2. Prevent postponing and procrastinating over treatment.	To model appropriate attention to treatment.
3. Provide accurate information about treatment.	To correct irrational thoughts, erroneous ideas or misinterpretations of facts.
4. Provide information about need for further long-term treatment even when symptoms are no longer evident.	To present a realistic picture of the importance of treatment, perhaps for the rest of client's life.
5. Provide information about medications, treatments, diagnosis, and disease process.	To help client understand his illness and need for treatment.
6. Provide information about risks and benefits of treatment.	To give client accurate information on which to make decisions about his treatment.
7. Provide information about controversies over treatment.	To state all the facts about differing opinions on client's treatment. Client is entitled to this information.
8. Promote client's participation in decision making about treatment.	To promote compliance. Client will generally adhere to treatment regimen when he has taken part in making the decision.
9. Provide information about client's right not to comply with treatment.	To inform client of rights.

IMPLEMENTATION—cont'd

NURSING ACTIONS	RATIONALE
10. Write out instructions for treatment of client with memory deficits.	To help client remember treatment.
11. Use few technical terms.	To ensure understanding.
12. Explore ways to help client remember to take medications, for example, keeping a record book or setting out daily doses in kitchen window.	To elicit ways client can be responsible for adhering to treatment regimen.
13. Prevent denial by reducing client's anxiety.	To lessen anxiety promotes clearer, more realistic thinking.
14. Increase anxiety to moderate level to motivate client to comply.	To promote a degree of discomfort can be motivating; for example, saying to client, "You have 10 more minutes to finish your project before your treatment" may motivate client to stop dawdling in order to get his treatment.
15. Provide information on medication package inserts.	To reduce emphasis on warnings and risks that client could use as a reason for noncompliance.
16. Have client make own appointments.	To promote autonomy and participation in making decisions about own care.
17. Send postcards or telephone regarding treatments.	To remind client of treatment.
18. Give feedback about consequences resulting from not following directions.	To present factual information about possible consequences of failure to follow directions.
19. Refrain from being punitive.	To prevent negativism about treatment regimen or caregiver that may result in noncompliance.
20. Develop a method for client to monitor own progress and report to caregiver.	To promote feelings of control and self-esteem.
21. Make a compliance contract with client.	To ensure compliance.
22. Foster client's motivation and willingness to participate in own treatment planning.	To promote self-responsibility for health care.

Social Dimension

1. Promote autonomy toward health-seeking behavior with positive reinforcement.	To encourage client to take responsibility for own health.
2. Promote recognition and respect for client by asking for client's preferences about treatment.	To be sensitive to client's preferences when possible.
3. Provide individualized care despite impersonal aspects of the setting.	To promote feelings of importance and worth.
4. Promote positive attitudes among family members toward client and illness.	To help client's family be supportive to client and treatment regimen.
5. Provide family with information about medications, treatment, diagnosis, and disease process.	To help family understand client's treatment regimen and be supportive.
6. Eliminate secondary gains client receives from symptoms by identifying behaviors eliciting it.	To stop all benefits and satisfactions client receives from illness.
7. Refer or provide care for family members who are ill and cannot be supportive to client.	To promote family health and indicate caring about total family.
8. Provide family therapy for family discord regarding client's illness.	To help reduce family conflicts that may contribute to noncompliance.
9. Reestablish therapeutic relationship with client.	To regain client's trust.
10. Promote positive attitudes in caregiver toward client with supportive relationship.	To enhance compliance. Negativism toward caregiver often results in noncompliance.
11. Avoid maternalistic relationship with client.	To prevent relating to client as a child who needs mothering.
12. Increase client's autonomy and independence by encouraging decision making.	To help client maintain control over own life.
13. Promote changes in life-style and habits slowly, beginning with one aspect at a time.	To allow time for client to adjust to change.
14. Give positive feedback as changes occur.	To reinforce compliance.
15. Prevent isolation of older clients.	To decrease likelihood of noncompliance.
16. Refer to social worker and community agencies when finances are inadequate to buy medications or treatment supplies or to pay for transportation to clinic.	To assist client in complying without excessive financial burden.

NURSING ACTIONS	RATIONALE
17. Collaborate with school or employer to arrange time off for appointments.	To encourage compliance.
18. Ensure privacy when discussing noncompliance.	To protect confidentiality.
19. Encourage "contracting" when behavior modification is indicated.	To form an agreement with client that spells out what client will do to comply with treatment regimen.
Spiritual Dimension	
1. Explore with client meaning of illness and its effects on client.	To determine possible reasons for noncompliance.
2. Promote a courageous and positive response to illness through reasoning and questioning.	To promote optimism about illness by client's compliance with treatment regimen.
3. Promote a sense of value to life despite illness.	To help client value life rather than give up on life.
4. Encourage others with similar illness to share experiences with client and offer optimism about outcome.	To provide encouragement and support.
5. Respect client's religious beliefs about illness.	To demonstrate sensitivity about client's religious beliefs.
6. When religious beliefs conflict with treatment, continue relationship with client and offer support.	To remain supportive even though you disagree with client's beliefs about treatment.
7. If client is a minor and parents' religious beliefs conflict with treatment, refer to physician.	To protect rights of minors. Parents cannot impose their religious beliefs about treatments on minor children.
8. Accept client's decision to refuse to comply with life-sustaining treatments.	To show respect for client's decision.
9. Provide continued support with client's pain as a result of noncompliance.	To remain supportive.
10. Refer to clergy to promote realistic faith in God or other power.	To sustain client's religious beliefs.
11. Use bibliotherapy that discusses problems of existence.	To enable client to explore issues about life and its meaning as a way to promote compliance.

EVALUATION

Measurable goals and outcome criteria provide the data for evaluating whether the client is complying with the treatment regimen. Observations by the nurse, other caregivers, members of the family, and persons significant in the client's life, as well as the client's self-report, provide additional data for evaluation. The following behaviors indicate a positive evaluation:

1. States accurate information about his illness or disability
2. Accepts his condition realistically
3. Seeks support from others
4. Has a positive relationship with a caregiver
5. Complies with treatment regimen

BIBLIOGRAPHY

Chiang B: Adherence to health care regimens among elderly women: selected components of nurse practitioner care, *Nurs Res* 34(1):24, 1985.

Dubinsky M: Predictors of appointment non-compliance in community mental health patients, *Commun Ment Health J* 22(2):142, 1986.

Eraker S, Kirscht J, Becker M: Understanding and improving patient compliance, *Ann Intern Med* 100(2):258, 1984.

Evans L, Spelman M: The problem of non-compliance with drug therapy, *Drugs* 25(1):63, 1983.

Kolton K, Piccolo P: Patient compliance: a challenge in practice, *Nurse Practit: Am J Prim Health Care* 13(12):37, 1988.

Molzhan A, Northcott H: The social bases of discrepancies in health/illness perceptions, *J Adv Nurs* 14(2):132, 1989.

Plawecki H, Mallory D: Compliance and health beliefs, *J Natl Black Nurses' Assoc* 2(1):38, 1988.

Pristach C: Medication compliance and substance abuse among schizophrenic patients, *Hosp Community Psychiatry* 41:1345, 1990.

Thiederman S: Ethnocentrism: a barrier to effective health care, *Nurse Practit: Am J Prim Health Care* 11(8):52, 1986.

Whiteside S, Harris A, Whiteside H: Patient education: effectiveness of medication programs for psychiatric patients, *J Psychosoc Nurs Ment Health Serv* 21(10):16, 1983.

Youssef F: Compliance with therapeutic regimens: a follow-up study for patients with affective disorders: the effect of patient education on medication compliance, *J Adv Nurs* 8(6):513, 1983.

Youssef F: Adherence in therapy in psychiatric patients: an empirical investigation on the impact of patient education, *Int J Nurs Stud* 21(1):51, 1984.

Obesity

Obesity is defined as an excessive proportion, 15% above the established norms, of fat or adipose tissue in the body mass. In the United States obesity is recognized as a major health problem with physical, emotional, intellectual, social, and spiritual components. Within the last decade obesity has been targeted as a national concern. Approximately 60 million Americans are considered obese. Childhood obesity is an increasing health problem in this country, and it is positively correlated with adult obesity.

Some of the most commonly held beliefs of health professionals are that obesity contributes to (1) life-shortening diseases, (2) biochemical and metabolic abnormalities, and (3) deficient social interactions.

The American public, especially women, values thinness. Thinness is seen as part of being attractive and healthy. Billions of dollars are spent each year pursuing the ideal physique. However, current treatment strategies for obesity have produced limited success, which suggests the existence of some unknown variables. Professional nurses have a definite role to play in helping individuals of various ages with the prevention and treatment of obesity. Nurses are in numerous situations where they can teach health and give clients assistance in dealing with this problem.

Related DSM-III-R disorders

Anorexia nervosa
Bulimia nervosa
Pica
Rumination disorder of infancy
Eating disorder not otherwise specified

Other related conditions

Anxiety
Anger
Depression

The original content for this section was contributed by Rita Gelazis, R.N., M.N.Ed. and Alice Kempe, R.N., M.S.N.

Guilt
Sexual dysfunction
Dependency
Negative self-concept or self-image or low self-esteem
Helplessness
Lack of control

PRINCIPLES

▶ Physical Dimension

1. Obesity occurs when an individual is more than 15% above established weight norms.
2. The obese person often reports being overweight for a number of years.
3. The person's diagnostic tests may reflect normal values.
4. The individual lacks interest in exercise programs and prefers passive, observer activities to participant sports.
5. Obesity increases the stress on the total body system, for example, cardiovascular system or respiratory system.
6. Failure to maintain weight loss over extended periods of time is a problem that continues to plague the obese individual.
7. The obese person tends to eat quickly, often reporting skipping meals or eating only one small meal a day.

▶ Emotional Dimension

1. If anxious, the dieter is likely to demonstrate negative or defensive behaviors.
2. The individual displays appropriate affect except in regard to the body and eating, in which case the obese person tends to overreact (for example, euphoria about an immediate meal).
3. Many obese clients deal with emotions or feelings by eating and report intense negative feelings and guilt toward themselves when deviating from a weight loss diet.

4. Weight loss groups serve to decrease feelings of helplessness and hopelessness about the weight problem and tend to mobilize the individual toward the goal of weight loss.
5. The obese person often displays unrealistic dependence on food for pleasure and meeting other emotional needs.
6. The obese client may display decreased sexual interest and activity.
7. Dieters report some fears of weight loss related to changes this loss may bring about in their lives:
   a. Relationship with spouse or significant others may change or end.
   b. More control and independence may be expected of the individual.
   c. Balance of power in relationships may be altered.
8. Obese clients report eating when faced with various emotions, feelings, and states such as anxiety, anger, guilt, fatigue, boredom, hopelessness, helplessness, inadequacy, ambivalence, indecisiveness, loneliness, or unattractiveness.
9. Obesity is a regression to an infantile orality to fill voids such as frustrated dependency needs represented by a wish to be loved.
10. Eating may be a way of decreasing anxiety, insecurity, worry, frustration, or monotony.
11. Obesity is a way of expressing hostility and rebellion against authority or is an attempt at independence.
12. Obesity is an expression of anger turned toward the self to punish.
13. Obesity is a way of avoiding competition in life and maturity.
14. A big body may represent strength or greatness achieved by becoming bigger and stronger than others.
15. Obesity may be an attempt to modify a depression.
16. Guilt is a frequent feeling experienced by the overweight person and is self-defeating if excessive.
17. The compulsive overeater uses food to deal with fear, pain, or other emotional issues. Obesity may occur secondary to compulsive overeating.

▶ **Intellectual Dimension**

1. The client may describe self as fat and doubts own ability to alter the overweight problem.
2. The obese client has difficulty accurately describing a usual dietary intake and is not able to give accurate dietary information regarding daily food requirements. The amount of food eaten and the appropriate size of portions are often underestimated.
3. The following irrational thoughts are often a part of the obese client's cognitive structure:
   a. It is important to have love and approval from all significant people.

b. It is important to be competent in everything you do.
c. Life is catastrophic when everything does not go perfectly.
d. People who harm you are wicked and you should blame or punish them.
e. Anything causing fear must occupy and upset you.
f. It is horrible if a good solution is found quickly to life's problems.
g. Misery comes from external sources and you have little ability to control feelings of hostility or depression.
h. It is easier to avoid life's difficulties than to be disciplined.
4. Obese individuals often report external factors as dominant motivators in eating behavior.

▶ **Social Dimension**

1. Obese individuals tend to perpetuate self-defeating overeating behaviors when feeling negative about themselves.
2. Success in weight loss depends to an extreme degree on external support.
3. Disturbed social and family relationships are often part of the weight problem.
4. Food is described by the client as a very important part of social activities.
5. The client may binge secretly and hide food from other family members.
6. Support from a spouse or significant other can be used positively by emphasizing the pair's joint effort in weight loss; the partner's role is primarily to serve as a monitor and to reinforce the dieting spouse's weight loss efforts.
7. Addressing the issue of negative attitudes or mixed reactions toward weight reduction treatment by both the spouse or significant other and the dieter may increase the effectiveness of the weight loss program. The tendency of some spouses or significant others to subtly and perhaps knowingly sabotage dieting is documented.
8. The obese individual's culture and ethnicity influence dietary intake and the value placed on various foods. This influence is so strong that changes are slow and difficult to maintain over time.
9. Patterns of eating are developed early in life based on family traditions and beliefs.
10. The child learns to eat when not hungry if the mother ignores his cues and feeds him when she thinks he is hungry.
11. The child learns to overeat if parents insist that the child eat everything on the plate.
12. Parents may teach the child to use food as a way of dealing with feelings.

13. The obese are stigmatized because they are held responsible for their lack of control and willpower.
14. The obese child may be the scapegoat for one or both parents when marital conflict is present.
15. Weight loss groups offer support to individuals so they can move toward their goal of weight loss and maintenance.
16. Obesity may be a way of justifying all interpersonal or career failures.
17. Dieters who have a high need for independence and self-achievement may be more threatened by aid than those whose need for independence is low.

▶ Spiritual Dimension

1. A spiritual focus can be used positively to assist the obese person in decreasing the importance of food in his life.
2. Eastern and Western religions sanction a healthy, physically toned body. The spiritual component of a healthy body as the "temple of the spirit" is seen, for example, in many Judeo-Christian religions. In Eastern religions a "balance" in life is favored, and ex- cesses of any kind, including those of the body, are not sanctioned.
3. The obese individual is often made to feel like a fail- ure for having a weak will or not having a strong character, since overeating is viewed as a weakness. Such a belief system can increase guilt, create in- creased anxiety, and lead to further overeating.
4. Religion can be a source of strength for the obese individual.
5. Some support groups use religious beliefs and sanc- tions as a source of help.
6. The spiritual teaching of loving oneself can be used to counteract negative feelings and ideas about obe- sity and oneself.
7. Existential theory provides an important dimension to consider in assisting the obese individual to deal with a weight problem. The significance of overeating alters the meaning of life for the individual.
8. Overeating can be self-destructive and eventually hasten a person's death.
9. The obese individual substitutes food for expressions of or acceptance of love.

ASSESSMENT

▶ Physical Dimension

I. History
  A. Activities of daily living
    1. Nutrition
      a. Eats when not hungry
      b. Eats quickly, does not savor food
      c. Skips meals or eats one small meal a day
      d. Binges secretly
      e. Hides food from family
      f. Has difficulty accurately describing di- etary intake
      g. Snacks
      h. Weight gain more than 15% above es- tablished norms
      i. Unable to maintain ideal body weight
  B. Habits
    1. Medications and drugs
      a. Appetite suppressants
      b. Phenothiazine
      c. Hormones [thyroxine, medroxyproges- terone acetate (Provera), conjugated es- trogens (Premarin, steroids)]
    2. Excessive alcohol intake
  C. Destructive behavior—systemic effects of obe- sity can result in increased chance of problems with the heart, circulatory system, liver, gall- bladder, and pancreas
  D. Health history
    1. Illnesses
      a. Endocrine disease
      b. Polycystic ovaries
  E. Genetic factors
    1. Has one or more obese parents
  F. Body image
    1. Attempts to hide body size
  G. Review of systems
    1. Cardiovascular
      a. Reports heart palpitations
    2. Respiratory
      a. Reports shortness of breath on exertion

II. Diagnostic tests
  A. ECG
  B. Chest x-ray examination
  C. Complete blood count
  D. Blood chemistry tests
  E. Urinalysis

▶ Physical Examination

CLIENT DATA	ANALYSIS	NURSING DIAGNOSIS
Weight 15% over recommended amount	One pound of body weight is the result of intake of 3,500 calories over the amount the body needs to maintain itself.	Altered nutrition: food intake more than body requirements
Triceps skinfold greater than 15 mm in men and 25 mm in women	Caloric needs differ based on age. Ideal weight at age 25 is best weight to maintain throughout life. In order to accomplish this, calories must be reduced 3% from 30 to 40 years of age, another 3% from 40 to 50 years of age, 7.5% from 50 to 60 years of age, and another 7.5% from 60 to 70 years of age.	Knowledge deficit: lack of information regarding caloric intake and body requirements
Problems with heart, circulatory system, liver, gallbladder, and pancreas	Systemic effects of obesity can result in increased chance of adult-onset diabetes, decreased activity, slowed metabolism, increased cholesterol levels, decreased vitamin and mineral absorption, increased risk of surgery, and complication of any disease process.	Altered health maintenance: related to obesity
Daily exercise limited or absent	All persons need moderate exercise to maintain physical well-being. Persons who are physically active are less likely to be overweight. Regular exercise is essential to maintain good muscle tone and achieve more attractive proportions. Most weight reduction efforts limited to attempts to decrease number of calories consumed. Weight reduction will occur more quickly if energy expenditures are increased because (1) more calories will be burned up and (2) basal metabolism will increase.	Altered health maintenance: related to lack of needed daily exercise
Takes appetite-suppressing drugs or hormones	Appetite suppressants may be habit forming and have a negative effect on other body systems. Dietary changes are needed on long-term basis to achieve and maintain weight loss.	Altered health maintenance: related to taking of appetite suppressants related to obesity Altered nutrition: less than body requirements related to drug use (thyroxine) Altered nutrition: more than body requirements related to drug use (Provera and Premarin)
Elevated blood pressure	Frequently seen in association with obesity.	Altered health maintenance: elevated blood pressure related to obesity

▶ **Emotional Dimension**

CLIENT DATA	ANALYSIS	NURSING DIAGNOSIS
Helplessness (lack of control)	Often the obese person feels out of control.	*Helplessness: overeating related to a loss of control
Anxiety	When an individual feels out of control, anxiety is increased, which may trigger overeating	Anxiety: increased food consumption related to loss of control
Anger	Overeating can be result of suppressed anger.	Ineffective individual coping: overeating related to suppressed anger
Hopelessness and depression	Feels that losing weight is hopeless. Hopelessness can lead to feelings of general depression.	Hopelessness: related to fears of inability to lose weight
Guilt	Felt when deviating from weight loss diet or when not able to control overeating.	*Guilt: related to loss of control, overeating

▶ **Intellectual Dimension**

CLIENT DATA	ANALYSIS	NURSING DIAGNOSIS
Lacks accurate information regarding food requirements	Does not know which foods are high in calories. Does not recognize that maintaining well-balanced schedule of meals throughout day provides an even source of energy.	Knowledge deficit: related to inaccurate information regarding basic nutrition
Unable to identify body signals of hunger	Eating is a way some obese persons have learned to cope with mood states. Eating substituted for other means of coping. Successful dietary program involves plan for lifetime changes, which when individualized, help client learn new coping behaviors.	Ineffective individual coping: eating related to altered mood states
Views self as weak willed or lacking a strong character	Irrational beliefs associated with overeating.	Altered thought processes: related to irrational views of self as weak-willed or lacking a strong character

▶ **Social Dimension**

CLIENT DATA	ANALYSIS	NURSING DIAGNOSIS
Has low self-esteem	Feels inadequate. Has intense negative feelings about self when overeats or goes off diet. Feels out of control.	Self-esteem disturbance: situational, related to feelings of inadequacy for overeating or going off diet
Avoids looking in mirrors and makes self-deprecating remarks about body	Unaware of self-perceptions about body. Behavior reflects thinking, feelings, value system, and cultural and spiritual orientation of an individual.	Self-esteem disturbance: chronic, related to poor self-perceptions
Wears loosely fitting clothing	Selects clothes that he believes will mask true size.	Personal identity disturbance: negative body image related to obesity
Has decreased sexual interest	Frequently accompanies obesity and can relate to distortions in body image and lowered self-esteem.	Sexual dysfunction: related to lower self-esteem

▶ **Social Dimension—cont'd**

CLIENT DATA	ANALYSIS	NURSING DIAGNOSIS
Skips meals and eats quickly without social interaction	Food has intrinsic value. It may be substitute for love, affection, and friendliness. Individual may focus on food rather than on relationships.	Impaired social interactions: related to skipping meals and eating quickly without social interaction
Describes high reward value attached to food at social occasions	Intrinsically high reward value of eating, along with unavoidable necessity of ingesting food daily, promotes universal problem with maintenance.	Altered thought processes: related to high intrinsic reward value of food
Spouse or significant other sabotages dieting	Subtle and knowing sabotage of dieter's plan occurs because of fear of change by significant other. May be critical of eating behavior of spouse but introduces food-related topics and offers food to spouse.	Ineffective family coping: related to sabotage of diet by spouse or significant other because of fear of change in dieter
Increases food intake during holiday and special events	Social pressures to eat and cultural values and beliefs learned from family result in overeating at holidays.	Ineffective individual coping: related to increased food intake at holidays due to social pressures, values, and beliefs
Environmental cues trigger overeating	Obese persons are stimulus bound; they are more apt to eat in response to external food cues such as taste, sight, smell, availability of food, and time of day than their more slender peers.	Ineffective individual coping: related to overeating caused by environmental stimuli

▶ **Spiritual Dimension**

CLIENT DATA	ANALYSIS	NURSING DIAGNOSIS
Lacks motivation to adhere to weight loss plan	Lack of faith, spiritual values, or an organized religion. Spiritual teachings related to individual's faith or belief system can aid in finding motivation to begin and sustain changes needed for weight loss. Eastern and Western religions sanction healthy, physically toned body.	Spiritual distress: related to inability to use spiritual values for motivation to lose weight
Describes self as unworthy and unlovable	Self-respect and self-love are bases for ability to give love to others. Healthy self-respect is incorporated into most forms of faith and religious groups.	Spiritual distress: related to perception of self as unworthy and unlovable
States that meaning of life is often unclear or forgotten, thereby overemphasizing importance of eating and food in life	Overweight individual often overstates importance of eating and food in life. Insufficient gratification in life comes from food-related activities rather than from spiritual and other sources.	Spiritual distress: related to lack of meaning in life associated with obesity
Relates frequent or recurrent instances when feeling guilty or weak willed if diet plan is not strictly followed	Negative beliefs about lack of control can be part of religious beliefs. Support groups with a religious basis can be useful for some individuals.	Spiritual distress: related to guilty feelings about self-regulation of behavior associated with obesity

PLANNING

Long-Term Goal

To regain control over dietary intake by integrating concepts of a balanced, low calorie diet for achievement of desirable weight for life

SHORT-TERM GOALS	OUTCOME CRITERIA
Physical Dimension	

To eat only when physically hungry	1. Describes individual physiological response to hunger
	2. Eliminates identified impulse eating
	3. Implements behavioral changes into life-style:
	   a. Carries no change for the snack machine
	   b. Shops for food after eating
	   c. Buys and prepares food in smaller quantities
	   d. Shows love in ways other than giving food
	   e. Prerecords what will be eaten during the day and sticks to that plan

To eat a diet that includes the basic foods in the food pyramid	1. Client stays within planned daily intake 2. Caloric intake is based on reduced amount appropriate to age, sex, body size, and activity level

To maintain or achieve optimum physiological functioning of each body system	1. Has decreased physical symptoms
	   a. Improvement in ECG
	   b. Improved blood pressure
	   c. Improved lipid and cholesterol levels
	   d. Improvement in blood chemistry
	   e. Describes no intolerance to fat intake
	   f. Describes increased energy
	   g. Fewer or no signs of difficulty with venous return in extremities
	   h. Healing occurs following surgery or trauma within normal time limits
	   i. Complications to any disease process reversed or improved
	   j. Blood sugar levels maintained within normal range

To increase daily exercise to balance food intake with body requirements for age and sex	1. Uses appropriate form of daily exercise 2. Chooses from activities such as walking, swimming, cycling, or any activity that progresses to aerobic exercise
To limit drug ingestion to only those necessary to maintain normal functioning of body systems	1. Uses no appetite suppressants 2. Takes only medication(s) prescribed for diagnosed system deficiencies
Emotional Dimension	
To decrease anxiety	1. Uses relaxation techniques when experiencing moderate to high anxiety 2. Relieves tension by using a planned exercise 3. Communicates feelings to significant others in an assertive way (see Anxiety, p. 48)
To identify and express anger at appropriate times, places, and persons	1. Labels anger as a personal feeling and accepts it as own 2. Selects appropriate responses to feelings of anger from repertoire of possible responses 3. States source of anger using "I" statements 4. Deals with source of anger rather than using other passive-aggressive responses such as overeating
To increase feelings of hope regarding ability to lose weight and to decrease feelings of depression	1. Demonstrates loving, caring behavior toward self and significant others 2. States that several pleasurable activities are engaged in daily without feelings of guilt 3. Shows improved personal hygiene and appearance 4. Communicates positive feelings in regard to self and daily activities 5. Displays less need to overeat 6. States achievement of balance in life activities

SHORT-TERM GOALS	OUTCOME CRITERIA
Intellectual Dimension	
To maintain a feeling of self-control in activities of daily living	1. Uses food exchange list in making appropriate dietary decisions 2. Substitutes other activities such as a walk when feeling out of control rather than eating 3. Eats slowly and focuses attention while eating on taste and quality of food 4. Sips water between bites; uses napkin frequently 5. Talks between bites 6. Cuts food one piece at a time 7. Chooses a designated time and place for eating and eats only then at that place 8. Does not eat while doing other activities (watching television) 9. Prepares only small portions on a small plate
To incorporate knowledge of basic nutrition into daily eating patterns	1. Loses 1 pound per week through decreased caloric intake 2. Adjusts weight loss goal to just maintenance during holidays or special events by saving calories that can be used during the event 3. Lists foods to be avoided, such as foods high in fat and in carbohydrates and refined sugars 4. Adheres to individualized dietary weight loss plan
To replace irrational beliefs associated with eating with rational thinking	1. Uses relaxation techniques to get in touch with positive thoughts about self 2. Periodically reviews rational thoughts that he can focus on and continues to incorporate positive thoughts into his life
To regulate eating according to plans made	1. Adheres to plan 2. Uses positive methods to deal with feelings about self, such as exercising instead of feeling guilty when deviations occur
To reward self in nonfood-related ways	1. Lists nonfood rewards 2. Develops a reward system for maintaining diet
Social Dimension	
To increase self-esteem	1. Exhibits increase in positive statements about self, body, and own capabilities 2. Is able to look into mirrors and see self realistically 3. Shows increased interest in clothes and in wearing current styles 4. Avoids using food to feel better about self
To establish a plan to increase social interactions with others to decrease overeating	1. Identifies methods to interact in a positive way with significant others 2. Develops an individual plan for change in interpersonal responses 3. Implements plan in appropriate social situations
To appreciate the value of friends and significant others in life	1. Identifies ways of fostering growth in relationships with others without including food in plan 2. Carries out plan and includes personal reward for achievement of goal
To become responsible for own thoughts, feelings, and behaviors	1. Uses "I" statements to describe personal experiences related to family interactions 2. Accepts negative thoughts and feelings toward and from others as natural 3. Recognizes forms of dysfunctional communication as part of change process 4. States that it is possible to change only one's own behavior 5. Ceases trying to change others 6. Seeks support from individual or group counseling to support new patterns of communication

PLANNING—cont'd

SHORT-TERM GOALS	OUTCOME CRITERIA
To make food choices based on body needs rather than on tradition or cultural influences	1. Identifies cultural beliefs, values, and traditions that influence food choices 2. Encourages family to help plan activities not linked with food for traditional holidays and special events
To reduce response to food-related environmental stimuli	1. Monitors own eating patterns to identify individual cues to eating 2. Develops own plan to eliminate usual response to food cues 3. Plans strategies to substitute for eating: a. Call a friend b. Exercise c. Recognize situations or people that trigger certain feelings and either avoid or use assertive techniques to deal with the particular situations d. Label the feeling and whenever that particular feeling occurs, have a substitute ready so food intake is no longer the response
Spiritual Dimension To identify and express faith in oneself and one's ability and make needed behavioral changes related to eating	1. Uses spiritual teachings such as scriptural passages to assist with motivation in weight loss process if appropriate
To recognize own strengths and positive attributes	1. Shares positive attributes with another individual or group 2. Identifies a strength each time he has an irrational thought
To describe personal meaning in life unrelated to food	1. Plans daily activities focusing on significant aspects of life that are not related to food 2. Describes food as essential to life but not connected to meaning of life

Discharge Planning

The following client behaviors demonstrate readiness for discharge:

1. Knows medications or treatments prescribed for related physical and emotional problems
2. Recognizes that control of obesity will involve lifetime effort and therefore makes appropriate plans for future
3. Knows of several alternative methods that are available to assist with control of obesity: support groups in the community (Overeaters Anonymous), eating disorder clinics in community, and facilities and organizations where client can exercise
4. Makes appropriate decisions about how to carry out weight control plan for self
5. Has an awareness of dangers of any future weight gains and takes steps to prevent this at gain of first several pounds
6. Knows what factors will contribute to maintenance of desirable weight and takes steps to plan for such maintenance
7. Recognizes that emotional, intellectual, social, and spiritual changes accompany any physical change
8. Knows where to go for additional help to integrate changes in personality and life-style

IMPLEMENTATION

NURSING ACTIONS	RATIONALE
Physical Dimension	
1. Assist client in monitoring and recording weekly food intake and activity and exercise pattern.	To assess usual eating and activity patterns.
2. Derive weekly realistic weight loss goals, striving for a weight loss of 1 to 2 pounds per week.	To provide a baseline for measuring progress in weight reduction.
3. Help client identify factors that contribute to overeating.	To learn more adaptive behavior, to lose weight, and to keep it off.
4. Help client reestablish a balanced nutritional diet including basic four groups.	To ensure adequate nutritional intake.
5. Help client establish and maintain an age-appropriate weight that is in proportion to height.	To promote overall health.

6. Teach client to modify rate and amount of eating by:
  a. putting utensils down between bites
  b. talking between bites and increasing social pleasures of eating
  c. chewing food more thoroughly
  d. designating a place for eating and then always eating there.
	To help client adopt healthy eating habits.

7. Focus discussions, as much as possible, away from food and toward pleasure from other sources such as identifying personal rewards, exercising, and finding balance in life.	To lessen importance of food in client's life.
8. Increase awareness of improved physical appearance and well-being.	To reinforce benefits of decreased weight.
9. Develop an individualized exercise regimen taking into account occupation, interests, and physical and medical needs.	To burn excess calories and promote weight loss.
10. Discourage use of any drugs (such as appetite suppressants) that client may have used.	To educate client about negative effects.
11. Help client recognize individual physiological response to hunger.	To promote awareness of physical sensations associated with hunger and differentiate sensations from hunger associated with psychological hunger.
12. Encourage client to keep food out of sight.	To prevent easy access to food and impulse eating.
Emotional Dimension	
1. Help client develop new patterns of coping with emotions or feelings such as anxiety, boredom, fatigue, stress, and anger without eating.	To promote alternatives to eating that are pleasant and contribute to a decreased emphasis on food.
2. Record feelings and make a structured individualized plan to follow in dealing with identified problem emotions.	To facilitate client's awareness of feelings associated with eating.
3. Recognize emotions that trigger overeating.	To promote awareness of feelings and plan interventions.
4. Help obese individual show love in other ways than through giving or taking food.	To provide client with other pleasurable methods and showing love and affection that are not related to food.
5. Facilitate expression of client's feelings of anger, guilt, depression, anxiety, hopelessness, and helplessness.	To help client identify feelings that may trigger overeating.
6. Redirect emotions to appropriate sources.	To help client link the feeling with the event or situation and cope effectively with the event or situation rather than avoiding the event or situation and eating.
7. Encourage self-exploration of eating habits.	To increase awareness and ownership of feelings.
8. Encourage appropriate methods of expressing feelings (relaxation, exercise, sports, art, writing, music, and assertive techniques).	To prevent avoidance or denial of feelings that may result in eating.
9. Convey empathy and understanding at times of weight loss plateaus or with weight gain.	To support client in disappointments, as well as successes.
10. Allow client to select foods from an exchange list.	To help client exert control and increase independence.
11. Discuss situations in which it is inappropriate to express anger, and find substitutions other than eating.	To prevent client from having other negative feelings that result from expressing anger, for example, guilt, self reproach.

IMPLEMENTATION—cont'd

NURSING ACTIONS	RATIONALE
12. Explore relationship between suppressing anger and overeating.	To increase client's awareness of eating habits.
13. Encourage client to assume responsibility for feelings of anger.	To promote ownership of feelings.
14. Encourage client to have a substitute ready for overeating when angry.	To avoid intake of food as a response to anger or other uncomfortable feeling.
Intellectual Dimension	
1. Assist client in setting a realistic weight loss goal.	To promote success in achieving an appropriate weight.
2. Direct education toward learning about high-calorie foods.	To teach client foods to avoid.
3. Teach client the calorie count of favorite fast foods.	To accommodate client's life-style and weight reduction program.
4. Teach client basic nutritional facts including food exchange system.	To increase client's feelings of control over foods.
5. Help client learn new ways to deal with holidays, special events, and social pressures to eat from family and friends. (See box below.)	To prevent overeating, to receive pleasure from other events or activities that are less food related.
6. Give positive feedback to client for weight loss of 1 to 2 pounds per week.	To reinforce appropriate weight loss.
7. Involve client in developing assertive skills.	To help client deal with social and environmental cues that hinder the weight loss program.
8. Discuss various irrational thoughts that are common to many people. Help client identify irrational beliefs related to overeating. (See Principles—Intellectual Dimension, p. 261.)	To determine client's irrational beliefs about food and help client question those beliefs.
9. Encourage continuation with daily diet plan even if it has not been followed perfectly.	To maintain consistency in following diet plan, to help client incorporate plan into overall life-style.
10. Assist client in recognizing that weight change is a slow process requiring continuous effort by the individual.	To prevent discouragement.
11. Teach client that there are basic food groups in daily requirements: milk, vegetables and fruits, breads, meat and other proteins.	To educate client about basic nutrition.

SPECIAL HOLIDAY WEIGHT CONTROL TIPS

When you're a guest:

1. Think ahead. Attending a brunch and dinner the same day? Don't use up all your calories at the first party—save some for the next social event.
2. Don't deprive yourself completely—sample just a sliver of a rich dessert, a spoonful of creamed vegetables.
3. Snacks and hors d'oeuvres: Nibble at one or two of the lower-calorie choices to take the edge off your appetite. Leave some on your plate so you won't be offered more.
4. Watch where you stand or sit. Stay away from the hors d'oeuvres tray or dessert cart. Concentrate on conversation with guests to keep your mind off the plum pudding.
5. If dinner is buffet style, stand last in line. By the time you get to the table, others will be midway through eating and you'll finish your smaller serving at the same time.
6. At a sit-down dinner? You may feel compelled or encouraged by your hostess to try everything that's passed to you. Eat half-portions and savor every bite. Eat slowly—you'll be less apt to be offered seconds.
7. Choose your "holiday cheer" with care. A half cup of eggnog, with rum or whiskey, is a whopping 335 calories! Opt for a fruit punch or one of the new low-calorie light wines, at 60 to 70 calories per 4-ounce serving. Another good choice is a half and half spritzer of club soda and red or white wine. Substitute also low-calorie sodas and sparkling water for mixers such as tonic water and ginger ale. Want something spicy? Ask for a tomato juice cocktail or Bloody Mary mix with a celery stirrer (about 50 calories per cup).
8. When the party is over, help the hostess empty ashtrays or fold up chairs, but stay out of the kitchen. Politely decline take-home leftovers.
9. Whether you're the hostess or guest: If you overeat during the holidays, cut back on calories the next day and exercise more. A "check and balance" system will help keep those extra pounds off.

NURSING ACTIONS	RATIONALE
12. Teach client to use these food groups and to select appropriate quantities from each food group.	To promote client's understanding of well-balanced, nutritious meals in appropriate quantities.
13. Assist client in recognizing cues, people, or situations that affect feelings about eating.	To increase awareness of cues from people or situations that trigger eating.
14. Help client label feelings that act as stimulus for eating.	To help client respond to stimulus without eating.
15. Teach client to use substitutes for eating, such as taking a nap, reading, or exercising.	To prevent impulsive eating by planning substitute responses.
16. Individualize dietary program so that lifetime changes occur as a result of client learning new coping behaviors.	To help client maintain appropriate weight loss over time.
17. Present reality to client regarding mortality rates and obesity.	To increase client's awareness of health hazards associated with obesity.
18. Teach client to maintain journal to monitor eating patterns and note cues that stimulate eating.	To increase client's awareness of eating patterns.
19. Encourage substitution of rational thoughts for irrational thoughts about eating.	To present reality.
20. Encourage client to practice use of rational thoughts.	To help client change focus of thinking from irrational to rational.
21. Help client develop plan of substitute activities in response to environmental stimuli that contribute to overeating.	To motivate client to assume responsibility for changing eating patterns.
22. Teach client to eat only when physically hungry.	To prevent client from eating for psychological reasons.
23. Explore with client problem times or situations that stimulate overeating.	To help client identify time and situations that stimulate eating and plan alternative responses.

24. Teach client to use techniques that will reduce eating as a response to environmental stimulus:
   a. Carry no change for the snack machine.
   b. Shop for food after eating.
   c. Buy and prepare highly nutritious food in smaller quantities.
   d. Show love in ways other than giving food.
   e. Prerecord what will be eaten during day and stick to plan.
   f. Stock no "empty calorie" foods.
	To promote self-control and feelings of success.

25. Promote realistic approach to dieting on holidays and special events. (See box on p. 270.)	To help client integrate diet plan into special events in life.
26. Acknowledge that client will generally eat more calories on holidays.	To present reality, to prevent discouragement and guilt.
27. Encourage development of plan to keep caloric intake within limits over holidays.	To promote client's participation in decisions about diet plans, thus fostering compliance with the plan.
28. Adjust weight goal to maintaining weight rather than losing weight during holidays.	To provide client with realistic diet plan.
29. Help client develop a plan to save up calories the day before the holiday.	To help client keep total caloric intake within limits.
30. Assist client in planning a personal nonfood-related reward system for achievement of specific goals.	To provide client with pleasures that are not related to food, for example, going to a movie, buying a new plant.
31. Discuss the relationship between avoidance of problems and overeating.	To increase client's awareness of reasons for overeating.
32. Discuss what thoughts client uses to excuse overeating.	To gain an understanding of client's defenses related to overeating.
33. Explore with client underlying assumptions that place blame on others for feelings that lead to overeating.	To gain an understanding of client's defenses, to identify anxieties.
34. Explore with client the relationship between catastrophic expectations when things don't go well and overeating.	To increase client's awareness of eating behaviors.
35. Explore concept of change, how change occurs, and how to assume responsibility for self-change.	To increase client's understanding of behavior change and how it is accomplished.

IMPLEMENTATION—cont'd

NURSING ACTIONS	RATIONALE

36. Assist client in employing one or more of the following techniques:
  a. Self-monitoring of weight and food intake
  b. Implicit or explicit goal setting
  c. Nutritional, exercise, and health counseling
  d. Social reinforcement (family support)
  e. Cognitive restructuring strategies
  f. Stimulus control procedures
  g. Rewards and punishments for weight change.
	To help client change eating behaviors.

Social Dimension	
1. Assist client in developing a social network of significant others. (See box below.)	To give client support through weight loss process.
2. Encourage client to develop a regular plan of eating revolving around the basic food groups and to avoid snacks of empty calories when social interactions do not meet client's expectations.	To prevent overeating following disappointments with social interactions.
3. Discourage eating when client is feeling lonely, bored, frustrated, or fatigued.	To prevent eating associated with negative feelings.
4. Focus discussion with client on the importance of social functions without viewing food as main event.	To help client receive satisfaction and rewards through interpersonal relationships and lessen the importance of food.
5. Encourage spouse or significant others to assist in developing for client a reward system that does not revolve around food. Reward can be a trip or an evening out with spouse or significant others.	To help client find new meaning to life through inexpensive daily nonfood-related rewards.
6. Assist spouse or significant others in viewing weight loss process in a positive way, pointing out positive aspects of change.	To help client focus on positive aspects of weight loss, thereby increasing self-esteem and confidence in ability to change.
7. Help client recognize and change dysfunctional communication in family, which may provoke overeating.	To prevent client from coping with frustrations of miscommunication in family with overeating, to increase client's feelings of mastery, self-control, and independence.

SUGGESTIONS FOR FAMILY MEMBERS AND FRIENDS

Help the weight watcher with generous verbal *praise* for successes, record keeping, practice of target behaviors, good eating habits.

Ignore any errors the weight watcher makes. Nagging and criticism are only detrimental!

Each day go over the weight watcher's records and graphs with client. Praise good records and any successes; *ignore* any errors.

Have at least one meal a day with the weight watcher so you can directly praise efforts toward learning new eating habits.

Develop a system with the weight watcher that provides some rewards for meeting long-term goals, for example, going to a movie together as a reward for a successful week, a weekend trip for three consecutive successful weeks.

Help the dieter avoid tempting situations by not bringing high-calorie food into the house, by finding other pleasurable activities and presents other than those involving food and eating.

Discuss together how the weight watcher's weight loss might affect your relationship, both positively and negatively.

NURSING ACTIONS	RATIONALE
8. Serve as role model in accepting negative aspects of self ("Let me tell you about my clay feet" or "Let me tell you about a mistake I made yesterday.")	To acknowledge to client that perfection may not be possible or necessary.
9. Explore with client activities that can replace food traditions.	To decrease overemphasis on food-related traditions.
10. Encourage involvement in a support group (Overeaters Anonymous and Weight Watchers).	To provide support and structure to achieve a successful weight loss.
11. Enlist aid of significant supportive others to develop new nonfood-related special days (a day at the zoo, a trip to view fall foliage).	To introduce events that are pleasurable and deemphasize food.
12. Explore client's unrealistic expectations of others and relationship to overeating.	To increase client's awareness of overeating patterns (for example, when disappointed with others).
13. Explore with client satisfaction gained from others' assistance or help. Discuss universal need of individuals for support in changing behavior such as overeating.	To help client feel understood and supported regardless of success or failure in losing weight.
14. Help restore and maintain a positive body image.	To increase self-concept.

Spiritual Dimension

1. Encourage client to assess own strengths.	To promote client's positive attributes.
2. Instill hope and confidence in client's ability to carry out plan for weight loss and maintenance.	To promote positive thinking about client's ability to change.
3. Convey attitude that weight loss can be part of an individual's self-growth.	To promote optimism about client's ability to enrich the quality of life.
4. Assist client in using strength obtained from religious leaders, friends, and family.	To strengthen support system and develop meaningful relationships with others.
5. Help client integrate weight control behaviors into a lifelong pattern.	To ensure weight maintenance throughout life and promote a healthy life-style associated with eating adequate amounts of nutritious meals.
6. Explore with client ways in which food consumption may have been substituted for a search for meaning in life.	To help client understand reasons for overeating and plan interventions.
7. Explore client's reactions to perceived failure to reach goals and relationship to obesity.	To help client connect feelings of failure to obesity and plan interventions.
8. Support positive plans and attempts to change life-style and eating patterns.	To provide encouragement to client to move toward a more healthy life-style without overeating.
9. Encourage client to seek, express, and accept love from sources other than through food.	To receive satisfactions from life that do not focus on food.

EVALUATION

Measurable goals and outcome criteria provide the data for evaluating the obese client's progress with weight reduction. The following behaviors indicate a positive evaluation:

1. States a realistic weight for self
2. Maintains an appropriate weight
3. Eats adequate amounts of food from the basic food groups
4. States calorie content of foods and avoid those with high calories
5. Exercises regularly
6. Identifies feelings and situations that contribute to overeating
7. Copes with feelings and situations without overeating
8. Rewards self with nonfood-related rewards for weight loss
9. Uses support groups (Weight Watchers, TOPS)
10. Enjoys social functions that do not focus on food
11. Verbalizes positive statements about self

BIBLIOGRAPHY

Allon N: The stigma of overweight in everyday life. In Wolman B, editor: *Psychological aspects of obesity*, New York, 1982, Reinhold Co.

Bagley CR et al: Attitudes of nurses toward obesity and obese patients, *J Perc Motor Skills* 68(3):954, 1989.

Blundell JE: Behavior modification and exercise in the treatment of obesity, *Postgrad Med* 60(suppl 3):37, 1984.

Brownell KD: Behavioral, psychological, and environmental predictors of obesity and success at weight reduction, *Int J Obes* 5:543, 1984.

Castiglia PT: Obesity in adolescence, *J Pediatr Health Care* 3(4):221, 1989.

Cecere MC: PIP (Positive Image Program): a group approach for obese adolescents, *Nurs Clin North Am* 18(2):240, 1983.

Cohen RY, Stunkard AJ: Behavior therapy and pharmacotherapy of obesity: a review of the literature, *Behav Med Update* 4(3):7, 1983.

Court J: Energy expenditure of obese children: techniques for measuring energy expenditures over periods of up to 24 hours, *Arch Dis Child* 47:153, 1972.

Cowell JM, Montgomery AC, Talashek ML: Cardiovascular risk assessment in school-age children: a school and community partnership in health promotion, *J Pub Health Nurs* 6(2):67, 1989.

DeJong W: The stigma of obesity: the consequences of naive assumptions concerning the cause of physical deviance, *J Health Soc Behav* 21:75, 1980.

Ellis A: *A guide to rational living*, North Hollywood, Calif, 1970, Wilshire Books Co.

Foreyt JP: Diet, behavior modification, and obesity: Nine questions most often asked by physicians, *Consultant* 30(6):53, 1990.

Gierszewski S: The relationship of weight loss, locus of control and social support, *Nurs Res* 32(1):43, 1983.

Jeffery RW, Adlis SA, Forster JL: Prevalence of dieting among working men and women: the healthy worker project, *Health Psych* 10(4):274, 1991.

Jonides LK: Childhood obesity: an update, *J Pediatr Health Care* 4(5):244, 1990.

Lazarus A, Fay A: *I can if I want to*, New York, 1975, Warner Books.

Leininger MM: Transcultural eating patterns and nutrition: transcultural nursing and anthropological perspectives, *Holistic Nurs Pract* 3(1):16, 1988.

Lustig A: Weight loss programs: failing to meet ethical standards? *J Am Dietetic Assoc* 91(10):1252, 1991.

Miller KD: Compulsive overeating, *Nurs Clin North Am* 26(3):699, 1991.

Morgan J: Behavioral treatment of obesity: the occupational health nurses' role, *Occup Health Nurs* 32(6):312, 1984.

Orbach S: *Fat is a feminist issue: the anti-diet guide to permanent weight loss*, New York, 1980, Jason Aronson.

Orr J: Obesity, *J Adv Nurs* 10(1):71, 1985.

Schlundt DG, Katahn M: Advances in the outpatient treatment of obesity: life-style changes part 1, *Physician Assist* 12(8):49, 1988.

Schroeder MA: Symbolic interactionism: a conceptual framework useful for nurses working with obese persons, *Image* 13(3):78, 1981.

Wardle J: Cognitive control of eating, *J Psychosom Res* 32(6):607, 1988.

White J: An overview of obesity: its significance to nursing, *Nurs Clin North Am* 17:191, 1982.

Obsessions

Obsessions are involuntarily produced, persistent, and recurring ideas, thoughts, images, and impulses that invade consciousness and usually are experienced as senseless and repugnant. Attempts are made to suppress or ignore them. The most common obsessions are repetitive thoughts of violence, contamination, and doubt. Rumination, brooding, and preoccupation are closely aligned to obsessions but are not true obsessions because they are generally regarded as meaningful by the individual.

Compulsions are commonly associated with obsessions. Compulsions are repetitive and seemingly purposeful behaviors or rituals performed according to certain rules or in a stereotyped fashion. The behavior is designed to produce or prevent some future event or situation. It is difficult to separate obsessions from compulsions. The two frequently occur together. However, to understand the dynamics of each, they are discussed separately (see Compulsions, p. 72).

Phobias are also related to obsessions. Phobias are persistent, irrational fears of a specific object, anxiety, or situation; the fear is recognized as excessive or unreasonable. Examples include fear of heights or snakes.

Obsessions are a means of dealing with excessive anxiety. The repetitive acts (compulsions) are attempts to control anxiety and deal with the obsessive thoughts. Generally, obsessive thoughts are symbolic of the client's conflict.

Obsessive thinking is valued in our society in areas of functioning where thoroughness, cleanliness, and attention to detail are required. It is when the person is obsessive to the point that he is unable to function that obsessions become pathological.

Related DSM-III-R disorders

Anxiety disorders
Phobic disorders
Obsessive-compulsive disorders
Compulsive personality disorder
Psychoactive substance use disorders
Pathological gambling
Kleptomania
Pyromania
Anorexia nervosa
Bulimia nervosa

Other related conditions

Obesity

PRINCIPLES

▶ Physical Dimension

1. Obsessions followed by a compulsion to act may influence the client's physical health, for example, nutrition or sleep.

▶ Emotional Dimension

1. Mounting anxiety is discharged through obsessions.
2. Obsessions represent a conditioned response to anxiety.
3. Obsessions are viewed as a source of threat and anxiety, not as deeply unconscious, primitive drives, but as unacceptable ideas and feelings that are close to an individual's conscious awareness.
4. The behavior of an obsessional person is designed to minimize anxiety and maintain interpersonal security.
5. Obsessions do not allow the person to feel satisfied, and they give rise to feelings of guilt that need to be expiated through self-punishment.
6. A feeling of anxious dread provokes the obsession and leads the individual to take countermeasures to reduce the anxious dread.
7. Obsessions result when an individual regresses to the pre-oedipal or anal-sadistic stage with the consequent emergence of earlier levels of functioning of the id, ego, and superego.
8. With fixation at a particular stage of development, the person maintains personality characteristics (obsessions) typical of that stage.

▶ **Intellectual Dimension**

1. Miscommunication is a common trait of the obsessional person.
2. Earlier levels of functioning combined with specific ego functions (isolation, undoing, or displacement) produce symptoms of obsession.
3. The individual has the insight to recognize the irrationality of the obsession and the distress it causes.
4. When the balance between control and expression leads to a decreased ability to function, the obsession becomes a liability.
5. Obsessions are viewed as a psychological conflict between impulses and controlling defensive forces.
6. Cognitive processes mediate any threat that creates anxiety; the threat becomes frightening if the individual perceives that he does not have the ability to cope.

▶ **Social Dimension**

1. Obsessions are responses the individual has learned and selected or has chosen to repeat.
2. Obsessive traits are highly valued in Western culture and are demonstrated in many successful businessmen and businesswomen.
3. When the number and range of behavioral activities that are taboo for the person with obsessive thinking are markedly increased, he becomes harsher in self-judgment.
4. Power struggles over bowel training between an impatient and demanding mother and a child with a stronger-than-average level of omnipotence may result in obsessive traits.
5. Obsessive thoughts give rise to a need for perfection in oneself and others.
6. Obsessions are ego alien to the individual's self-concept.
7. Obsessions substitute for relationships with others.
8. Obsessions are used in negotiating interactions and social roles.

▶ **Spiritual Dimension**

1. There is rigid adherence to beliefs and moral standards in obsessive persons.
2. There is little tolerance for differences of opinion about values and beliefs.
3. Prejudices are firmly fixed in persons with obsessive traits.
4. The individual may accept religious beliefs unquestioningly.
5. The obsessive individual may become depressed, hopeless, and disillusioned when high standards for self and others are not met.

ASSESSMENT

▶ **Physical Dimension**

I. History
  A. Activities of daily living
    1 Nutrition
      a. Obsessions about food preparation, germs, and contamination; possible deficits in nutritional intake
      b. Refusal to eat
      c. Weight loss
    2. Sleep
      a. Obsessions about sleep; getting up, dressing, and going to bed; possible result, actions that consume inordinate amounts of time
  B. Destructive behavior
    1. Obsessions that threaten health
      a. Concern about body image
      b. Concern about germs and contamination
      c. Concern about food

▶ **Emotional Dimension**

CLIENT DATA	ANALYSIS	NURSING DIAGNOSIS
Anxiety	Increased anxiety unapparent and discharged through obsessive thinking.	Altered thought processes: obsessive thinking related to increased anxiety
Distress and despair	Knows unreasonableness of the thought but unable to do anything about it.	Ineffective individual coping: despair and distress related to obsessive thinking
Fearfulness	Fears being harmed; may be associated with any object, situation, or activity, such as going out, dogs, germs, height, or darkness (phobias). Obsessions represent conditioned response to anxiety.	Altered thought processes: obsessive thinking related to fear of going out/dogs/germs/height/darkness
Limited ability to express emotions	Thinking dominated by obsessions.	Ineffective individual coping: inability to express emotions related to obsessive thinking
Guilt	Feels sinful; may attempt to repress hostile, aggressive feelings; psychological conflict between id impulses and controlling defenses.	*Guilt: related to obsessions

▶ **Intellectual Dimension**

CLIENT DATA	ANALYSIS	NURSING DIAGNOSIS
Irrational, bizarre thoughts of violence, contamination, or doubt	Symbolic of client's destructive thoughts, anxieties, and conflict; obsessions are ego alien to individual's self-perception.	Altered thought processes: obsessions related to irrational, bizarre thoughts
Impaired judgment and insight	Aware of irrational thought but unable to do anything about it; lacks ability to be insightful and introspective.	*Altered judgment: impaired insight related to obsessive thinking
Ethnocentricity	Prejudges others based on irrational thoughts.	Altered thought processes: prejudgment of others related to obsessions
Repetitive thoughts and ruminations	Unable to ignore or suppress thoughts; not under voluntary control.	Altered thought processes: ruminations related to obsessive thinking
Use of rationalization, symbolization, and isolation	Aim to have others unaware of their obsessions, to protect from impulses that are unacceptable.	Defensive coping: excessive use of defense mechanisms related to obsessions
Rigid, dogmatic thinking	Restricted interests and knowledge; closed mind.	Altered thought processes: rigidity in thinking related to obsessions
Overabundance of detail	Striving for accuracy and perfection; need to be correct; a "stickler" for details.	Altered thought processes: overabundance of detail related to obsessive thinking
Ambivalence and indecision	Dominated or incapacitated by doubt, indecisiveness, reluctance to take risks, and difficulty making and carrying out decisions.	Altered thought processes: ambivalence and indecisiveness related to obsessive thinking

▶ **Social Dimension**

CLIENT DATA	ANALYSIS	NURSING DIAGNOSIS
Dependency in relationships	Needs reassurance; loath to let go; compromises personal aspirations.	Ineffective individual coping: related to dependency
Decreased social contacts; self-isolation and avoidance of others	Obsessions are restrictive; client withdraws from others; obsessions substitute for relationships with others.	Social isolation: withdrawal or avoidance of others related to obsessions
Aloofness and superficial involvement with others	Has difficulty expressing feelings.	Impaired social interactions: superficiality and aloofness related to obsessions
Strained family relationships	Controls family with idiosyncratic needs; symptoms dominate interactions.	Ineffective family coping: strained family relationships related to obsessions
Impaired social roles	Obsessions interfere with role functioning; behavior is ritualistic, with need for certain procedures to be completed before individual can move to next procedure.	Altered role performance: related to obsessions

▶ **Spiritual Dimension**

CLIENT DATA	ANALYSIS	NURSING DIAGNOSIS
Deviation from rigidly following morally scrupulous standards	Conflict between impulses and controlling defenses; creates anxiety.	Spiritual distress: deviations from rigid adherence to moral standards related to obsessions
Conflict with prejudices	Unwilling to accept differing faiths; prejudice based on irrational thoughts.	Spiritual distress: questioning of prejudices related to obsessions
Unquestioning, blind obedience to religious principles	Religious principles, beliefs accepted literally; obeys without question.	Spiritual distress: blind obedience to religious principles and beliefs related to obsessions
Lack of comforting quality in religion	Rigid adherence prevents sense of comfort and serenity.	Spiritual distress: lack of comfort with religion associated with obsessive thinking
Distress	Ponders pros and cons of a religious or philosophical question in a prolonged, fruitless, inconclusive inner dialogue.	Spiritual distress: prolonged, inconclusive inner dialogue regarding religion or philosophical question related to obsessions
Despair	Rigid adherence to religious and ethical beliefs creates feelings of guilt and inadequacy; high standards, when not met, result in guilt, disillusionment, and despair.	Spiritual distress: despair related to unmet high standards

PLANNING

Long-Term Goals

To decrease obsessive thoughts so that client can function effectively
To cope with anxiety without use of obsessive behavior

SHORT-TERM GOALS	OUTCOME CRITERIA
Physical Dimension To identify causes of obsessive thinking	1. Describes events, concerns, life stressors, and situations that produce anxiety 2. Explores effects of events, concerns, life stressors, and situations on behavior
Emotional Dimension To express feelings about events, concerns, life stressors, and situations	1. Expresses feelings about stressors 2. States that anxiety evokes obsessive thoughts
Intellectual Dimension To decrease or eliminate obsessive thinking	1. Allows self a short period of time to focus on obsession (10 minutes every hour) 2. Attends to other thoughts and feelings remainder of the time 3. Decreases time for focusing on obsession gradually to as little as 5 minutes every 2 hours or less 4. Uses thought-stopping techniques
To identify other ways to cope with anxiety without obsessive behavior	1. Explores other ways to cope with anxiety
Social Dimension To increase self-esteem	1. Verbalizes feelings of adequacy, competence, and worth 2. Is successful in completing tasks 3. Demonstrates decreased anxiety 4. Tells jokes, uses humor, and laughs appropriately
To maintain supportive relationships	1. Seeks out friends 2. Participates in social activities 3. Is comfortable during social interactions, one on one and small groups
To function effectively in roles (family, work, school)	1. Describes situations/events that increase anxiety and interfere with role functioning 2. States methods for reducing anxiety 3. Uses anxiety-reducing methods 4. Functions effectively in role
Spiritual Dimension To live a satisfying life with less obsessive thinking	1. Functions independently 2. Communicates without alienating family 3. Maintains supportive relationships 4. Is flexible in interpreting values and moral standards 5. Is able to think abstractly 6. Is less prejudiced 7. Thinks with openness and flexibility 8. Has less need to be correct and perfect 9. Is able to take risks 10. Is curious about new knowledge and ideas 11. Receives comfort from religion 12. Accepts differing faiths

Discharge Planning

The following client behaviors demonstrate readiness for discharge:
1. Identifies own anxiety
2. Reduces anxiety level with stress-reduction techniques
3. Identifies the relationship between anxiety and obsessions
4. Copes effectively with obsessions
5. Is open to new ideas and experiences

IMPLEMENTATION

NURSING ACTIONS	RATIONALE
Physical Dimension	
1. Reduce demands when increased anxiety is evident.	To lessen anxiety.
2. Limit behavior when it threatens health, for example, excessive concern about germs.	To prevent harmful effects of obsessive-compulsive behavior.
3. Establish routine daily activities.	To increase feelings of security. This occurs when client knows what to expect each hour of the day.
4. Allow sufficient time to complete tasks.	To avoid increasing client's anxiety by hurrying.
Emotional Dimension	
1. Provide activities leading to positive accomplishments.	To increase self-concept and feelings of adequacy.
2. Encourage client to verbalize when anxious or fearful.	To help client talk about distress may decrease acting on it with compulsive behavior.
3. Provide diversional activities of interest to client.	To promote pleasurable experiences.
4. Accept client without scolding or criticism.	To prevent client from further devaluing self. Client can cope with this kind of behavior. When the nurse acts differently from others a change in behavior occurs.
5. Avoid hurrying client.	To prevent increasing anxiety that occurs when pushed.
Intellectual Dimension	
1. Assist client with new ways to solve problems by teaching problem solving.	To develop more effective coping skills.
2. Provide information and teaching when anxiety is at a low level.	To promote learning. Learning takes place best when anxiety is at a moderate level.
3. Avoid arguing or persuading about fears and anxieties.	To prevent client from holding on tighter to obsessions, which may occur when threatened.
4. Use a matter-of-fact approach.	To avoid responding emotionally.
5. Use systematic desensitization.	To help client control feelings in the presence of feared stimuli (phobias).
6. Use thought stopping and thought switching.	To help client change to a positive way of thinking.
7. Explore with client prejudices and stereotypes that hinder self-growth.	To help client consider other ways of perceiving people, ideas, beliefs. To be more open and accepting and to increase relationships with others who think differently.
8. Refrain from calling attention to client's obsession.	To avoid reinforcing the behavior.
9. Direct interaction in a positive direction when client is obsessing.	To distract with a positive experience and increase client comfort.
10. Give verbal support for attempts to lessen obsessive thinking and decrease frequency.	To reinforce appropriate behavior.
11. Talk about other symptoms (ambivalence, frustration, and rigidity).	To facilitate client's expression of feelings. Once identified, ways to cope with them can be explored.
12. Interject reality when obsessions are delusional by saying, for example, "I see it this way."	To present reality.
13. Identify a baseline frequency of obsessive thinking and keep a record to show a decrease in time used for obsessive thinking.	To measure progress.
14. Intervene when obsessive thinking becomes life-threatening.	To prevent self-harm.
15. Explore the differences between thoughts and actions.	To help client see that thinking is not the same as acting, that the social consequences are different, and that it is OK to think negative thoughts.

NURSING ACTIONS	RATIONALE
Social Dimension	
1. Improve client's self-concept.	To increase feelings of adequacy and competence.
2. Provide supportive relationships.	To decrease feelings of loneliness and isolation.
3. Encourage family to participate in client's treatment regimen.	To provide support to client.
4. Help client increase social skills; introduce self, carry on a conversation, accept a compliment.	To promote comfort in social interactions.
5. Demonstrate personal flexibility and explore with client his reaction to others who demonstrate flexibility in thinking.	To promote awareness of benefits of flexibility and openness.
6. Support client for participating in activities, treatment, and interactions.	To reinforce participation in activities, treatment, and interactions that, in turn, promote comfort with others and lessen time for obsessive thinking.
7. Propose change in behavior after a supportive relationship is established.	To establish trust first, then work on behavioral change.
Spiritual Dimension	
1. Help client question rigid beliefs and personal standards.	To help client be open to and accept other ways of believing or thinking.
2. Help client be curious about new information and knowledge.	To motivate client to consider new experiences with less anxiety.
3. Explore with client differing faiths.	To help client be more open and accepting of people of other faiths without feeling threatened.
4. Refer to clergy.	To help client receive comfort from religion.
5. Promote activities that client enjoys.	To add pleasurable quality to life.

EVALUATION

Measurable goals and outcome criteria provide the data for evaluating clients with obsessive behavior. Nurse observations and family reports provide additional data. The following behaviors indicate a positive evaluation:

1. Identifies own anxieties
2. Knows when anxiety is increasing
3. Uses stress-reduction measures to lessen anxiety
4. States the relationship between anxiety and obsessive thinking
5. Copes with anxiety without obsessive thinking

BIBLIOGRAPHY

Barlow D: *The anxiety disorders: the nature and treatment of anxiety and panic*, New York, 1988, Guilford Press.

Cronin D: *Anxiety, depression and phobias: how to understand and deal with them*, Englewood Cliffs, N.J., 1982, Prentice-Hall.

Dalton P: Family treatment of an obsessive compulsive child: a case report, *Family Process* 22:99, 1983.

DeVeaugh-Geiss J, Landau P, Katz R: Treatment of obsessive-compulsive disorder with clomipramine, *Psychiatr Annals* 19:97, 1989.

DiNardo P, Barlow D: *Anxiety disorders interview schedule—revised (ADISI—R)*, Albany, N.Y., 1988, Phobia and Anxiety Disorders Clinic, University of Albany, State University of New York.

Insel T: Obsessive-compulsive disorders, *Psychiatr Clin North Am* 8:105, 1985.

Jenike M: *Obsessive-compulsive disorders: theory and management*, St. Louis, 1989, Mosby–Year Book.

Knowles R: Positive self talk, *Am J Nurs* 81(3):35, 1984.

Laraia M, Stuart G, Best C: Behavioral treatment of panic-related disorders: a review, *Arch Psychiatr Nurs* 3(3):125, 1989.

Marks I: Behavioral aspects of panic disorder, *Am J Psychiatry* 144:1160, 1987.

Mercer S: Obsessive compulsive disorders, *Nurs Times* 80(35):34, 1984.

O'Conner J: Why can't I get hives: a brief strategic therapy with an obsessive child . . . feared he would vomit, *Fam Process* 22(2):201, 1983.

Runck B: Research is changing views on obsessive compulsive disorders, *Hosp Community Psychiatry* 34(7):597, 1983.

Passive-Aggressive Behavior

Passive-aggressive behavior is the indirect verbal or nonverbal expression of angry, hostile feelings. It may be seen in any situation in which assertive behavior or the expression of anger is discouraged or punished. It is also seen as a habitual or enduring pattern of behavior, a pattern of behavior that results in disrupted social relations and may interfere in occupational functioning. Hostility and aggression are often expressed in an indirect, passive, nonviolent way such as procrastination, forgetting, stubbornness, intentional inefficiency, and obstructionism. Individuals with passive-aggressive traits view themselves as blameless for their difficulties; consequently, they have difficulty learning from previous troublesome situations. Disturbances in social and occupational roles result in anxiety and depression and frequently precipitate entrance into the health care system.

The behavior is usually unconsciously motivated and is employed to punish, retaliate, gain attention, express displeasure, or diminish another's effectiveness. Passive-aggressive behavior can be employed infrequently and exclusively in relation to specific persons or circumstances. While considered unhealthy, the behavior also exists within certain groups of oppressed peoples.

Related DSM-III-R disorders

Passive-aggressive personality disorder
Major depression
Dysthymia

Psychoactive substance-use disorders
Borderline personality disorder
Noncompliance with medical treatment

Other related conditions

Superior-subordinate roles such as physician-nurse or nurse-patient
Repressive bureaucratic environments
Oppressive political, social, or economic environments

PRINCIPLES

▶ Physical Dimension

1. An instinctual aggressive drive is common to all animals.

▶ Emotional Dimension

1. The individual has two basic instinctual drives—Eros, the life drive, and Thanatos, the death drive, which is expressed through anger and aggression.
2. The infant is totally dependent at birth and remains dependent for an extended period of time.
   a. The child whose dependency needs are met feels relatively secure about being cared for, but the child with unmet dependency needs becomes anxious.
   b. Unmet dependency needs result in frustration, anger, and insecurity.
   c. Parenting that is threatening, tenuous, or harsh results in the young child not daring to express anger, frustration, and resentment.
   d. The child does not feel safe in the expression of anger and inhibits its direct expression; however,

---

The original content for this section was contributed in part by Ann Adams, R.N., M.N.Sc.

anger and rage persist and build and indirect means of expression are chosen, causing further anger, frustration, and irritation.

e. While the child avoids the consequences of his act, the behavior creates a series of failures that undermine self-esteem and contribute to the child's inability to develop a sense of competence that normally results from the assumption of responsibility for his actions.

f. The greater the dependency needs of the adult, the greater the likelihood of indirect expressions of anger.

3. Anxiety results from the fear that the inhibited anger will be discovered.

4. The behavior pattern is ego syntonic, and the individual is comfortable with the behavior, since there is no awareness of the hostile intent of the behavior.

▶ Intellectual Dimension

1. Passive-aggressive behavior is the result of faulty or distorted thought processes resulting from conclusions that the individual draws from life experiences.

2. Contradictory messages from parents may contribute to the formation of such conclusions as "It is not acceptable to express my anger; others will retaliate against me and destroy me."

3. There are distortions in beliefs:
   a. It is impossible to achieve valued goals; thwarted goal achievement is the result of the unfairness of others.
   b. People who block other people's goals deserve to have their goals blocked in return.
   c. It is wrong to express anger and other feelings and thoughts directly.
   d. Direct assertion or aggression involves too great a risk.

▶ Social Dimension

1. Positive reinforcement following appropriate experiences of anger reinforces or supports further and continued expression of such anger.

2. Negative reinforcement or punishment suppresses or eliminates overt angry behavior.

3. Behaviors that produce the most desired results, which are reinforced, will be adopted.

4. Learning is acquired from observing the behavior of others.

5. The child observes (probably in caregivers) passive-aggressive behavior in response to a disagreement or frustration. In a similar situation, the child uses passive-aggressive behavior that is positively reinforced.

6. Relationships and communications in family systems are conceptualized as circular rather than linear. Resistance or aggression indirectly expressed is communicated to and disturbing to family members.
   a. Passive-aggressive behaviors are viewed as interactions rather than isolated behaviors.
   b. These behaviors are both active and reactive and are reinforced by feedback loops affirming the behavior.

7. The cultural milieu may encourage the indirect expression of negative feelings.

▶ Spiritual Dimension

1. Passive-aggressiveness is an experience in which the individual views the world or someone in the world as a controlling authority.

2. The dominated, controlled person experiences self as a helpless victim who relates in a passive-aggressive manner to retaliate or further elicit controlling behavior in others; this in turn confirms or validates the manner in which the person experiences being.

ASSESSMENT

▶ Physical Dimension

I. History
  A. Destructive behavior
    1. Indirect aggressive or hostile behavior that often destroys relationships

▶ Emotional Dimension

CLIENT DATA	ANALYSIS	NURSING DIAGNOSIS
Anger	Anger and aggression unconsciously channeled into passive-aggressive behavior; has not developed assertiveness in expressing anger.	*Anger: related to inability to express anger in a conscious and constructive manner

▶ **Emotional Dimension—cont'd**

CLIENT DATA	ANALYSIS	NURSING DIAGNOSIS
Anxiety	Frustrated dependency needs among other demands create anger and resentment. Anger is inhibited but fear that it may be discovered results in anxiety. Rarely acknowledged that anger is reason for seeking help.	Anxiety: related to anger and the inability to meet dependency needs
Guilt	Anger is considered an unacceptable feeling and results in feelings of guilt.	Guilt: related to unacceptable feelings of anger
Helplessness	Feels like the victim and blames others for difficulties.	*Helplessness: related to inability to accept own feelings and responsibility for own actions
Superficially cordial, yet hostile (for example, "You look lovely today but that color doesn't do a thing for you")	Anger is pervasive and is expressed indirectly; fears retaliation if anger expressed directly.	Ineffective individual coping: hostility related to inability to assert self or express anger directly
Sullenness and moodiness	Discontented and frustrated.	Ineffective individual coping: sullenness and moodiness related to inability to express anger
Ambivalence	Vacillates between passive dependence and assertive independence; unable to gauge which strategy will achieve the rewards wished.	Ineffective individual coping: ambivalence related to obedient dependence versus assertive independence
Resentfulness	Expects others to meet client's needs.	Ineffective individual coping: resentful of others when dependency needs unmet

▶ **Intellectual Dimension**

CLIENT DATA	ANALYSIS	NURSING DIAGNOSIS
Little insight	Does not perceive behavior as contributing to unhappiness if habitual pattern of behavior. Behavior pattern is ego syntonic; individual is comfortable with it.	Altered thought processes: related to inability to evaluate the reality of the effect of behavior on others
Forgetfulness	Will forget appointments, birthdays, and special events; forgets to bring important documents to meetings; suffers distortions in beliefs, believing direct assertion or aggression involves too great a risk.	Altered thought processes: forgetfulness related to inability to express anger directly
Believes self to be victimized	Believes that he is blameless and that others are to blame for inability to achieve goals.	Altered thought processes: cognitive distortions related to belief that others are to blame for inability to achieve goals
Believes world unfair and unpredictable place	An underlying assumption that results in distorted beliefs.	Altered thought processes: cognitive distortions related to a negative view of the world
Views authority figures as unjust and tyrannical	An underlying assumption that results in distorted beliefs.	Altered thought processes: cognitive distortions related to belief that authority figures are unjust
Uses denial	A defense mechanism to reduce anxiety; hostility remains at unconscious level.	Ineffective denial: related to inability to accept own feelings of anger

▶ Intellectual Dimension—cont'd

CLIENT DATA	ANALYSIS	NURSING DIAGNOSIS
Uses projection	A defense mechanism to reduce anxiety; projects blame for misfortunes to others.	Ineffective individual coping: projection related to the inability to assume responsibility for own actions
Speaks softly or loudly	Can be a source of irritation to others.	Impaired verbal communication: speaking too softly or loudly related to inability to express anger directly
Unable to consider alternative forms of behavior	Persists in behavior even when more adaptive functioning is possible.	Ineffective individual coping: related to inability to consider alternatives to present behavior

▶ Social Dimension

CLIENT DATA	ANALYSIS	NURSING DIAGNOSIS
Fails to live up to potential	Lacks self-confidence. Passive-aggressive behavior creates series of failures that undermine self-esteem; sense of competence not developed.	Self-esteem disturbance: chronic, related to a series of life failures
Unable to maintain an effective, flexible relationship with others	Individual is comfortable with behavior; does not have insight necessary to change behavior.	Impaired social interactions: related to alienation of others
Smilingly sarcastic, friendly but cutting observations	Provokes anger in person who is target; confrontation with sarcastic humor results in denial of intent to hurt—"What's wrong? Can't you take a joke?"	Impaired social interactions: related to alienation of others by sarcasm
Sweetly nagging; critical and complaining	Has not developed ability to make needs known.	Impaired verbal communication: nagging, criticism, and complaining related to inability to make needs known
Withholds information	Anger demonstrated through resistant behaviors.	Ineffective individual coping: resistance related to withholding information
Dawdling—"Gee, sorry I'm late again, but . . . "	Indirect expression of resistance.	Ineffective individual coping: dawdling related to resistance in response to social and role responsibilities
Stubbornness	Indirect expression of resistance.	Ineffective individual coping: stubbornness related to resistance in response to social and role responsibilities
Procrastinates—"Next time I'll be sure to bring that material."	Indirect expression of resistance.	Ineffective individual coping: procrastination related to resistance in response to social and role responsibilities
Intentionally inefficient—"No, I just didn't have time to make those arrangements."	Indirect expression of resistance.	Ineffective individual coping: intentional inefficiency related to resistance in response to social and role responsibilities
Dependency demonstrated by questions such as "What should I do?" and "Why do I do that?"	Failure to understand how to help self; unwillingness to assume responsibility for successes or failures; asks others for assistance.	Ineffective individual coping: passive dependency related to subordinating one's needs to decisions of others

▶ **Spiritual Dimension**

CLIENT DATA	ANALYSIS	NURSING DIAGNOSIS
Pessimistic about the future	Believes that life is unpredictable and difficult.	Spiritual distress: related to pessimism about future
Finds little reward in life	Ineffective socially and occupationally because of passive-aggressive behaviors.	Spiritual distress: related to unrewarding life
Experiences being a helpless victim	Relates in passive-aggressive manner to retaliate, eliciting behavior in others that in turn validates the helplessness.	Spiritual distress: related to experience of being a helpless victim

PLANNING

Long-Term Goals

To develop more efficient, direct, and effective means of expression of hostility and anger

To become more adequate in social and occupational role performance by demonstrating less resistance and more self-determination

SHORT-TERM GOALS	OUTCOME CRITERIA
Emotional Dimension	
To become aware of feelings of hostility or anger	1. Identifies the subjective experience of anger or hostility 2. Identifies the physical sensation of anger or hostility 3. Labels the experience as anger or hostility
To express feelings of anger or hostility	1. Expresses anger or hostility directly 2. Verbalizes acceptance of feelings of anger or hostility in self
Intellectual Dimension	
To increase the capacity to judge the effects of passive-aggressive behavior on others	1. Identifies situations that cause irritation or anger 2. Identifies response or behavior in irritating or anger-producing situations 3. Discusses the effects of indirect expression of anger on others 4. Becomes more assertive
Social Dimension	
To become more cooperative in social and role functioning	1. Completes work on time 2. Keeps appointments and is on time 3. Is willing to compromise and cooperate 4. Increases efficiency 5. Reduces procrastination
To increase self-esteem	1. (See Negative Self-Concept, p. 231)
To become more independent	1. Makes own decisions 2. Expresses differences in opinions 3. Looks beyond self and helps others
Spiritual Dimension	
To experience being in a new open and direct way	1. Discusses choices 2. Learns to explore body reactions to situational experiences 3. Discusses effects of anger on the total experience
To become more conscious of self	1. Examines conflicting emotions and integrates into conscious self 2. Becomes more accepting of self
To decrease estrangement from others	1. Expresses genuine care and concern for others 2. Becomes more adept in relating to others in an effort to understand them

Discharge Planning

The following client behaviors indicate readiness for discharge:
1. Identifies anger-producing situations
2. Reduces the frequency of hostile remarks
3. Assumes responsibility for meeting own dependency needs
4. Is assertive
5. Uses less resistance to and more cooperation with others

IMPLEMENTATION

NURSING ACTIONS	RATIONALE
Physical Dimension	
1. Encourage physical activities.	To decrease restlessness associated with anxiety and anger.
2. Assist client in identifying physical manifestations of anxiety.	To promote awareness of bodily sensations of anxiety and plan interventions.
3. Use relaxation techniques.	To reduce effects of anxiety and become more open to change.
4. Assist client in identifying physical manifestations of anger.	To promote awareness of bodily sensations of anger and plan interventions.
Emotional Dimension	
1. Focus on client's feelings.	To help client identify feelings since unacknowledged and unexpressed feelings are the root of client's problems in living.
2. Assist client in labeling feelings of irritation, resentment, anger, or hurt.	To increase client's awareness of negative feelings and ability to express them openly.
3. Discuss relationship between feelings of irritation, hurt, resentment, and behavior.	To help client connect identified feelings with behavior and consider options for change.
4. Suggest that client may be hurt, irritated, or upset rather than angry, since those feelings are more acceptable than anger.	To help client accept negative feelings in self.
5. Encourage client to discuss uncomfortable feelings of hurt, irritation, or being upset.	To determine degree and duration of uncomfortable feelings and help client to know that talking about negative feelings with a trusted person is therapeutic.
6. Convey to client that irritation, anger, and resentment are normal responses.	To help client accept self with feelings, both negative and positive.
7. Use fantasy in a nonthreatening situation.	To help client express anger appropriately.
8. Observe nonverbal cues that indicate anger.	To give client feedback about nonverbal behaviors.
9. Use self-disclosure to share experiences that cause irritation and anger.	To help client understand that it is normal to get irritated or angry.
10. Explain how your own unawareness of feelings of resentment or anger resulted in passive-aggressive behavior.	To model self-disclosure and help client feel comfortable in self-disclosing.
11. Discuss interactions in situations or with persons that result in feelings of resentment.	To determine reasons for feelings of resentment.
12. Encourage expression of guilt feelings (see Guilt, p. 155).	To determine degree of guilt and plan interventions.
13. Note that feelings of guilt do not mean that a person has done something bad.	To help client understand guilt feelings and relationship to behavior.
Intellectual Dimension	
1. Involve client in activities that encourage or require self-responsibility such as goal setting, and carefully explain client's responsibilities.	To elicit client's participation in making decisions about self, thereby increasing compliance with treatment goals and feelings of control and independence.
2. Be aware that client will attempt to have you do much of the work and will find ways to withdraw from the contract while blaming you.	To increase awareness of client's ability to manipulate.
3. Hold client accountable for keeping appointments, arriving on time, and completing assignments.	To promote client's accountability for own behavior.
4. Involve client in assertiveness training.	To learn to be direct and open in expressing self, to decrease passivity.

IMPLEMENTATION—cont'd

NURSING ACTIONS	RATIONALE
5. Model assertiveness.	To help client see assertive skills and the effects on others.
6. Provide opportunities for client to practice and express assertive behavior or anger.	To gain confidence in the skill of asserting self and expressing anger appropriately.
7. When client asks for permission such as, "Is it OK if I go to the rec room now?" ask client to change request to statement, "I am going to the rec room now."	To help client express self directly.
8. Teach problem-solving techniques (see Appendix C).	To help client discover appropriate methods for the expression of anger.
9. Encourage negative and positive feedback from client, such as "Have I said anything that has hurt your feelings?" or "Have we talked about something that was particularly helpful?"	To help client be sensitive to others and learn to ask for feedback.
10. When client is assertive, respond empathetically, not defensively or argumentatively; for example, say "I hear you saying that I can't ever understand how you feel in that situation. Tell me more."	To provide support, to help client by letting him know you want to understand what he is feeling.
11. Ask client to make a list of the advantages and disadvantages of expressing anger in a situation.	To consider best options for handling anger, to demonstrate problem-solving skills.
12. Discuss ways that anger expression will be hurtful or harmful to client and others.	To increase awareness of effects of anger expression on self and others.
13. Examine with client appropriate expressions of anger, for example, how to keep his language from being excessively hostile or blaming.	To promote expressions of anger that do not hurt others and that help client accept responsibility for feeling angry.
14. Examine motivations associated with the expression of resentment or anger.	To determine underlying reasons for anger or resentment.
15. Discuss with client that expression of anger can be a way of sharing feelings and negotiating problems or a way of getting revenge.	To help client understand underlying reasons for anger.
16. Role play or rehearse behaviors that provide client the opportunity to examine passive-aggressive behavior.	To help client develop more effective coping and communication styles.
17. Assist client in identifying situations that are upsetting and cause negative feelings, and identify thoughts that are associated with those feelings.	To help client gain insight about negative feelings by connecting them to situations.
18. Assist client in identifying distortions in beliefs that result in unrecognized anger or hostility.	To present reality, to help client identify anger and hostility.
19. Teach client to substitute thoughts that are more objective and realistic.	To promote realistic thinking.
20. Examine with client fears of retaliation for expression of anger.	To discuss fears openly and plan strategies to handle them often reduces the fear.
21. Provide positive feedback for successful expression of anger.	To reinforce appropriate behavior.
22. Ignore client when he is argumentative, complaining, or sarcastic.	To argue with client induces further stubbornness, resentment, and passive-aggressive behavior.
23. Provide positive reinforcement when client is on time.	To give feedback and acknowledge appropriate behavior.
24. Provide positive reinforcement when client makes effort to compromise.	To give feedback and acknowledge appropriate behavior.
25. Identify alternative ways to express anger.	To help client have knowledge of several methods of expressing anger, for example, verbally expressing it or physically expressing it.
26. Call attention to tone of client's voice when client complains or whines.	To promote awareness of verbal tones.
27. Interrupt blaming others or using the past as justification for present behavior.	To help client examine angry behavior, assume responsibility for it, explore anxiety and need for defenses.

NURSING ACTIONS	RATIONALE
Social Dimension	
1. Involve client in group therapy.	To promote confrontation with passive-aggressive behavior, stubbornness, and procrastination, to model assertive behavior.
2. Encourage client to express differences of opinion with group members.	To promote active, direct communication, to decrease passivity and indecisiveness.
3. Enhance self-esteem (see Negative Self-Concept, p. 231).	To increase client's confidence in self and ability to change behavior.
4. Encourage independence; when client asks, "What should I do?" reply with "What do you want to do?"	To decrease dependence and passivity, to help client rely on own resources.
5. Clarify with client the feelings, both negative and positive, that accompany dependency.	To identify secondary gains associated with dependence, to reinforce independence.
6. Involve family or significant others in family therapy.	To interrupt the circular pattern of passive-aggressive behavior within the family.
Spiritual Dimension	
1. Encourage client to experience feelings of situations or events as a means of experiencing total self.	To promote a sense of wholeness and harmony within one's total self that includes both positive and negative feelings associated with life events.
2. Guide client in the discovery of a more satisfying life with less anger and resentment.	To motivate client to be curious about his behavior as a basis for change.
3. Provide opportunities for creative expression of anger and hostility.	To help client express anger openly in new ways that are appropriate for client.
4. Assist client in assuming responsibility for own actions and behavior.	To increase feelings of worth and respect that are associated with assuming responsibility for own self.

EVALUATION

Measurable goals and outcome criteria provide the data for evaluating the client with passive-aggressive behavior. Nurse observations and family reports provide additional data. The following behaviors indicate a positive evaluation:

1. Identifies situations that evoke anger and resentment
2. States when angry and resentful to appropriate person
3. Is aware of effects of anger and resentment on others
4. Makes fewer sarcastic, critical comments
5. Expresses differences of opinions to others
6. Refrains from blaming others
7. Uses physical activity to reduce feelings of anger and resentment
8. Tolerates anger and resentment in self
9. Has an increased self-concept
10. Increases independence in thinking and actions

BIBLIOGRAPHY

Abstracts from the fifth biennial meeting of the International Society for Research on Aggression, *Aggress Behav* 9(2):103, 1983.

Averill JR: Studies on aggression: implications for theories of emotions, *Am Psychiatry* 38(11):1145, 1983.

Bassoff EL: Healthy aspects of passivity and Gendlin's focusing. *Personnel Guidance J* 62(5):268, 1984.

Blashfield RK, McElroy RA: Ontology of personality disorder categories, *Psychiatr Ann* 19(3):126, 1989.

Bonds-White F: The special it: treatment of the passive-aggressive personality, *Transact Anal J* 14(3):180, 1984.

Burns D, Epstein N: Passive-aggressiveness: a cognitive-behavioral approach. In Parsons R, Wicks R, editors: *Passive-aggressiveness: theory and practice*, New York, 1983, Brunner/Mazel.

Chinisci RA: Transient oxygen deficiency dementia or passive-aggressive personality disorder? *Clin Gerontol* 7(3–4):78, 1988.

Cole M: How to make a person passive-aggressive: or the power struggle game, *Transact Anal J* 14(3):191, 1984.

Davidhizar RE: Managing the passive-aggressive student nurse, *Nurse Educ* 8(2):34, 1983.

Davidhizar R, Giger J: When subordinates go over your head: the manipulative employee, *J Nurs Admin* 20(9):29, 1990.

Eichelman B: The limbic system and aggression in humans, *Neurosci Behav Rev* 7(3):391, 1983.

Evans D: Problems in the decision-making process: a review, *Intensive Care Nurs* 6(4):179, 1990.

Hedlund BL, Linquist CA: The development of an inventory for distinguishing among passive aggressive and assertive behavior, *Behav Assess* 6(4):379, 1984.

Jaffe DS: Aggression: instinct, drive, behavior, *Psychoanal Inq* 2(1):77, 1982.

Johnson-Saylor MT: An exploratory study of the experience of resentment, *West J Nurs Res* 8(1):49, 1986.

Kaplan AG, Yasinki L: Conflict and conflict inhibition in women: theoretical considerations and clinical applications, *J Am Acad Psychoanal* 12(1):13, 1984.

Karli P: Human aggression and animal aggression: a unifying view of the brain-behavior relationships involved, *Aggress Beh* 9(2):94, 1983.

Kaslow F: Passive-aggressiveness: an intrapsychic, interpersonal, and transactional dynamic in the family system. In Parsons R, Wicks R, editors: *Passive-aggressiveness: theory and practice*, New York, 1983, Brunner/Mazel.

King M: Look back in anger, *Nurs Mirror* 155:52, 1982.

Korenblum M et al: The classification of disturbed personality functioning in early adolescence, *Can J Psychiatry,* 32(5):362, 1987.

Lanza ML: Origins of aggression, *J Psychosoc Nurs Ment Health Serv* 21(6):10, 1983.

Lerner HE: Female dependence in context: some theoretical and technical considerations, *Am J Orthopsychiatry* 53(4):697, 1983.

Lorenz K: *On aggression* (translated by M.K. Wilson), New York, 1966, Harcourt Brace & World.

Maher A: An existential-experimental view and operational perspective on passive aggressiveness. In Parsons R, Wicks R, editors: *Passive-aggressiveness: theory and practice,* New York, 1983, Brunner/Mazel.

McCann JT: Passive-aggressive personality disorder: a review, *J Pers Dis* 2(2):170, 1988.

Musiker H, Norton R: The medical system: a complex arena for the exhibition of passive-aggressiveness. In Parsons R, Wicks R, editors: *Passive-aggressiveness: theory and practice,* New York, 1983, Brunner/Mazel.

Ober L: The analysis of a passive young man involved in fleeting relationships, *Issues Ego Psych* 11(2):79, 1988.

Parsons R: The educational setting: a cultural milieu fostering passive-aggressiveness. In Parsons R, Wicks R, editors: *Passive-aggressiveness: theory and practice,* New York, 1983, Brunner/Mazel.

Peterson C, Seligman ME: Learned helplessness and victimization, *J Soc Issues* 39(2):103, 1983.

Roberts S: Oppressed group behavior: implications for nursing, *Adv Nurs Sci* 5(4):21, 1983.

Rosenberg MS: Characteristics of the passive-aggressive personality disorder: males, *J Training Pract Prof Psych* 1(1):29, 1987.

Steketee G: Personality traits and disorders in obsessive-compulsives, *J Anxiety Dis* 4(4):351, 1990.

Weeks GR, L'Adate L: *Paradoxical psychotherapy: theory and practice with individuals, couples, and families,* New York, 1982, Brunner/Mazel.

Zerwekh J: Undoing the habit of hostility, *J Prof Nurs* 7(5):265,1991.

Phobias

Phobias are persistent and irrational fears of a specific object, activity, or situation that result in a compelling desire to avoid the dreaded object, activity, or situation. The individual recognizes the fear as excessive and out of proportion to the actual dangerousness of the object, activity, or situation. Phobias range from harmless to exceedingly dysfunctional.

The phobic object symbolizes an underlying conflict that usually is not recognizable to the client. Personal perceptions, life experiences, and cultural values provide the basis for the meaning of the symbolization to the client.

Phobias vary in degree of disability and discomfort. Mild phobias require less psychic energy and can be adapted to everyday living; others are so severe that the person is disabled.

Persons with phobias are not usually hospitalized. Many people seek help from a health professional when they become aware that the fear is interfering with their personal growth and functioning. At this time they are willing and motivated to change their behavior. When a person is hospitalized, the phobia is often seen in combination with severe anxiety. Relief from the anxiety is provided before the individual can work on the phobia. Many also get help from special phobia treatment clinics that have become available.

Related DSM-III-R disorders

Separation anxiety disorder
Obsessive-compulsive disorder
Anorexia nervosa
Simple phobias
   Acrophobia (height)
   Agoraphobia (open places)
   Ailurophobia (cats)
   Anthophobia (flowers)
   Anthropophobia (people)
   Aquaphobia (water)
   Arachneophobia (spiders)
   Astraphobia (lightning)
   Aviophobia (flying)
   Brontophobia (thunder)
   Claustrophobia (closed spaces)
   Cynophobia (dogs)
   Equinophobia (horses)
   Herpetophobia (lizards and reptiles)
   Maniaphobia (insanity)
   Microphobia (germs)
   Musophobia (mice)
   Mysophobia (dirt, germs, contamination)
   Nyctophobia (darkness)
   Ochlophobia (crowds)
   Ophidiophobia (snakes)
   Pyrophobia (fire)
   Thanatophobia (death)
   Trichophobia (loose hair)
   Xenophobia (strangers)
   Zoophobia (animals)
Social phobias

Other related conditions

Panic attack

PRINCIPLES

▶ Physical Dimension

1. Specific objects or situations form the basis of a phobia, for example, dogs, heights, flying.
2. Phobias may cause serious problems in day-to-day functioning.

▶ Emotional Dimension

1. Anxiety is a central component of a phobia.
2. Phobias may originate in the oedipal stage of development (3 to 5 years of age) when sexual impulses need to be repressed and denied conscious expression.

3. When repression fails, the original source of anxiety is displaced (symbolically attached) to some other object, person, or situation.
4. The symbolism is highly personal and determined by perceptions, life experiences, and cultural values.
5. A phobia is a disguised representation of a unconscious impulse.
6. Phobias control anxiety by providing a specific object to attach to it.
7. The individual controls the intensity of the anxiety by avoiding the object that is feared.
8. Mild fears (phobias) are common in children during the oedipal stage of development.
9. Aggression and sexual drives contribute to phobic reactions.
10. Phobias may become chronic disorders with frequent recurrence of symptoms that are resistant to treatment.
11. The degree of severity of the symptom and the incapacity resulting from it depends on the practical significance for the individual.

▶ **Intellectual Dimension**

1. Displacement is the essential feature in phobias.
2. Displacement keeps the relationship between the self and the forbidden impulse out of awareness.

▶ **Social Dimension**

1. Anxiety is aroused by a naturally and inherently frightening stimulus and can produce a conditioned reflex, a phobia.
2. Anxiety is viewed as a drive that motivates the individual to learn actions that avoid the stimulus of anxiety and subsequent pain.
3. Avoidance behavior becomes effective in preventing the individual from anxiety.
4. When the dreaded object cannot be avoided, intense anxiety is felt and panic may result.
5. Agoraphobia (fear of open places) is the most common phobia.
6. Phobias are learned behaviors.
7. Phobic behaviors can be unlearned and new behaviors learned.
8. The phobic client feels helpless to do anything about his phobia even though he recognizes it as excessive and out of proportion to the situation.
9. Systematic desensitization that presents anxiety-provoking cues in a climate of pleasure and relaxation reduces anxiety arousal.
10. Behavioral therapy effectively treats mild phobias.

▶ **Spiritual Dimension**

1. The quality of life becomes impoverished with certain phobias.
2. Escalation of imagined disasters chokes rational thinking and leads to despair and depression.

ASSESSMENT

▶ **Physical Dimension**

I. History
  A. Activities of daily living
    1. Inadequate nutrition if fears include germs, dirt, contamination, getting fat, or eating in the presence of others
    2. Impaired sleep if darkness is feared
    3. Termination of usual activities if fears dominate life
    4. Sexual dysfunction if sexual intimacy is feared
    5. Severely restricted average day if going out is feared

▶ **Physical Examination**

CLIENT DATA	ANALYSIS	NURSING DIAGNOSIS
Dyspnea Palpitations Chest pain Choking or smothering sensations Dizziness Vertigo Feelings of unreality Tingling in hands or feet Hot and cold flashes Sweating Faintness Trembling or shaking	Overwhelming fear contributes to symptoms similar to severe anxiety or panic attacks.	Severe anxiety related to fear of specific object, situation, or activity

▶ **Emotional Dimension**

CLIENT DATA	ANALYSIS	NURSING DIAGNOSIS
Intense fear of specific object, situation, activity	Anxiety is symbolically displaced onto object, situation, or activity.	Fear: related to specific object, situation, or activity
Fear is out of proportion to dreaded object	Client recognizes unreasonableness and excessiveness of fear but is unable to do anything about it.	Fear: disproportionate, related to specific object, situation, or activity
Depression	Distress and despair associated with symptoms (for example, fear of going out). Hopeless to do anything about it.	Ineffective individual coping: depression related to fear of going out (agoraphobia)
Fear of losing control	Anxiety and fear of unknown threatens personal security.	Fear: of losing control related to phobia

▶ **Intellectual Dimension**

CLIENT DATA	ANALYSIS	NURSING DIAGNOSIS
Disturbed perception	Objects, activities, or situations are perceived as more frightening than appropriate.	Altered thought processes: disturbed perception related to intense fear of object, situation, or activity
Insightful (to a degree)	Is aware of unreasonableness of fear, unaware of original anxiety-producing stimulus.	Altered thought processes: unaware of source of anxiety related to intense fears
Preoccupation with fears	Phobias dominate thinking.	Altered thought processes: preoccupation related to intense fear
Use of displacement, repression	Protects individual from overwhelming anxiety and reduces intensity of anxiety.	Defensive coping: related to intense fear
Rigid thinking	Unable to see alternatives as responses to fears ("closed mind"); anxiety acts as a drive so that client continues to use avoidance.	Altered thought processes: rigid thinking related to intense fears

▶ **Social Dimension**

CLIENT DATA	ANALYSIS	NURSING DIAGNOSIS
Lowered self-esteem	Fears being weak, cowardly, ineffective, or incapable.	Self-esteem disturbance: related to intense fears
Dependent, demanding obligatory companion	Passive in relationships; infantile clinging and demanding if afraid of being alone.	Ineffective individual coping: related to intense fear of being alone
Impaired or incapacitated social roles	Fears scrutiny by others, fears actions may humiliate or embarrass self. Avoidance of feared object results in dysfunction in social role.	Altered role performance: related to intense fears
Affected by environmental factors (heights, open places, cats, spiders, flowers, people, water, lightning, thunder, closed spaces, dogs, insanity, horses, lizards and reptiles, germs, mice, dirt, contamination, numbers, darkness, fire, death, hair, strangers, and animals)	Any environmental factor has potential for causing intense fear, depending on person's personal perception, life experiences, and cultural values; anxiety may be displaced to any object or situation.	Fear: intense, related to environmental factors

▶ **Spiritual Dimension**

CLIENT DATA	ANALYSIS	NURSING DIAGNOSIS
Lack of ability to move beyond phobia, stuck and distressed with situation	Distress and despair over phobia and inability to deal with it satisfactorily.	Spiritual distress: despair related to inability to deal with phobia
Impoverished life	Phobias are restrictive to client and prevent full enjoyment of life.	Spiritual distress: life restrictions related to phobia
Phobia-dominated life	Phobias are chronic disorders and resistant to treatment.	Spiritual distress: related to phobia-dominated life

PLANNING

Long-Term Goal

To cope adaptively with anxiety and stress without irrational fears

SHORT-TERM GOALS	OUTCOME CRITERIA
Physical Dimension	
To identify physical signs and symptoms of anxiety	1. Verbalizes physical sensations associated with anxiety 2. States relationship between anxiety and phobia
To use relaxation techniques	1. Uses relaxation techniques: deep breathing, muscle relaxation, guided imagery
Emotional Dimension	
To confront and feel anxiety directly	1. Identifies conflict situations and fears about them 2. Discusses factors contributing to fears and anxiety that may be related to phobia 3. Identifies physical sensations indicative of anxiety 4. States anxious feelings
To reduce or eliminate phobia	1. Controls fear of dreaded object 2. Is no longer fearful of dreaded object 3. Uses relaxation techniques when feeling anxious
Intellectual Dimension	
To develop alternative ways of responding to anxiety without phobias	1. States other ways to respond to anxiety 2. Demonstrates other ways to respond to anxiety 3. Verbalizes satisfaction with new ways to respond to anxiety 4. Participates in therapy (e.g., desensitization therapy)
To gain insight about relationship of anxiety to phobia	1. Identifies fears and anxieties 2. States relief measures for fears and anxieties 3. Uses other ways to cope with fears and anxieties without phobias 4. States relief measures are effective
Social Dimension	
To relate to others without anxiety	1. Learns social skills 2. Forms relationships with others 3. States a sense of comfort in relationships with others 4. Verbalizes anxiety to others 5. Accepts feedback from others about behavior
Spiritual Dimension	
To seek ways to enjoy pleasures of life	1. Asks for help with phobia 2. Cooperates with treatment methods 3. Participates in activities that formerly were feared

Discharge Planning

The following client behaviors demonstrate readiness for discharge:
1. Identifies own anxiety
2. Is able to control phobia
3. Uses relaxation techniques
4. Can desensitize self with help of supportive person
5. Discusses fears with significant person so that teaching can be reinforced

IMPLEMENTATION

NURSING ACTIONS	RATIONALE
Physical Dimension	
1. Provide adequate nutrition when phobia interferes with food and fluid intake.	To maintain adequate nutritional status and fluid balance.
2. Provide night lights.	To lessen fear of dark.
3. Encourage participation in activities.	To lessen restrictions in life.
4. Provide or refer for sex therapy if indicated.	To help client with problems with sexual functioning.
5. Refrain from forcing client to confront feared object.	To prevent increasing anxiety or panic attack.
6. Use supportive physical measures (warm bath, massage, or whirlpool) to reduce anxiety.	To reduce anxiety.
7. Promote vigorous physical activity.	To use the energy of anxiety and direct client's attention away from self.
8. Establish routine activities for daily living.	To avoid anxiety associated with change.
Emotional Dimension	
1. Help client face and feel anxiety, not avoid it.	To help client identify anxiety and discuss new ways to handle it.
2. Reduce anxiety-producing situations that stimulate phobia, using stress reduction methods, relaxation, deep breathing.	To provide client with protection, to allow time to adapt or adjust to situation.
3. Assist client in dealing with depression and despair associated with phobic symptoms.	To help client work through phobia requires helping with the despair first. Depressed clients have difficulty with attention and concentration and thus have difficulty learning new ways to cope with phobias.
4. Facilitate verbalization of feelings of anxiety.	To increase client's awareness of anxiety and plan interventions.
5. Monitor for signs of mounting anxiety; restlessness, tenseness.	To prevent severe anxiety or panic attack.
Intellectual Dimension	
1. Help client identify stress and anxiety.	To help client connect feeling of anxiety to phobia.
2. Refrain from ridiculing or belittling phobia.	To prevent increasing client's anxiety with behavior that is threatening, thus increasing need for phobia.
3. Refrain from attempting to argue or reason client out of phobia.	To prevent client from defending phobia more strongly.
4. Set limits, over time, on client's behavior.	To protect client from harmful effects of phobia or from others who may not understand client's behavior.
5. Refrain from pressuring client to change prematurely.	To prevent increasing client's anxiety with behavior that is threatening, thus increasing need for phobia.
6. Assist client in distinguishing between harmless and harmful fears.	To allow client to keep his harmless fears and help him find ways to deal with harmful fears.
7. Avoid reinforcing phobia.	To lessen focus on phobia.
8. Assist client in understanding that phobia is a symbolic representation of anxiety.	To increase client's awareness of causes of phobia.
9. Teach relaxation techniques.	To help client reduce anxiety.
10. Provide behavioral modification techniques (desensitization, reciprocal inhibition, flooding, and implosion).	To reduce or eliminate phobias.

IMPLEMENTATION—cont'd

NURSING ACTIONS	RATIONALE
11. Reinforce and support client at each step of behavior change.	To help client trust those helping him and have confidence in himself that he can overcome his phobias.
12. Refrain from reinforcing secondary gains obtained from phobia.	To prevent client from receiving benefits or satisfaction from phobia.
13. Teach alternative coping strategies.	To prevent other symptoms from developing.
14. Teach stress management.	To motivate client to reduce own anxiety and assume responsibility for doing so with specific techniques.
Social Dimension	
1. Encourage participation in activities and interests.	To limit time for phobias.
2. Reinforce socially productive behavior.	To increase feelings of adequacy, competence, and self-esteem.
3. Include family as source of support for client with phobias.	To help client increase support system.
4. Promote independence in relationships with assertiveness skills.	To decrease ambivalence and fear of being alone or without a supportive person.
5. Teach social skills.	To reduce anxiety from social situations, to prevent embarrassment or humiliation.
6. Reduce environmental factors that cause anxiety and subsequent phobia.	To provide protection while client works on and adjusts to new behaviors.
7. Provide psychotherapy or behavioral therapy.	To treat the incapacitating effects of phobia and promote self-growth.
Spiritual Dimension	
1. Assist with participation and enjoyment in other aspects of life (art, piano, and reading).	To reduce despair and depression, to maximize client's capabilities.
2. Help client deal with phobia so that client becomes less constrained and life is more pleasurable.	To help client live a more fulfilling, productive, and pleasurable life without the self-imposed constraints and restrictions associated with phobias.

EVALUATION

Measurable goals and outcome criteria provide the basis for evaluating the client with a phobia. Client self-reports, nurse observations, and family reports provide additional data. The following behaviors indicate a positive evaluation.

1. Identifies own anxiety
2. Links anxiety to phobia
3. Uses anxiety-reduction techniques to deal with phobia
4. Asks for help from a supportive person to desensitize self
5. Is able to control phobia
6. Attends self-help group for persons with phobias

BIBLIOGRAPHY

Adler J: The fight to conquer fear, *Newsweek* 103(17):66, 1984.

Bandura A: Modeling approaches to the modification of phobic disorders. In Forter R, editor: *The role of learning in psychotherapy,* Boston, 1968, Little, Brown, & Co.

Carper J: How phobias can be healed, *Reader's Digest* 125(48):102, 1984.

Fife B: The resolution of school phobia from family therapy, *J Psychiatr Nurs Ment Health Serv* 18(2):13, 1980.

Holm M: The case of the fearful flyers, *Your Life Health* 97(12):9, 1982.

Jones I: When the going gets tough . . . emotional casualities: victims of depression, anxiety, phobias, or self-harm, *Nurs Times* 83(38):46, 1987.

King N: The management of medical related phobias: strategies for nurses and allied health professionals, *Aust J Adv Nurs* 1(1):26, 1983.

Liebowitz M: Anxiety and phobias: dealing with disabling fear, *McCall's* 114(1):82, 1986.

MacPhail D, McMillan I: Fighting phobias, *Nurs Mirror* 157(7):8, 1983.

Mitchell R: Breakdown: anxiety states and phobias, part 5, *Nurs Times* 79(7):50, 1983.

Perrine S: Phobias: the facts about fears, *Parents* 64(9):208, 1989.

Rape Trauma Syndrome

Rape is a forced, violent sexual assault on an individual against her will and without her consent. According to legal criteria, three essential elements define an act of rape: the use of force, threat, or intimidation; vaginal penetration; and a lack of consent. Although men can be raped, this chapter focuses on women as victims of rape.

The incidence of rape has increased over the last decade and is rapidly becoming the fastest rising violent crime in the nation. Many women choose not to report rape because of unclear legal definitions and fear that the courts will decide that they did not resist the attack hard enough and therefore were not legally raped. Other women fear the publicity and humiliation of being a rape victim and prefer not to relive the experience through a court procedure.

Rape trauma syndrome occurs in two stages: disorganization and reorganization. Disorganization occurs during the acute phase immediately following the assault in which the victim's life is disrupted by the crisis. Reorganization is a long-term process during which the victim mobilizes her physical, emotional, and behavioral reactions to the rape and integrates them into her life experiences.

Responses to rape include an expressed style, a controlled style, and a compounded style of responding. A victim who expresses feelings of anger, fear, anxiety, who cries and is restless and shaking, is using an expressed style of response. Victims using a controlled style mask their feelings with a calm, subdued, and composed manner. A reaction is compounded when the victim has a previous history of psychiatric, physical, or social problems. Frequently, a woman who does not report the assault suffers a silent rape trauma syndrome and carries this psychological burden alone.

The nurse may be the first person with whom the victim of a rape comes in contact. Her support immediately following the rape and during the medical and legal proceedings that follow may determine how well the victim reorganizes and reintegrates into the community. It is essential for the nurse to be aware of her own biases and myths about rape and to be skillful in crisis intervention and rape counseling to support the victim throughout the crisis and assist her in returning to her previous level of functioning.

Related DSM-III-R disorders

Posttraumatic stress disorder

Other related conditions

Anxiety
Anger
Depression
Fears and phobias
Guilt
Obsessions
Sexual dysfunction
Suicide

PRINCIPLES

▶ Physical Dimension

1. Rape is an act of physical violence rather than sexual passion.
2. All women are vulnerable to rape (reports include females 5 months to 91 years of age).
3. The composite picture of the rape victim is a young, black, single female student from a lower socioeconomic group.
4. Many rape victims develop psychiatric symptoms following the rape.
5. The victim can become pregnant or develop sexually transmitted diseases as a result of the rape.
6. The greater the force and brutality the victim experiences, the greater the psychological harm produced.
7. In 50% of rape cases weapons are used.
8. Physical resistance often increases the violent behavior of the offender.
9. Rape is not a crime of impulse, usually having been planned in advance.

10. Most rapes occur in the victim's home.
11. Reports concur that in most rapes the man and woman are the same race.
12. Victims are not responsible for their victimization.
13. The rape victim may experience sexual dysfunction following the assault.

▶ Emotional Dimension

1. Reactions to rape are similar to reactions to any great stress, from cool and composed to hysterical and from verbal and talkative to quiet and guarded.
2. Many rape victims blame themselves for the attack and experience feelings of guilt, shame, and embarrassment.
3. Victims with pre-existing emotional problems need more extensive psychiatric treatment.
4. Every rape has elements of anger and power in it.
5. Responses to life-threatening situations such as rape include severe anxiety.
6. Intense fears or phobias may develop when personal safety and security have been threatened.
7. Victims of rape feel a loss of power and a loss of control of their lives.

▶ Intellectual Dimension

1. Rape trauma syndrome encompasses two phases:
   a. An acute phase of disorganization, which usually lasts a few days to several weeks
   b. A long-term process of reorganization
2. The victim's loss of control undermines her confidence and ability to maintain control and care for herself.
3. Psychological defenses (repression and rationalization) are used to block out unbearable feelings.
4. Disbelief and denial are early reactions to rape.
5. Victims of rape may suffer from nightmares and violent dreams.
6. Victims of rape may obsess about the assault.
7. Traditional society may place blame on the rape victim.

▶ Social Dimension

1. Rape victims experience social consequences: a financial loss as a result of medical expenses, damaged property, a change in housing, and loss of time at work because of injury or court proceedings.
2. Rape places a strain on any relationship.
3. Legal consequences include reporting the rape, court testimony, and involvement with the criminal justice system for several months.

4. Press releases and newspaper accounts of the rape may further humiliate the victim.
5. Implications of wantonness and ostracism may occur among family, friends, and neighbors of the victim.
6. Rape has an impact on the victim and on her significant others.
7. In many cases the victim is acquainted with the offender.
8. Once husbands of rape victims have resolved the incident in their own minds, they become impatient with the victim, whose resolution is much slower.
9. Society's attitudes, which often blame or hold the victim responsible, play a major part in the outcome of a rape crisis.
10. Sexual behavior, normal or deviant, is the product of socialization.
11. Reactions from police, courts, medical and legal persons, family members, and spouses may have a long-lasting effect on the victim's self-concept.
12. When interactions with others are abusive and painful, as in rape, the person may blame herself.
13. When the assailant is an acquaintance, the victim may have difficulty integrating the reality of the rape.
14. Often a mistrust of men follows rape.
15. Families of rape victims frequently respond with overprotection of the victim and increase her dependence.
16. Families of rape victims may respond with vengeance.

▶ Spiritual Dimension

1. Rape affects the individual's life to her very core of existence.
2. Long-term reactions include mental illness, marital problems, and suicide.
3. Reactivation of previously existing symptoms such as heavy drinking or drug abuse may reflect the victim's devaluation of herself.
4. A victim may be unable to integrate the situation into her total life and to continue functioning at her usual level of emotional health.
5. Rape influences a victim's self-worth and self-respect.
6. Rape promotes feelings of spiritual emptiness.
7. Religious beliefs may be shaken by rape.
8. Rape victims frequently question their personal faith.
9. A sense of hopelessness—that men are basically evil and society is inhumane—may pervade the victim's thinking.

ASSESSMENT

▶ Physical Dimension

I. History
- A. Activities of daily living
  1. Nutrition
     - a. Loss of appetite
     - b. Vomiting
     - c. Gagging
     - d. Nausea
     - e. Loss of weight
  2. Sleep
     - a. Sleep disturbances
     - b. Nightmares
     - c. Violent dreams
  3. Sexual activity
     - a. Dysfunction
       1. Aversion to sexual activity
       2. Reduction in vaginal lubrication
       3. Loss in sensation in genital area
       4. Vaginismus
       5. Loss of orgasmic ability
- B. Habits
  1. May misuse or abuse alcohol
  2. Uses medications and drugs excessively
  3. May smoke excessively
- C. Destructive behavior—suicide
- D. Physical abuse
  1. Trauma from the rape
     - a. Lacerations
     - b. Abrasions
     - c. Contusions
     - d. Bites
     - e. Burns
     - f. Fractures
  2. Previous unreported rape
- E. Review of systems
  1. Breasts
     - a. Bruises
     - b. Bites
     - c. Burns
  2. Gastrointestinal
     - a. Irritability
     - b. Nausea
     - c. Vomiting
     - d. Anorexia
  3. Genitourinary
     - a. Pain
     - b. Pruritus
  4. Reproductive
     - a. Date of last menstrual period
     - b. Date of last sexual contact
     - c. History of sexually transmitted disease
  5. Musculoskeletal
     - a. Headache
     - b. Joint or soft tissue pain

II. Diagnostic tests
- A. Blood values
  1. Drug and alcohol screening
  2. Blood typing
  3. VDRL
  4. Pregnancy test
- B. Wet mount test for motile sperm
- C. Wood's light for sperm presence
- D. Hair samples from head and pubic area
- E. Fingernail clippings or scrapings

III. Legal evidence
- A. Documentation
- B. Safekeeping of physical evidence

▶ Physical Examination

CLIENT DATA	ANALYSIS	NURSING DIAGNOSIS
Any injured area is examined with particular attention to head, neck, throat, and mouth—bruises, lacerations, and abrasions	Rape is an act of physical violence.	Rape trauma syndrome: related to injury to head, neck, throat, and mouth
Back and buttock area injuries	Resisting victims suffer back and buttock injuries because of force of assailant.	Rape trauma syndrome: related to injury to back and buttock area
Pelvic examination—internal and external injuries	Force and violence result in internal and external injuries. To collect specimens for evidence of assault.	Rape trauma syndrome: related to injury to vaginal area
Rectal examination—internal and external injuries	Force and violence result in internal and external injuries.	Rape trauma syndrome: related to injuries to rectal area

▶ **Emotional Dimension**

CLIENT DATA	ANALYSIS	NURSING DIAGNOSIS
Severe anxiety	A response to life-threatening situation.	Rape trauma syndrome: related to anxiety
Fears and phobias of being alone, in crowds, going out of the house, people walking behind her, being rejected by partner	Personal safety and security have been threatened. Fears losing significant other as result of rape.	Rape trauma syndrome: related to intense fears and phobias
Guilt	Society may hold victims responsible for their sexual assaults.	Rape trauma syndrome: related to guilt
Anger Resentment	Victims express anger and rage at assailant for having used them for violent sexual attack and are frustrated that society encourages aggressive behavior from men.	Rape trauma syndrome: related to anger and resentment
Sadness	A sense of personal loss is felt, of self, of respect, of virginity, of self-esteem.	Rape trauma syndrome: related to intense sadness
Humiliation and embarrassment	Victim may think she is to blame for rape because of society's attitude.	Rape trauma syndrome: related to humiliation and embarrassment
Emotional numbness	A coping response produced by intense stress of rape.	Rape trauma syndrome: related to emotional numbness

▶ **Intellectual Dimension**

CLIENT DATA	ANALYSIS	NURSING DIAGNOSIS
Disbelief and denial	Victim has difficulty integrating reality of rape, particularly if assailant is an acquaintance.	Rape trauma syndrome: related to disbelief and denial
Nightmares, violent dreams, obsessions	Major stressful events are frequently followed by obsession, an attempt to maintain control.	Rape trauma syndrome: related to nightmares, violent dreams, or obsessions
Loss of control, powerlessness	Rape is a stressor over which victim has no control.	Rape trauma syndrome: related to loss of control
"If only" thinking	A form of magical thinking—belief that if a person wishes, dreams, or says something, it will come true. Frequently expressed as self-imposed guilt.	Rape trauma syndrome: related to magical thinking
Self-blame	Society traditionally holds victim responsible for assault, resulting in victim blaming herself.	Rape trauma syndrome: related to self-blame

▶ **Social Dimension**

CLIENT DATA	ANALYSIS	NURSING DIAGNOSIS
Negative self-concept	Feels used, dirty, less than whole, damaged by assault.	Rape trauma syndrome: related to negative self-concept
Marital or couple problems	Spouse or partner misunderstands assault and blames victim. Victim is sexually dysfunctional.	Rape trauma syndrome: related to marital or couple problems
Mistrust of men	Stress of being raped, along with rejection and loss of control, promotes a fear of men in general. Feeling of safety with men is decreased.	Rape trauma syndrome: related to mistrust of men

▶ **Social Dimension—cont'd**

CLIENT DATA	ANALYSIS	NURSING DIAGNOSIS
Overprotection from family	Response to feelings of helplessness with infantalizing. Disservice to victim because family assumes she cannot cope.	Rape trauma syndrome: related to overprotection from family
Disrupted relationships, loss of partner or husband	Traditional view of rape sees woman as property of man, and he is victim or injured party.	Rape trauma syndrome: related to disrupted relationships
Brutal court process	Symbolic repetition of rape.	Rape trauma syndrome: related to brutal court process
Vengeance-seeking behavior	Response to feelings of helplessness.	Rape trauma syndrome: related to vengeance-seeking behaviors

▶ **Spiritual Dimension**

CLIENT DATA	ANALYSIS	NURSING DIAGNOSIS
Feels alone and isolated from significant other, God, or supreme power (particularly when rape is kept secret)	Lack of assurance of self-worth; feeling of spiritual emptiness.	Rape trauma syndrome: related to feeling alone and isolated
Questions faith	Faith and beliefs are shaken for "allowing" rape to happen.	Rape trauma syndrome: related to questioning of faith
Lacks inner strength to cope with assault	Response to stress and rape and inability to understand the "why" of the rape.	Rape trauma syndrome: related to lack of inner strength
Feels hopeless, feels that world is evil	Despair; no hope seen for a more safe and humane society or for things to ever change.	Rape trauma syndrome: related to despair and hopelessness
Vulnerable to hostile environment	Society's attitudes have an impact on victim, often blaming or holding her responsible rather than assisting.	Rape trauma syndrome: related to vulnerability to hostile environment

PLANNING

Long-Term Goal

To regain control over own life by integrating the rape event into life experiences and resuming her optimal level of functioning

SHORT-TERM GOALS	OUTCOME CRITERIA

Physical Dimension
To decrease physical symptoms
	1. Has decreased physical symptoms
	  a. Sleeps without interruptions
	  b. Has no nightmares
	  c. Has no violent dreams
	  d. Has an increased appetite
	  e. Has no nausea, vomiting, or gagging
	  f. Has no need to misuse alcohol or drugs

To prevent pregnancy and sexually transmitted disease	1. Takes a morning-after pill 2. Has VDRL test done 3. Monitors self for sexually transmitted diseases (AIDS), lesions, burning on urination

PLANNING—cont'd

SHORT-TERM GOALS	OUTCOME CRITERIA
Emotional Dimension	
To express feelings about rape	1. Expresses feelings of resentment, anger, sadness, guilt, and anxiety 2. Does not mask feelings with a composed or subdued manner 3. Responds with appropriate affect 4. Uses art, dance, poetry, and music to express feelings 5. Cries
To express feelings about sexual adequacy and identity	1. Expresses feelings about sexual adequacy and identity 2. Sets a realistic time frame for working through sexual concerns
Intellectual Dimension	
To reduce self-blame	1. Refrains from blaming herself 2. Verbalizes using poor judgment (e.g., hitchhiking) if applicable 3. Acknowledges that not responsible for the rape 4. Makes statements indicating improved self-worth
To regain a sense of control over life	1. Requests assistance from others 2. Makes requests of others 3. Makes decisions regarding herself at work, school, and home 4. Verbalizes concerns about loss of control
To perceive the rape realistically	1. Sees rape as a violent, rather than sexual, crime 2. Sees rape as an indiscriminate act 3. Resolves doubt that she was responsible 4. Knows that she may have a reactivation of feelings at times in relation to the rape
Social Dimension	
To receive support from family and friends	1. Receives support from family and friends 2. Stays with others following the rape or others stay with her
To report the rape to authorities	1. Reports to police 2. Undergoes court testimony
To use rape counseling	1. Seeks rape counseling
Spiritual Dimension	
To increase feelings of self-respect and self-worth	1. Verbalizes feelings of self-respect and self-worth 2. Is able to return to work or school and pursue usual activities 3. Uses supportive persons to discuss feelings and concerns
To integrate the rape into life experiences	1. Sees the impact of the rape and emotional responses diminishing over time 2. Continues to pursue activities that bring pleasure to life 3. Becomes more empathic with others in similar situations

Discharge Planning

The following client behaviors demonstrate readiness for discharge:
1. Leaves clinic or hospital with a supportive person
2. Knows telephone number of a rape crisis center
3. Verbalizes signs and symptoms of stress related to the rape
4. Makes some decisions about her own health care, for example, going home, changing door locks, and telephone number
5. Knows the results of rape (possible pregnancy, possible sexually transmitted disease, and reactivation of emotions related to rape during other stressful times)

IMPLEMENTATION

NURSING ACTIONS	RATIONALE
Physical Dimension	
1. Encourage client to eat small amounts of nutritional food frequently.	To maintain adequate nutrition.
2. Remain with client when she is gagging or vomiting.	To offer comfort and support.
3. Use comfort measures to promote sleep.	To ensure client is getting adequate sleep.
4. Prevent from being alone at home initially.	To promote feelings of safety.
5. Encourage client to discuss sexual concerns.	To identify problem areas and plan interventions.
6. Refer for sex counseling if needed.	To help client treat sexual dysfunctioning as a result of rape.
7. Monitor alcohol and drug intake for possible misuse as a response to the stress of rape.	To determine coping skills, to prevent excessive intake of alcohol or drugs.
8. Be alert for clues of possible suicide attempts.	To prevent self-harm as a result of rape.
9. Chart trauma sites.	To depict areas of injury for legal purposes.
10. Treat injuries, lacerations, bruises, and somatic symptoms resulting from the rape.	To promote comfort and caring, to prevent infections.
11. Assist with physical examination, explaining each procedure and test that is done and the reason.	To promote comfort, physical and emotional, to decrease anxiety about examination.
12. Provide care in a private, quiet environment.	To ensure privacy, confidentiality.
13. Do not allow client to go home alone after the rape.	To prevent client from being without a supportive person, to provide anticipatory guidance to avert alarm about response to rape.
14. Avoid overfocusing on the sexual activity and focus on the violence of the rape.	To help client see rape as an act of violence.
15. Provide care that demonstrates utmost respect for the individual.	To promote emotional healing.
16. Elicit information on the specifics of the assault (where, when, description of assailant, and weapons used).	To collect data for legal purposes.
Emotional Dimension	
1. Help client express feelings of anger, fear, guilt, resentment, and sadness by listening actively, reflecting, and clarifying.	To talk about the painful feelings helps to lessen the intensity of the feeling and enables client to view event in a more rational manner.
2. Assure client that feelings are normal and appropriate responses to the rape.	To help client accept feelings as appropriate for the situation.
3. Avoid hurrying client through procedures.	To allow client time to tell her story as she wants to tell it.
4. Help client redirect anger for rape toward rapist.	To prevent client from directing anger at herself.
5. Encourage crying and expression of feelings of loss and hurt.	To help client express her anger and grief.
6. Remain calm if victim is abusive or demanding toward you or other staff.	To allow client to vent her anger, knowing that you may be the target but not the source.
7. Recognize client's abusive behavior as an angry, vengeful response to rape and an attempt to regain some control of her life.	To increase your awareness of client's abusive behavior and enable you to respond empathically.
8. Recognize client's demanding behavior as a response to rape and an attempt to regain some control of her life.	To increase your awareness of client's demanding behavior and enable you to respond empathically.

IMPLEMENTATION—cont'd

NURSING ACTIONS	RATIONALE
9. Encourage other methods of expressing anger (art, poetry, music, and sports).	To offer other options for expressing anger appropriately.
10. Encourage physical activity.	To release the energy of anxiety and anger.
11. Convey empathy and understanding to victim.	To provide support, to establish trust.
12. Be patient while dealing with client's fears.	To allow time for client to adjust to changed life-style.
13. Be nonjudgmental in approach to client.	To maintain supportive relationship.
14. Acknowledge client's psychological trauma even when victim is outwardly calm.	To prevent client from attempting to keep the rape secret and bearing the burden alone.
15. Encourage client's self-exploration.	To increase client's self-awareness and ownership of feelings.
Intellectual Dimension	
1. Help client acknowledge that rape is difficult to accept and that shock and disbelief are normal responses.	To help client feel normal about her responses to rape.
2. Assist client with options for health decisions.	To help client regain a sense of control of her life by making decisions about her health care.
3. Encourage client to talk about dreams, nightmares, and obsessive thoughts that follow the rape.	To lessen the intensity of the painful feelings associated with rape and the memory of it.
4. Help client understand that dreams, nightmares, and obsessive thoughts are stress related and disappear in time.	To give client information, to decrease anxiety over continued dreams.
5. Refer to mental health professionals if dreams, nightmares, and obsessive thoughts last more than 6 weeks.	To provide client with more in-depth treatment.
6. Encourage client to make own decisions.	To regain control of life.
7. Explain reasons for procedures, tests, and preserving evidence (do not wash clothes, do not use gargles, do not douche).	To prevent increased anxiety over unfamiliar procedures, to preserve evidence for legal proceedings.
8. Help client perceive rape realistically, that she may have used poor judgment (for hitchhiking, walking alone at night), but she was *not* responsible for the rape.	To prevent client from blaming herself and feeling guilty.
9. Intervene when client's logic is faulty.	To present reality.
10. After emotional energy is lessened, talking about the rape allows for cognitive processing and factual information about rape can be presented.	To refute myths.
11. Set limits on client's expressions of blame and worthlessness.	To prevent client from focusing on perceived negative aspects of herself.
12. Convey belief that client is not to blame for the rape.	To help client understand that no woman can be blamed for being raped, that it is a violent act that no woman deserves.
13. Refrain from moralizing or preaching.	To establish and maintain a helping relationship. Moralizing and preaching are not helpful communication techniques.
14. Encourage client's adaptive strategies (moving or changing telephone number).	To support client's decisions, to help her regain control.
15. Listen attentively when client wants to talk about the rape.	To help client know you are listening to her and trying to understand her feelings.
16. Be aware that she may need to retell the rape many times.	To be sensitive to client's needs.
17. Inform client of legal rights (collection of evidence and prosecution).	To provide legal information to client about rape.
18. Provide written material for medical care, legal advice.	To ensure client's understanding. Recall may be poor because of high anxiety.
19. Promote verbalization of thoughts, feelings, and actions.	To enable client to clarify her thoughts, feelings, and actions.
20. Explore with client causes of and reasons for particular concerns.	To plan a course of action.

NURSING ACTIONS	RATIONALE
Social Dimension	
1. Help client find ways to increase self-esteem and self-worth.	To promote positive self-concept.
2. Refer for or provide marital or couples therapy when problems result from the rape.	To help client and partner to resolve problems associated with rape.
3. Encourage resumption of usual pursuits (work, school, and at home).	To prevent client from becoming incapacitated by the rape and begin to integrate rape into her life experiences.
4. Be aware of client's continued need for support from family, friends, and spouse.	To be sensitive to client's needs.
5. Help client explore reasons for mistrust of men.	To prevent client from applying one negative life situation to all others that may inhibit her ability to relate and enjoy intimate relationships with other men.
6. Be aware that family and friends may be overprotective of client following rape as a response to feelings of helplessness.	To increase awareness of family response and plan interventions.
7. Discuss with family ways to provide support.	To provide family with information on ways to be supportive.
8. Discourage overprotectiveness from family and friends.	To prevent dependence.
9. Help client explore broken relationship resulting from rape.	To increase client's awareness that some people cannot or will not deal with rape situations.
10. Explore with client society's traditional views and the cultural implication of rape (men are socialized to be aggressive and women are the property of men).	To present facts, to explain some of client's feelings of powerlessness and degradation.
11. Assist client in expressing thoughts and feelings about court process and legal implications.	To determine client's perception and plan interventions.
12. Support client when court process reactivates symbolically a repeat of the rape.	To provide continuing understanding and empathy.
13. Help client and family refrain from seeking vengeance on the rapist.	To prevent client and family from destructive acts, to encourage them to use energy to cooperate with legal agencies.
14. Help client and family to see vengeance-seeking behaviors as a response to feelings of helplessness.	To enable client and family to understand their behavior.
15. Help client and family find healthy ways to respond to helplessness.	To plan more effective ways to cope with rape.
16. Encourage client to call a rape crisis center within 1 hour after the rape.	To help client use resources for support and understanding, as well as for medical and legal information.
17. Assist client in disclosing the rape to others.	To help client regain a sense of control of life.
18. Offer support to family of victim.	To prevent family disorganization from the crisis of rape.
19. Offer support for health decisions that client makes, even though they differ from your health decisions.	To help client regain control of life by making decisions.
20. Avoid imposing own decisions regarding health on client.	To remain sensitive to personal, family, and cultural influence on decisions about health.
21. Assist client in identifying supportive friends and family members.	To increase network of supportive persons.
Spiritual Dimension	
1. Help client find ways to assure her worth and value as an individual.	To promote a positive self-concept. Persons who have been raped often feel less valued.
2. Include religious leader as a member of health care team.	To provide religious and spiritual comfort, if appropriate for client.
3. Refer to clergy or religious leader if client sees rape as a sin or religious failing or begins to question faith.	To prevent conflicts with religious faith.
4. Help client deemphasize the *why* of rape and focus on health and healing the trauma.	To help client place rape in perspective over time.

IMPLEMENTATION—cont'd

NURSING ACTIONS	RATIONALE
5. Promote sense of hope and confidence that in time the impact of the rape will diminish in intensity.	To restore client's faith in herself, others, and the world in general.
6. Explore with client reasons for feeling abandoned by God.	To plan intervention, for example, refer to clergy.
7. Help client gain optimism about future relationships with other men.	To prevent overgeneralizing feelings associated with rape to all men.
8. Help client integrate rape event into her life and grow from the experience (be more assertive and value herself).	To promote increased mental health and ability to handle life circumstances.
9. Convey an attitude of hope that the event can be integrated into her life.	To enable client to feel optimistic, that she can handle the rape with positive outcomes in time.

EVALUATION

In both the acute state of crisis and the long-term reorganization process, measurable goals and outcome criteria provide the basis for evaluating the client who has been raped. Client self-reports, nurse observations, and family reports provide additional data. The following behaviors indicate a positive evaluation:

1. Has physical wounds treated
2. Leaves clinic or hospital with a supportive person
3. States telephone number of rape crisis center
4. States symptoms of possible later reactions to rape
5. Expresses feelings about rape
6. Uses methods to handle feelings that promote mental health
7. Distinguishes facts from myths about rape
8. Talks about rape to appropriate others
9. States legal requirements for collecting evidence, testifying in court, identifying offender
10. Resumes sexual relationships
11. Resumes usual life activities
12. Seeks help with problems in sexual relationships

BIBLIOGRAPHY

Belden L: Why women do not report sexual assault, *Aegis* 1:5, 1980.

Brownmiller S: *Against our will: men, women and rape*, New York, 1975, Simon and Schuster.

Burgess A: Rape trauma syndrome: a nursing diagnosis, *Occup Health Nurs* 33(8):405, 1985.

Campbell J, Alford P: The dark side of marital rape, *Am J Nurs* 89:946, 1989.

Cornman J: Group treatment for female sexual abuse victims, *Issues Ment Health Nurs* 10:261, 1989.

Damrosch S: Nurses' attributions about rape victims, *Res Nurs Health* 10:245, 1987.

Davis L: Rape and older women. In Warner G, editor: *Rape and sexual assault: management and intervention*, Germantown, Md., 1980, Aspen Systems Corp.

DiVasto P: Measuring the aftermath of rape, *J Psychosoc Nurs Ment Health Serv* 23(2):33, 1985.

Foley T, Davies M: *Rape: nursing care of victims*, St. Louis, 1983, Mosby—Year Book.

Heinrich L: Care of the female rape victim, *Nurse Pract* 12(11):9, 1987.

Lew M: *Victims no longer*, New York, 1988, Nevraumont Publishing.

Moynihan B, Duggan K: The rape crisis team: consultation to critical care, *Dimens Crit Care Nurs* 1(6):354, 1982.

Sanday P: The socio-cultural context of rape: a cross-cultural study, *J Soc Issues* 37:5, 1981.

Schultz L, DeSavage J: Rape and rape attitudes on a college campus, In Schultz L, editor: *Rape victimology*, Springfield, Ill., 1984, Thomas.

Schwendinger J, Schwendinger H: *Rape and inequality*, Beverly Hills, Calif., 1983, Sage Publications.

Swift C: The prevention of rape, In Burgess A, editor: *Rape and sexual assault: a research handbook*, New York, 1985, Garland Publishing Co.

Walsh D, Liddy R: *Surviving sexual abuse*, Dublin, Ireland, 1989, Attic Press.

Sleep Disorders

A sleep disorder is a condition in which an individual undergoes a change in the quality or quantity of rest patterns. These changes are associated with an individual's rhythmic cycles and represent various stages of neural functioning. The changes can be identified by electroencephalogram patterns.

The need for sleep is universal, and normal sleep patterns are similar throughout the world. The average adult expects to sleep 6 to 9 hours a night, regardless of race, location, or vocation. Environmental, emotional, or physical stimuli may interrupt this pattern, causing a sleep disorder. The disorder may be primary in origin, meaning that the individual has never experienced normal restful sleep, or may be secondary, occurring for some reason after the individual has experienced normal sleep.

Individuals who are chronically fatigued or who suffer from abnormal sleep patterns are affected by maladjustments in all phases of their lives. The inability to experience normal restful sleep results in excessive daytime sleepiness, inappropriate napping, and subsequent disruption of social, cultural, and vocational roles. In some instances, an underlying physical condition, such as respiratory obstruction, may actually be life threatening during sleep. Suicidal ideation may result from despair over chronic sleeplessness and fatigue, which dramatically decrease the quality of life.

Depending on the severity of the loss of sleep, the individual may exhibit progressive loss of motor and cognitive skills. In most cases, resumption of normal sleep patterns quickly reverses these losses, and functions return to normal.

When providing care for a client with a sleep disorder, the nurse collects data from significant others, as well as from the client. Frequently, the client may experience but not remember sleep actions or behavior that may be specific to a particular diagnosis.

The original content for this section was contributed by Marilyn Henderson, R.N., M.S.N.

Related DSM-III-R disorders

Sleepwalking disorders
Sleep terror disorders
Functional enuresis

Other related conditions

Insomnia
Impaired elimination
Respiratory disorder
Pregnancy
Jet lag
Pain
Intense feelings: anxiety, fear, anger, guilt, obsessions

Association of Sleep Disorders Center (ASDC) nosology diagnostic classification of sleep and arousal disorders

Disorders of initiating and maintaining sleep (insomnia; DIMS)
Disorders of excessive somnolence (narcolepsy; DOES)
Disorders of the sleep and wake schedule
Dysfunctions associated with sleep, sleep stages, and partial arousals (parasomnias)

PRINCIPLES

▶ Physical Dimension

1. Little variation exists worldwide in the organization of work and rest activities synchronized by light.
2. Disruptions of predictable rhythms of sleep and wake, stress and relaxation, and work and play, which synchronize vocational activities of most industrial countries, lead to sleep disorders.
3. General guidelines for sleep requirements are:

Infants	16 to 20 hours
Young children	10 to 14 hours
Adolescents	8 to 10 hours
Adults	6 to 9 hours
Older adults	5 to 8 hours

Individuals who normally require significantly shorter periods of sleep tend to be hyperactive but are productive and well adjusted. Those who require more sleep are usually low key, underachieving, and mildly depressed.

4. A sleep disorder is a response to interruption of the 24-hour circadian rest activity rhythm and the 90-minute ultradian sleep cycle of nonrapid eye movement (NREM) sleep and rapid eye movement (REM) sleep.
   a. NREM and REM sleep are classified as electrophysiological and behavioral phenomena.
   b. NREM sleep is nondreaming sleep; REM sleep is dreaming sleep.
   c. Alterations in the length of stages 3 and 4 of REM sleep interfere with the most restful and physiologically restorative phases of sleep.
   d. A decrease in the interval of NREM sleep is a biological sign that the individual is in a pathological depression.
   e. In alcoholics the ratio of NREM sleep to REM sleep is greatly increased for long periods of time because of the depressive effect of alcohol on the central nervous system. On or about the third day of alcohol withdrawal, this effect is reversed. Then the excessive amount of REM sleep contributes to delirium tremens.
5. The person who experiences jet lag, change in work shifts, or disorganization of rest-activity schedules may suffer sleep disorders related to disruption of biological rhythms.
6. Physiological sleep disorders are:
   a. Narcolepsy, or excessive daytime and/or daily sleepiness and abnormal manifestations of REM sleep. The narcoleptic tetrad consists of:
      (1) Excessive sleepiness, regardless of sleep obtained, resulting in sleep attacks at inappropriate times, such as while at work, driving, or eating. The attacks, which can be treated with medication, may last from 10 to 15 minutes or from 2 to 3 hours.
      (2) Cataplexy, or rapidly occurring attacks of loss of muscle tone, which seem to be the result of onset of REM sleep directly from wakefulness. Attacks, which may affect all or part of the body, are usually triggered by intense emotion or surprise and may last from a moment to several minutes. Individuals learn to control emotional responses to prevent the attacks.
      (3) Sleep paralysis, or the sensation of being unable to move just before falling asleep or just after waking up.
      (4) Hypnagogic hallucinations, or dreamlike images, that occur during the transition from wakefulness to sleeping.

b. Sleep apnea is a disorder characterized by frequent and repeated pauses in breathing during sleep. Three types are recognized:
   (1) Central apnea. Air flow across nostrils and mouth stops, and respiratory efforts cease. Infant apneas and Sudden Infant Death Syndrome (SIDS) may be facets of this syndrome.
   (2) Obstructive apnea. Air flow from nostrils and mouth stops, but respiratory efforts continue.
   (3) Mixed apnea. A combination of central and obstructive disorders. The sleep apnea episode begins with brief periods of central apnea, followed by return of respiratory efforts but no air flow because of obstruction. Cardiovascular disorders, such as right ventricular hypertrophy, hypertension, and cardiac arrhythmias, are common complications of sleep apnea.
c. Parasomnias. Sleep-dependent or sleep-associated disorders characterized by some loss of neural control during sleep. They appear to be age, sex, and sleep-stage related.
   (1) Enuresis. Bed wetting. This may be the result of very deep sleep and difficult arousal.
   (2) Night terrors. Fearful dreams. The individual may scream and exhibit extreme terror but have amnesia for the episode after waking. These differ from nightmares, which are frightening dreams the individual remembers.
   (3) Somnambulism. Sleepwalking. Automatic purposeful movements and actions may be performed. The individual does not remember what happened during the sleepwalking episode.
   (4) Bruxism. Grinding of teeth. Dental appliances have limited benefit when used to stabilize jaws during sleep.

▶ Emotional Dimension

1. Clients with depression often state that sleeplessness is a major cause or precipitating event in suicidal attempts.
2. Sleep disorders are the most consistent symptoms of depressive illness and may continue even after the psychiatric condition improves.
3. Difficulty or inability to fall asleep may be caused by fear, nervousness, feelings of guilt, or inability to exclude unwanted thoughts from the mind.
4. Hypersomnia (excessive sleeping) may occur as the result of boredom, discomfort, anxiety, fear, pain, delirium, depression, or failure of coping mechanisms.

▶ Intellectual Dimension

1. A client's response to therapy for a sleep disorder depends on his perception of the problem, its symbolic meaning, speculations about its cause, and his hopes for the future regarding continuance or resolution of the problem.
2. The client's concern for achieving effective sleep-wake patterns is influenced by his view of sleep as either a necessary feature of daily living or an activity to be indulged in only when time and circumstances permit.

▶ Social Dimension

1. Sleep disorders may occur when primary relationships are disturbed.
2. Individuals learn culturally derived sleep patterns:
   a. Afternoon siesta
   b. Blurring of night-rest and day-work activities, which occurs in urban, industrialized countries with round-the-clock activities
   c. Sleep-wake patterns of inhabitants of locations where prolonged periods of total light and total darkness occur (for example, Alaska).

▶ Spiritual Dimension

1. Chronic fatigue decreases the quality of life by lessening the sense of hope that the sleep disturbance can be overcome.
2. Ineffective sleep patterns deprive client of energy and motivation to strive for high levels of achievement or self-actualization.
3. Excessive sleepiness throughout normal waking hours prevents client from full participation in activities that add pleasure to life.
4. Clients may interpret disturbed sleep patterns as punishment of a vengeful God and doubt their ability to endure the suffering.

ASSESSMENT

▶ Physical Dimension

I. **History**
   A. Activities of daily living
      1. Sleep
         a. Development of complaints over time
         b. Fluctuation with stress
         c. Excessive sleepiness (hypersomnolence)
         d. Lack of sleep (insomnia)
         e. Sleep rituals
         f. Sleepwalking
         g. Sleep terrors
         h. Bedwetting
         i. Loud snoring
   B. Habits
      1. Alcohol
         a. Ingestion produces a rebound wakefulness as soon as it is metabolized in the body
         b. Lack of REM sleep during alcoholic binges leads to excessive REM sleep 2 to 3 days after withdrawal
      2. Medications and drugs
         a. Paradoxical action of some medications may cause sleep disruptions
      3. Caffeine
         a. Prevents sleep by stimulating the nervous system
      4. Nicotine
         a. Smoking may disrupt sleep
   C. Destructive behavior
      1. Suicide
         a. Irregular sleep patterns often precede suicide attempts
   D. Review of systems
      1. General
         a. Chronic fatigue
         b. Sleep habits
            (1) Rarely experiences satisfactory sleep
            (2) Has difficulty falling asleep
            (3) Wakes early and cannot go back to sleep
            (4) Exhibits excessive daytime sleepiness
      2. Nose and throat
         a. Hypertrophied tonsils or adenoids
         b. Tongue too large for oral cavity
      3. Cardiovascular
         a. Edema
         b. High blood pressure
         c. Right ventricular hypertrophy
      4. Respiratory
         a. Orthopnea
         b. Shallow breathing
         c. Apnea
      5. Gastrointestinal
         a. Gastroesophageal reflex associated with reclining position
         b. Constipation with use of sedatives
      6. Genitourinary
         a. Enuresis
         b. Nocturia

7. Musculoskeletal
  a. Muscle weakness with sleep paralysis
  b. Excessive musculature of neck contributes to obstructive apnea
8. Endocrine
  a. Many hormones are released during sleep, which may result in endocrine imbalances that may possibly be associated with sleep disorders
  b. Inadequate production of growth hormone may produce failure to thrive syndrome in infants and small children
  c. Anxiety associated with insomnia stimulates production of adrenalin

II. **Diagnostic tests**
  A. EEG—brain waves
  B. Electromyelogram (EMG)—muscle tone
  C. Electrooculogram (EOG)—eye movement
  D. ECG—heart actions
  E. Naso-oral airflow—respirations
  F. Oximetry—oxygen concentration of blood
  G. Multiple Sleep Latency Test (MSLT)—daytime sleep and wakefulness measurements
  H. Nocturnal Penile Tumescence—to evaluate impotence
  I. Swallowing—occurs approximately 73 times per hour while awake and 7 times per hour while sleeping
  J. Temperature

▶ **Physical Examination**

CLIENT DATA	ANALYSIS	NURSING DIAGNOSIS
Appearance (sleepy, yawning, edema around eyes, and dark circles under eyes)	Appearance reflects inadequate sleep.	*Altered sleep/arousal patterns: related to inadequate sleep
Tremors	Muscle incoordination from lack of sleep.	Sleep pattern disturbance: related to impaired muscle coordination
Incoherent speech	Inadequate speech contributes to disturbed thought processes and affects muscle tone necessary for speech.	Sleep pattern disturbance: related to impaired phonation
Hypertrophied adenoids	Impaired respirations resulting from obstruction of adenoids.	Sleep pattern disturbance: related to obstruction of adenoids
Small oral cavity, large tongue, or hypertrophied tonsils	Anatomic features that interfere with respiratory efforts.	Sleep pattern disturbance: related to obstruction of respiratory tract
Short, thick, and muscular neck	Contributes to obstructive apnea.	Sleep pattern disturbance: related to obstructions of trachea
Hypertension, orthopnea, dyspnea, pulmonary edema, and peripheral edema	Cardiovascular symptoms resulting from obstructive apnea.	Sleep pattern disturbance: related to cardiovascular symptoms

▶ **Emotional Dimension**

CLIENT DATA	ANALYSIS	NURSING DIAGNOSIS
Exhaustion	Feels too tired to participate in daily activities. Lack of adequate sleep in all stages to restore energy.	Sleep pattern disturbance: related to inadequate sleep
Embarrassment at excessive daytime sleepiness	Goes to sleep at inappropriate times and places. Possibly a functional insomnia or a chronic failure to allow sufficient time to sleep.	Sleep pattern disturbance: related to excessive daytime sleepiness
Fear (sleep apnea, enuresis, encopresis, or sleep terrors)	Fear of not waking up or dying in sleep, of loss of bladder or bowel control or frightening dreams.	Sleep pattern disturbance: related to fears of sleep behaviors
Nightmares	Avoids falling asleep to prevent terrifying dreams.	*Altered sleep/arousal patterns: related to nightmares
Depression, anxiety, and anger	Responses to stress that interfere with sleep. May precipitate suicidal ideation or activity.	*Altered sleep/arousal pattern: related to depression, anxiety, and anger

▶ Intellectual Dimension

CLIENT DATA	ANALYSIS	NURSING DIAGNOSIS
Distorted perceptions (hallucinations and delusions)	Unable to evaluate reality in severe sleep deprivations.	Altered thought processes: related to severe sleep deprivation
Hypnagogic	Dream images occurring immediately after falling asleep.	Sleep pattern disturbance: related to dreams
Hypnopompic	Dream images occurring just before waking.	Sleep pattern disturbance: related to dreams
Impaired memory	Less alert and more forgetful when fatigued.	*Altered memory: related to fatigue
Judgment and insight lacking	Ability to make decisions decreases as fatigue increases. Can be brainwashed at this time, as may occur with prisoners of war.	Altered thought processes: impaired judgment and insight related to fatigue
Suspiciousness	Increases as sleep deprivation increases.	Altered thought processes: suspiciousness related to sleep deprivation
Dwelling on real or imagined sleep loss	Preoccupation with sleep loss.	Altered thought processes: related to real or perceived loss of sleep
Diminished concentration	Concentration decreases as sleep deprivation increases.	Altered thought processes: diminished concentration related to sleep deprivation
Delusions of persecution	Has lost touch with reality. Possible response to prolonged sleep deprivation and hypnotic experience.	Altered thought processes: delusions of persecution related to sleep deprivation
Slurred speech	Coordination of fine motor tasks is diminished as fatigue and sleep deprivation increase.	Impaired verbal communication: slurred speech related to sleep deprivation

▶ Social Dimension

CLIENT DATA	ANALYSIS	NURSING DIAGNOSIS
Distressed, disgruntled when unable to sleep	Sets goal of 7 to 9 hours of normal sleep; feels anxious and disgruntled when unable to achieve desired goal.	Ineffective individual coping: related to inability to achieve adequate sleep
Lacks support during sleep disturbances	Dependent on family to provide support during sleep disturbances such as nightmares, sleep, terrors, somnambulism, and apnea.	Social isolation: related to lack of support during sleep disturbances
Family history of narcolepsy	Disease tends to be familial. Males more often affected than females.	Sleep pattern disturbance: related to possible genetic transmission of narcolepsy
Reduced ability to perform social role	Sleep disturbance and fatigue may impair ability to perform usual roles.	Altered role performance: related to sleep disturbance
Unable to participate in social activities	Inappropriate napping or sleepiness prevents social participation.	Impaired social interaction: related to inappropriate sleep behavior
Excessive stimuli	Environmental stimuli interrupts sleep.	Sleep pattern disturbance: related to excessive environmental stimuli
Lack of safety	Locked doors and sense of security promote sleep.	Sleep pattern disturbance: related to lack of safety

▶ **Spiritual Dimension**

CLIENT DATA	ANALYSIS	NURSING DIAGNOSIS
Conflict in beliefs about sleep	Ambivalence: recognition that body needs rest but unwillingness to curtail activities.	Spiritual distress: related to ambivalence about sleep
Belief that sleeplessness is punishment	Belief that any deviation from usual sleep habits is a form of punishment.	Spiritual distress: related to beliefs about sleeplessness
Despair over sleeplessness	Lack of hope that sleeplessness will improve.	Spiritual distress: related to despair over sleeplessness
Lack of participation in religious activity because of excessive sleepiness	Separation from religious activity because of excessive sleepiness may cause guilt.	Spiritual distress: guilt related to inability to stay awake to participate in religious activities
Belief that God is vengeful because he cannot sleep	Rationalization of beliefs to decrease anxiety over sleeplessness.	Spiritual distress: related to anger with God over inability to achieve desired sleep
Inability to be creative caused by sleeplessness	Use of energy to promote or prolong sleep.	Spiritual distress: related to inability to be creative because of sleeplessness
Inability to enjoy life	Preoccupation with sleeplessness prevents enjoyment of life's pleasures.	Spiritual distress: lack of joy in life related to sleep disorder

PLANNING

Long-Term Goals

To develop a sleep pattern that allows for age-appropriate hours of sleep nightly, with minimal interruptions

To accept the fact that there may be occasional nights of wakefulness without becoming anxious

SHORT-TERM GOALS	OUTCOME CRITERIA
Physical Dimension	
To identify causes of sleep disturbance	1. Discusses situations or activities that produce disturbance 2. Verbalizes anxieties related to sleep disturbance
To determine what activities produced sleep before disturbance occurred	1. Describes usual bedtime ritual 2. Explains usual sleep schedule 3. Expresses understanding of personal control over sleep habits 4. Engages in problem solving to determine effective sleep activities
To increase daytime activities	1. Engages in stimulating activities during customary nap times 2. Maintains schedule of activities throughout all waking hours 3. Exercises enough to become physically tired
To implement a regular sleep schedule	1. Gains knowledge from nurse of chronotherapy necessary to reset biological clock 2. Explains bedtime activities conducive to sleep 3. Finds a safe, comfortable resting place 4. Promotes nonstimulating bedtime ritual 　a. Dim lights 　b. No strenuous bedtime activities 　c. No stimulating conversation or beverages
To reduce environmental distractions and interruptions	1. Avoids sleeping locations near airports, trains, and whistles 2. Installs dark window coverings to shield from external lights 3. Posts notices not to telephone or knock on door 4. Enlists aid of family to protect from disturbances

SHORT-TERM GOALS	OUTCOME CRITERIA
Emotional Dimension	
To reduce anxieties, worries, and stress that interfere with sleep	1. Expresses anxieties, worries, and stress 2. Accepts that life is not always stress-free 3. Accepts that minor interruptions to sleep may always exist and not dwell on them
Intellectual Dimension	
To learn comfort measures that promote sleep	1. Drinks a warm, not hot, nonalcoholic or decaffeinated drink 2. Takes a warm bath, no stimulating rubdown 3. Reads a boring book 4. Watches boring TV program 5. Learns techniques to reduce tension
Social Dimension	
To participate in social activities that promote fatigue and tiredness	1. Participates in social activities 2. Verbalizes no episodes of sleep during social activities 3. Verbalizes good feelings from social activities with no focus on sleep problems
Spiritual Dimension	
To feel fresh and invigorated and enjoy each day after a good night's sleep	1. Verbalizes renewed strength and enthusiasm for life 2. Demonstrates less dependency 3. Expresses hope that this problem will be overcome and quality of life will improve

Discharge Planning

The following client behaviors demonstrate readiness for discharge:
1. Identifies situations that cause sleep disturbance
2. Knows methods to promote sleep
3. Accepts occasional sleep disturbance without becoming anxious
4. When possible, synchronizes natural body rhythms with actual pattern of daily living to avoid stress-related factors such as jet lag, shift change, and disrupting weekend activities

IMPLEMENTATION

NURSING ACTIONS	RATIONALE
Physical Dimension	
1. Monitor daily schedule of light-dark cycle with sleep activities.	To help client determine sleep-wake cycle and plan interventions.
2. Encourage client's involvement in deciding what activities promote normal sleep.	To identify activities that client thinks will promote sleep, to promote self-responsibility.
3. Encourage client to get out of bed for alternative activities when unable to fall asleep.	To do something positive, for example, read or watch TV, until sleepy.
4. Encourage client to reestablish desired circadian rhythm by carefully advancing biological clock over time (chronotherapy).	To help client balance day with internal sleep-wake cycle.
5. Establish nonstimulating bedtime ritual such as reading a book, drinking a warm drink, and being in a quiet room with low lights, a comfortable temperature, and no television.	To reduce stimuli and promote sleep.
6. Avoid stimulating foods such as caffeine and alcoholic drinks.	To decrease stimulating effects of caffeine.
7. Identify possible food allergies or medicine that potentiate sleeplessness.	To increase awareness of other possible causes of sleeplessness.
8. Provide medication if ordered.	To promote sleep.
9. Avoid taking hypnotics or sedatives for longer than 1 month.	To avoid rebound wakefulness.
10. Recognize paradoxical action of drugs, which may cause wakefulness.	To increase awareness of other possible causes of sleeplessness.
11. Encourage use of relaxation techniques.	To relax body and nerves and promote sleep.

IMPLEMENTATION—cont'd

NURSING ACTIONS	RATIONALE
12. Provide a comfortable, safe environment.	To increase feelings of comfort and safety that promote sleep.
13. Encourage physical activity during waking hours.	To produce fatigue.
14. Discourage daytime naps.	To promote tiredness and help client sleep at night.
15. Limit fluids for 3 hours before bedtime.	To prevent full bladder that may interfere with sleep.
16. Empty bladder before going to bed.	To help client avoid waking up to empty bladder.
17. Eliminate or diminish environmental factors such as whistles, squeaking doors, and traffic noises, that may disturb sleep.	To prevent distractions that interfere with sleep.
18. Be aware that persons suffering from illness require extra sleep.	To be sensitive to ill person's need for extra sleep for healing.
19. Refer for biofeedback.	To learn to relax.
20. Refer to sleep disorder clinic if necessary.	To treat severe sleep problems.
Emotional Dimension	
1. Encourage expression of emotions that may affect sleep (fear, anger, worries, and guilt) by listening actively, reflecting, clarifying.	To plan interventions that help client manage negative emotions.
2. Help client reduce anxiety, anger, guilt, or worries that prevent sleep, with stress-reducing measures or by talking with another person.	To prevent negative emotions from interfering with sleep.
3. Encourage acceptance of occasional sleep disturbances.	To help client accept realistic goals.
4. Encourage awareness of pleasure experienced in the achievement of a good night's sleep.	To increase client's awareness of good feelings associated with a good night's sleep.
Intellectual Dimension	
1. Discuss reasons for disturbances in sleep.	To determine client's perception of cause of sleep disturbance.
2. Encourage recognition of client's contribution to sleep disorder; negative feelings, excessive stimulation.	To increase client's awareness of behavior contributing to sleep disturbance.
3. Assist client in assuming responsibility for disruption of circadian rhythm or stimulating bedtime activity or ritual.	To promote self-responsibility and encourage client to take charge of behavior that restores disrupted circadian rhythm.
4. Limit client's self-punishing statements regarding sleep disturbance.	To prevent client from decreasing self-esteem.
5. Use problem-solving techniques.	To determine effective sleep behavior.
6. Use paradoxical intention (ask client to stay awake as long as possible).	To help client with resistive personality to sleep using an oppositional approach.
7. Explore client's attitudes about sleep.	To determine client attitudes (for example, "I should sleep 8 hours") and plan interventions.
8. Promote self-management of sleep by planning with client sleep-inducing activities.	To help client gain control over factors related to promoting good sleep.
9. Provide information about sleep.	To decrease anxiety about sleep.
10. Promote conditioning that allows client to associate the bed with sleep only.	To help client associate bed with sleep, to avoid associating bed with activity such as reading or watching TV.
11. Provide a variety of stimuli during waking hours.	To prevent naps, to decrease preoccupation with sleep disturbance.
12. Provide guided imagery.	To help client relax and induce sleep.
13. Encourage meditation.	To relax body and mind.
14. Explore rational and irrational aspects of client's beliefs about sleep disorder.	To determine client's beliefs about sleep, to question irrational beliefs, and to reinforce rational beliefs.
Social Dimension	
1. Enhance self-concept by helping client sleep.	To increase client's feelings of competence in self that he can overcome sleep disturbance.
2. Increase client's confidence in self.	To promote optimism that client can achieve desirable sleep habits.
3. Encourage independence by teaching client strategies to wake self according to specific clues to avoid bed wetting, night terrors, bruxism, and other undesirable sleep activities.	To help client assume responsibility for responding to clues that indicate undesirable sleep activities.

NURSING ACTIONS	RATIONALE
4. Promote participation in social activities to diminish preoccupation with sleeplessness.	To change emphasis of client thinking from preoccupation with sleep to enjoyment of social activities.
5. Encourage positive interactions with other individuals who have sleep disorders.	To share possible solutions to problem.
6. Improve relationships with significant others.	To lessen stress and promote peace of mind that comes with satisfying relationships, thus enhancing a good night's sleep.
7. Provide an environment free of stimuli at bedtime.	To promote relaxation and induce sleep.
8. Assess work, social, and environmental factors that have the potential to disrupt circadian rhythm, such as shift work or international travel.	To determine variations in client's life that disrupt usual sleep-wake cycle.
Spiritual Dimension	
1. Promote creative activities for client when unable to sleep, such as writing or reading.	To help client use time in endeavors that contribute to a positive result and enhance feelings of worth and value.
2. Promote hope that sleep patterns can be improved and quality of life enhanced.	To promote confidence and optimism in client's ability to change sleep patterns.
3. Explain alternative ways to view sleep disorder rather than as the punishment from a vengeful God.	To help client perceive sleep disturbance more realistically but without shattering faith.
4. Help client enjoy achievements and experience satisfactions in life even though he has sleep disturbances.	To lessen emphasis on sleep disturbance.
5. Refer to appropriate clergy for reassurance when client becomes despondent and questions faith because of lack of sleep.	To help client receive strength from faith through the clergy.
6. Encourage setting up a pattern of reflection, meditation, or prayer.	To help client use appropriate methods to induce relaxation and inner peace that contribute to sleep.

EVALUATION

Measurable goals and outcome criteria provide the data for evaluating the client's ability to achieve a good night's sleep. Nurse observations and family reports provide additional data. The following behaviors indicate a positive evaluation:

1. Identifies factors that disrupt sleep
2. Uses methods and techniques that promote sleep
3. Accepts some disturbances in sleep as normal
4. States resources available for help with sleep disturbances
5. Achieves a good night's sleep

BIBLIOGRAPHY

Barndt-Maglio B: Sleep pattern disturbance . . . the pediatric ICU, *Dim Crit Care Nurs* 5(6):342, 1986.

Davis D, Dickhoff J, Walsh J: Sleep apnea syndromes, *Focus Crit Care* 11(2):30, 1984.

Guilleminault C: *Sleep-waking disorders: indications and techniques,* Menlo Park, Calif., 1982, Addison-Wesley Publishing.

Guilleminault C, Lugaresi E, editors: *Sleep wake disorders: natural history, epidemiology, and long-term evaluation,* New York, 1983, Raven Press.

Kales A, Kales J: *Evaluation and treatment of insomnia,* New York, 1984, Oxford University Press.

Kellerman H: *Sleep disorders: insomnia and narcolepsy,* New York, 1981, Brunner/Mazel.

Knab B, Engle R: Perception of waking and sleeping: possible implications for evaluation of insomnia, *Sleep* 11:265, 1988.

Morgan H, White B: Sleep deprivation . . . in intensive care, *Nurs Mirror* 157(14):58, 1983.

Orr W: Altshuler K, Stahl M: *Managing sleep complaints,* Chicago, 1982, Mosby–Year Book.

Phillips E: *Get a good night's sleep,* Englewood Cliffs, N.J., 1983, Prentice-Hall.

Richards K: Techniques for measures of sleep in critical care, *Focus Crit Care* 14(4):34, 1987.

Rosekind M, Schwartz G: The perception of sleep and wakefulness 1: accuracy and certainty of subjective judgments, *Sleep Research* 17:89, 1988.

Ruler A, Lack L: Gender differences in sleep, *Sleep Research* 17:244, 1988.

Slots M: Implications of sleep deprivation in the pediatric critical care unit, *Focus Crit Care* 15(3):35, 1988.

Spiegel R: *Sleep and sleeplessness in advanced age,* New York, 1981, SP Medical and Scientific Books.

Webster R, Thompson D: Sleep in hospital, *J Adv Nurs* 11(4):447, 1986.

Wilhoit E, Brown E, Suratt P: Treatment of obstructive sleep apnea with continuous nasal airflow delivered through nasal prongs, *Chest* 85(February):2, 1984.

Wotring K: Using research in practice . . . what effects do drugs given in critical care have on patients' sleep? *Focus AACN* 9(5):34, 1982.

Suicidal Behavior

Suicide or overt self-destructive behavior is the act of voluntarily and intentionally taking one's life. Committing suicide involves the individual's conscious wish to be dead and the accompanying action required to carry out that wish. Suicidal behaviors are those overt gestures, attempts, or verbal threats that result in death, injury, or pain consciously inflicted upon the self. The term *suicide* may refer to an attempted suicide, a threatened suicide, or suicidal ideas.

Conservative estimates of suicide in the United States range from 25,000 to 50,000 per year. For every suicide completed, approximately ten suicides are attempted.

Indirect self-destructive behavior, or unconscious, latent, or covert actions or behaviors that cause harm to the individual and hasten death are not to be confused with the term *suicide*. Examples of indirect self-destructive behaviors include alcohol and drug addiction, self-mutilation, antisocial behavior, and polysurgery (numerous surgeries).

The incidence of suicide varies from one cultural group to another. Hungary, Finland, Denmark, Switzerland, and Austria rank highest of 43 nations reporting suicide death statistics, whereas countries such as New Guinea and the Philippines report very low rates. Suicide rates tend to increase during periods of social unrest.

Suicidal prevention centers have been established throughout the United States to assist individuals through suicidal crises. These centers have developed specific protocols for dealing with troubled clients on an outpatient basis. The guidelines presented in this manual are directed toward inpatient care.

Related DSM-III-R conditions

Bipolar disorder
Major depression
Cyclothymia
Dysthymia
Schizophrenia
Delusional (paranoid) disorders
Psychoactive substance-use disorders

Other related conditions

Accident proneness
Confusion
Crisis situations
Hemodialysis
Terminal illness
Aging

PRINCIPLES

▶ Physical Dimension

1. Biochemical changes associated with suicide are similar to the biochemical changes of clinical depression.
2. Indications are that changes occur in the biogenic amines of suicidal persons.
3. Methods preferred by men in suicide attempts are gunshot, hanging, carbon monoxide inhalation, drowning, barbiturates, jumping, other drugs, and cutting or stabbing.
4. Methods commonly used by women in suicide attempts are barbituates, hanging, gunshot, carbon monoxide inhalation, other drugs, jumping, and cutting or stabbing.

▶ Emotional Dimension

1. Life (Eros) and death (Thanatos) instincts are present in all individuals.

2. The life instinct functions to maintain life and has constructive aims.

3. The death wish is exhibited through anger and aggression toward others.

4. When anger is repressed and turned inward, self-destructive behaviors may result.

5. The life and death instincts are in constant conflict and interaction with each other.

6. The aggressive-hostile drive in suicide consists of three basic elements: the wish to kill, the wish to be killed, and the wish to die.

7. Loss, depression, fears of abandonment, rejection, and rage are a part of the suicide dynamic.

8. Self-directed rage is a reaction to frustrated dependency.

9. Expiation of guilt is an important motivational factor in suicide.

10. Feelings of hopelessness are a significant clue in persons at risk for suicide.

▶ Intellectual Dimension

1. Intense emotional suffering results from the irrational ways people construe the world and the assumptions they make.

2. Assumptions may lead to self-defeating internal dialogue that has an adverse effect on behavior.

3. Distorted thinking may produce a depressive episode and contribute to the risk of suicide.

4. Three identifiable cognitive patterns emerge:
   a. Devaluation of self
   b. Negative interpretation of life and experiences
   c. Negative and pessimistic view of the future

▶ Social Dimension

1. Individuals with suicidal tendencies depend on the achievements and the support of others and expect and demand that others fulfill their wishes.

2. Self-esteem from childhood on is low, and efforts are made to achieve importance. Inferiority feelings interfere with the development of social interest. Thinking is self-centered rather than problem- or other-centered.

3. Suicide is an act of reproach or revenge. It may be combined with aggression and may then be preceded by murder.

4. The well-adjusted person may commit suicide in situations in which he can find no other way out (fear of discovery of disgraceful or criminal acts, incurable or painful diseases, or cruel and inhuman acts resulting in endless suffering).

5. Three times as many men as women complete suicide, but females attempt more suicides.

6. The incidence of suicide in men increases as age increases; in females it increases up to age 40 to 60 and then decreases.

7. Suicide among young black individuals 25 to 34 years old and among adolescents is increasing.

8. Divorced, widowed, and single persons have higher suicide rates than married persons.

9. Certain occupational groups, such as physicians (particularly psychiatrists), lawyers, dentists, psychologists, policemen, college students, and those with low employment security, have a higher than average incidence of suicide.

10. The intent to commit suicide is frequently communicated beforehand by giving away personal possessions, threats, discussion of suicide methods, a developing depression, or suicide notes.

11. The more violent the planned method for suicide, the more serious is the intent.

12. There are no suicidal people, only individuals engaged in specific suicidal behaviors.

13. Suicidal behaviors are learned and can be unlearned.

14. Rewarding and/or punishing suicidal behavior will initially increase suicidal responses.

15. Reinforcement of nonsuicidal behaviors will increase alternative tension-reducing responses.

16. Helplessness is a prominent feature of a suicidal person.

17. Suicide is sometimes based on an individual's ties to society.
   a. Altruistic suicide results when the individual is closely bound to his society, and suicide may be required in certain circumstances.
   b. Egoistic suicide results when an individual is not integrated into a group and has too few ties to the community.
   c. Anomic suicide occurs when the accustomed relationship between an individual and society is shattered.

▶ Spiritual Dimension

1. Death is a dilemma of existence.

2. Suicide is a primary ethical issue.

3. Reponding to life's meaninglessness and despair is a primary task for individuals.

4. Different cultural value systems vary in attitudes toward suicide.

5. The Judeo-Christian view is that human life has great value.

6. In Judeo-Christian cultures suicide is a violation of the divine injunction against killing.

7. In Judeo-Christian cultures control over death is forbidden to human beings and retained by God.

8. Some Oriental cultures approve of suicide to prevent dishoner to self or family.

ASSESSMENT

▶ Physical Dimension

I. History

A. Identifying information
  1. Age—prevalent in all ages
  2. Sex
     a. Females—more attempts
     b. Males—more completions
  3. Living arrangements
     a. Recent widower or widow, divorced, separated, or person living alone—higher risk
     b. Married person—lower risk
  4. High-risk occupation
     a. Dentist
     b. Policeman
     c. Physician
     d. College student
     e. Psychologist
     f. Person with low employment security

B. Activities of daily living
  1. Loss of appetite
  2. Changes in sleep patterns
  3. Decreased physical activity
  4. Decreased sexual activity
  5. Hobbies
     a. Discontinued previous activities
     b. Has dangerous hobbies, such as mountain climbing, car racing

C. Habits
  1. Alcohol
     a. Excessive use
     b. Misuse
  2. Medications
     a. Prescribed antianxiety medication or antidepressant
     b. Drug abuse or dependence

D. Destructive behavior
  1. Past suicide attempts
  2. Accident-prone
  3. Violence-prone
  4. Risk-taking activities

E. Health history
  1. Illnesses
     a. Acute or chronic physical illness
     b. Intractable pain
     c. Hemodialysis
     d. Consultation with physician in last 6 months (research indicates that majority of those who committed suicide had seen a physician)
     e. Counseling or psychiatric treatment
     f. Recovering from a major depression

F. Past hospitalizations
  1. Psychiatric problems or suicide attempts

G. Coping strategies
  1. Assess client's coping with past crisis
  2. Which coping method used in the past are helpful in current situation and how are they helpful
  3. What would be helpful now

H. Family history
  1. Depression

II. Physical examination (see Depression, p. 133). While all potential suicides are not depressed, many are.

▶ Emotional Dimension

CLIENT DATA	ANALYSIS	NURSING DIAGNOSIS
Anxiety	High level of anxiety or panic state increases risk.	High risk for violence, self-directed: related to high level of anxiety
Depression, grief	Moderate to severe depression increases risk; may indicate that anger has been turned inward.	High risk for violence, self-directed: related to moderate or severe depression
	If client coming out of severe depression, risk is increased.	High risk for violence, self-directed: related to lifting depression
Hostility	Marked hostility increases risk. The aggressive-hostile drive includes the wish to kill, the wish to be killed, and the wish to die.	High risk for violence, self-directed: related to hostility
Guilt	Results of loss of or low self-esteem. Reparation is important motivational factor in suicide.	High risk for violence, self-directed: related to need to make reparation for feelings of guilt
Anger or rage	May be covert or overt. If covert, depression likely to be predominant affect.	High risk for violence directed at others: related to anger or rage
Hopelessness	Accurate indicator of seriousness of suicidal risk.	High risk for violence, self-directed: related to feelings of hopelessness

▶ **Intellectual Dimension**

CLIENT DATA	ANALYSIS	NURSING DIAGNOSIS
Helplessness	Belief that nothing will change, which is a learned response.	High risk for violence, self-directed: related to feelings of helplessness
Ambivalence	Plans made for suicide while entertaining fantasies of rescue and intervention. Life and death instincts are in constant conflict and interaction.	*Suicidal ideation: related to ambivalence
Reality-based perception	Decision to commit suicide may be rational decision based on situational circumstances (persons with intractable pain or incurable diseases). Person who is more aware of realistic implication of self-destructive behavior is the more serious risk.	High risk for violence, self-directed: related to rational decision to take own life
Narrow focus	Inability to see things that will lead out of suicidal state; inability to see alternatives.	High risk for violence, self-directed: related to inability to see alternatives to present situation
Hallucinations	Individuals whose hallucinations command them to commit suicide are at risk.	High risk for violence, self-directed: related to response to hallucinations
Fragmentation, spacey feeling, feeling of floating away	Indication of depression and increased suicidal risk. Suicidal thinking may reduce process of fragmentation.	*Suicidal ideation: related to depression with increased risk for suicide
Recent memory impairment	Seen in individuals whose suicidal attempt is part of chronic organic brain syndrome.	High risk for violence, self-directed: related to memory impairment
Disorientation, disorganization, and confusion	If marked, client is high suicidal risk.	High risk for violence, self-directed: related to marked disorientation, disorganization, and confusion
Poor impulse control	Use of alcohol or drugs to solve emotional problems and violent acting out against self and others increase risk.	High risk for violence, self-directed: related to poor impulse control associated with substance abuse
Awareness of effect of threats and attempts on others	Manipulative element indicates lower risk.	High risk for violence, self-directed: related to suicide attempts and threats related to efforts to control behavior of others
Inability to think abstractly	Ability reduced, particularly if in crisis or high level of anxiety.	High risk for violence, self-directed: related to anxiety
Inability to concentrate and difficulty in solving problems	Heightened emotional state with decreased mental productivity.	*Altered problem-solving: related to emotional instability
Fantasies	When death represents nirvana, reincarnation, paradise, rescue, fantasies of self-injury or injury to others, risk is increased.	*Suicidal ideation: related to fantasies of self-injury, injury to others
Suicidal plan	The more detailed the plan, the greater is the risk. Interrelation of four areas indicates increasing risk.	High risk for violence, self-directed: related to clear, specific, and lethal plan
a. Method	More lethal method increases risk (pills, shooting, or other method).	
b. Availability	More available method increases risk. Is gun available? Does person have access to pills?	
c. Specificity	Plan that is concretely detailed and accessible increases risk. If method unclear, with no reference to practical details or access, risk is decreased.	

▶ **Intellectual Dimension—cont'd**

CLIENT DATA	ANALYSIS	NURSING DIAGNOSIS
d. Lethality	Certain methods are associated with successful suicides (firearms and explosives, jumping from high places, hanging, drowning, poisoning, and cutting wrists). When person has detailed plan involving lethal method, risk is high. Less lethal methods (overdosing on pills) allows time for rescue.	
Suicide notes and letters, diaries, and verbal threats	Direct actions indicating exact intentions. Feelings of conflict may be expressed, and behavior may be plea for help. Suicidal act considered a cry for help; client is seeking removal from intolerable situation.	High risk for violence, self-directed: a perceived intolerable situation
Giving away personal possessions or settling accounts	Risk increased.	High risk for violence, self-directed: related to giving away personal possessions
Train of thought difficult to follow; rambling and disorganized	Result of psychological stress, drug or alcohol abuse, physical illness, or mental disturbance.	Altered thought processes: related to psychological stress, substance abuse, physical illness, or mental disturbance
Rigid thinking	Limited number of reactions to environment. If exhausts them, defenses begin to deteriorate.	Altered thought processes: rigid thinking related to limited number of reactions to environment

▶ **Social Dimension**

CLIENT DATA	ANALYSIS	NURSING DIAGNOSIS
Low self-esteem	Failure to live up to expectations. Low self-worth is correlated with depression. Devaluation of self occurs, and suicide becomes a solution. Self-esteem lowered when love is lost or approval is not received from others. Self-esteem is low from childhood on and efforts are made to achieve importance.	Self-esteem disturbance: chronic, related to failure to live up to expectations
Feelings of inferiority	Inferiority feelings interfere with development of social interest. Client feels that whether he lives or dies is not important.	Self-esteem disturbance: chronic, related to feelings of worthlessness
Significant loss in life (death, separation, or divorce)	Thoughts center on loss. Loss, fears of abandonment, rejection, and rage are part of suicide dynamic.	High risk for violence, self-directed: related to significant loss (death, separation, or divorce)
Decline in number and quality of relationships with significant others	If communication open and interpersonal needs gratifying, lethality decreased. Some people vulnerable to interpersonal frustration and tend to direct aggression inward; have history of interpersonal problems.	Social isolation: related to lack of meaningful relationships

▶ **Social Dimension—cont'd**

CLIENT DATA	ANALYSIS	NURSING DIAGNOSIS
Alienation, isolation, and loneliness	Alone and isolated; may see no point in going on. May have alienated others, or others may have alienated client. When feels that no one cares, risk increased. Loneliness that results from loss of significant others or self-esteem is stressor related to suicide.	High risk for violence, self-directed: related to social isolation, alienation, loneliness
Negative attitude of significant other toward client	If open and accepting of client, less risk. If angry, rejecting, and wishing to get out of relationship, lethality increases.	High risk for violence, self-directed: related to rejection by significant other
Dependency	Individuals with suicidal tendencies are dependent upon achievements and support of others; they expect and demand that others fulfill their wishes. Self-directed rage is a reaction to frustrated dependency.	High risk for violence, self-directed: related to frustrated dependency
History of suicides in family	Suicidal behaviors may be learned. Biochemical changes associated with suicide also associated with clinical depression. Risk is increased when family history of suicide exists.	High risk for violence, self-directed: related to history of suicide in family
Sporadic work record; loss of job, prestige, or status	Increased suicidal risk. Anomic suicide occurs when the accustomed relationship between an individual and society is shattered.	Altered role performance: related to loss of job, prestige, or status
Threat of prosecution, criminal involvement or exposure	Suicide may be socially or culturally condoned to spare family dishonor; considered rational suicide.	High risk for violence, self-directed: related to threat of prosecution, criminal involvement, or exposure
Living in subculture (such as skid row) where social cohesion is lacking; living alone or with few community ties	Egoistic suicide results when individual is not integrated into a group and has too few ties to community.	High risk for violence, self-directed: related to loose ties to community
Financial problems; no sources of support (family, friends, or agencies); no food, clothing, or shelter	The fewer resources available to client, the higher the suicide risk.	High risk for violence, self-directed: related to financial problems and few sources of social support High risk for violence, self-directed: related to inability to meet basic needs
Stressors (sickness, serious injury, surgery, accident, loss of any kind, or crisis)	Persons's perception of event or situation may increase suicide risk (see Crisis, p. 99).	High risk for violence, self-directed: related to crisis situation (sickness, serious injury, surgery, accident, or loss)

▶ **Spiritual Dimension**

CLIENT DATA	ANALYSIS	NURSING DIAGNOSIS
No meaning or purpose in life; questioning meaning of life's suffering	Death is dilemma of existence. Suicide is primary ethical issue for the human race. Responding to life's meaninglessness and despair is the main task of client.	Spiritual distress: suicide risk related to meaninglessness and purposelessness in life

▶ **Spiritual Dimension—cont'd**

CLIENT DATA	ANALYSIS	NURSING DIAGNOSIS
Feeling of hopelessness	Hopelessness is indicator of seriousness of suicidal threat. Client's inability to project into future and make plans indicates high degree of risk. Has negative and pessimistic view of future.	Spiritual distress: suicide risk related to feelings of hopelessness
Feelings of despair and powerlessness	Feels loss of control over life. Taking own life is one way to gain control.	Spiritual distress: suicide risk related to feelings of powerlessness and despair
Feelings of separation and isolation from spiritual resources	Alienation and remoteness from God or supreme power.	Spiritual distress: suicide risk related to isolation and separation from God or supreme power or other spiritual resources
May view death as peaceful sleep or way to be reunited with dead loved one	Death seen as release; risk of suicide increased.	High risk for violence, self-directed: related to inability to evaluate reality of death

PLANNING

Long-Term Goals

To develop a more positive attitude toward self so that physical well-being is maintained

To develop coping skills that will replace self-destructive behavior

SHORT-TERM GOALS	OUTCOME CRITERIA
Physical Dimension	
To assume responsibility for self in a safe environment	1. Verbalizes acceptance of close observation 2. Verbalizes acceptance of protective measures 3. Makes verbal contract to make no suicidal attempts 4. Delays self-destructive impulse while calling for help 5. Carries out activities of daily living (see Depression, p. 133)
Emotional Dimension	
To identify anxiety and prevent acceleration	1. Discusses situations that increase anxiety and consequent suicidal thoughts (see Anxiety, p. 48)
To develop acceptable ways of expressing anger, rage, and hostility	1. Describes physical feeling of these emotions 2. Identifies situations, persons, and events that precipitate feelings of anger and hostility 3. States ways to reduce anger and hostility (see Anger, p. 28)
To become more competent, hopeful, and optimistic	1. Discusses ways that problems may be resolved 2. Expresses confidence in capacity to change 3. Makes decisions 4. States that future will be better or different 5. Improves ability to establish situational and self-control
To identify source of guilt	1. (See Guilt, p. 155)
Intellectual Dimension	
To alter ineffective coping skills related to self-destructive behavior	1. Is able to determine which situations can be changed and which cannot 2. Identifies past successful coping mechanisms 3. Identifies alternative coping mechanisms 4. Applies new coping behavior to problems 5. Discusses judgments and seeks consensual validation for them from family and friends

SHORT-TERM GOALS	OUTCOME CRITERIA
To increase cognitive organization	1. States time and location correctly 2. Is able to increase attention span
To reduce suicidal ideation	1. Is able to list alternatives to suicide 2. Expresses an awareness of consequences of suicidal behavior 3. Is able to use problem-solving techniques
To determine goals for life	1. Sets realistic goals and a schedule for achieving life goals
Social Dimension	
To mobilize social support systems	1. Communicates care and concern for others 2. Focuses on others rather than on self 3. Learns social skills 4. Becomes involved in group activities 5. Recognizes effect of suicidal behavior on others 6. Acts more responsible for family and friends 7. Asks for help when needed 8. Listens to others and responds with interest
To increase self-esteem	1. (See Negative Self-Concept, p. 231)
Spiritual Dimension	
To discover meaning in own life	1. Discusses difference in fantasies and reality of death 2. Discusses meaning and meaninglessness of life 3. Discovers purpose and meaning in suffering 4. Is able to make choices regarding suicidal and other behaviors 5. Verbalizes the value of life
To determine purpose of life	1. Discusses expectations and values 2. Discusses future life goals
To discover the destructive and creative depths of self	1. Expresses and is conscious of reaction patterns 2. Makes associations between words, behavior, and mental images 3. Defines what is considered bad about self and accepts shortcomings 4. Defines and accepts the creative self
To develop a will to live	1. Discusses ambivalence about life and death 2. Verbalizes the wish to live 3. Identifies reasons for living

Discharge Planning

The following client behaviors demonstrate a readiness for discharge:
1. Demonstrates no evidence of self-destructive behavior
2. Client and family know early signs and symptoms of self-destructive behavior
3. Knows agencies to contact in the event of suicidal feelings
4. Uses techniques for anxiety reduction
5. States the value of life

IMPLEMENTATION

NURSING ACTIONS	RATIONALE
Physical Dimension	
1. Establish a contract with client, asking him to make statement that he will not do anything to harm himself intentionally or unintentionally.	To prevent client from acting impulsively. Most clients are willing to make an agreement and abide by it.
2. Determine appropriate level of suicide precautions for client.	To determine the seriousness of client's intent.

IMPLEMENTATION—cont'd

NURSING ACTIONS	RATIONALE
3. Assess client's suicidal potential and evaluate level of suicidal precautions on a daily basis.	To determine changes in seriousness of client's intent.
4. Provide client with one-to-one contact at all times.	To observe client and prevent self-harm.
5. Accompany to bathroom and stay with client.	To observe client and prevent self-harm.
6. Seclude client if confused and disorganized until able to control own behavior.	To provide safety and protect client.
7. Search client's personal belongings and remove dangerous objects, including such things as pantyhose and neckties.	To prevent client from using personal clothing in a lethal way.
8. Reassure client that objects will be returned when appropriate.	To promote a sense of hope that client will feel better, to motivate client to cooperate with treatment.
9. Decrease observations as suicidal risk decreases.	To allow client privileges associated with appropriate behavior.
10. Provide client with centrally located room near nurses' station.	To ensure close observation.
11. Make sure that windows are locked or shatterproof and that utility and storage rooms are locked.	To protect client.
12. Check client at frequent and irregular intervals during night.	To prevent suicide attempts during night when client is alone and awake.
13. Maintain close supervision of client during shift changes, mealtimes, weekends, or when fewer staff members are working.	To prevent suicide at times when staff responsibilities are greatest.
14. Give medication in liquid form when possible.	To ensure client is taking medication, not hoarding it.
15. Provide for release of tension, anger, and guilt through physical activities.	To use emotional energy in physical activity is therapeutic.
16. Refrain from accepting requests for confidentiality regarding suicide or suicidal thoughts. ("There are some things that I cannot keep secret, those things that involve your plans about killing or harming yourself.")	To prevent client from manipulating you, to let client know that you are part of the treatment team and the team needs information about suicide intent.
17. Emphasize delaying self-destructive act and calling for help.	To prevent impulsive acts of self-harm.
18. Assist client in maintaining proper nutrition, elimination, and rest if depressed (see Depression, p. 133).	To promote general physical and mental health.

Emotional Dimension

1. Assist client in focusing if anxiety level is high.	To prevent scattering, disorganized thinking.
2. Repeat information in simple language.	To ensure that client understands.
3. Assist client in identifying subjective experience of anxiety.	To increase awareness of feelings and plan interventions.
4. Explore with client situations that result in anxiety (see Anxiety, p. 48).	To identify causes of own anxiety.
5. Facilitate expression of angry, sad, or hostile feelings.	To determine intensity of feelings, to help client express feelings appropriately.
6. Assist client in identifying subjective experience of sadness, anger, or hostility.	To increase awareness of feelings and plan interventions.
7. Explore with client those situations that precipitate feelings of sadness, anger, or hostility.	To identify causes of sadness, anger, and hostility.
8. Jointly develop alternatives that reduce feelings of anger, hostility, and sadness and decide on ways to implement those strategies (see Anger, p. 28).	To involve client in plans for treatment and promote feelings of control of life.
9. Respond warmly and empathically and convey a hopeful attitude.	To convey understanding and confidence that client can feel better.
10. Observe client for changes in depression that indicate increased suicidal potential (see Depression, p. 133).	To revise treatment goals and plan interventions.
11. Explore client's ambivalence.	To focus on positive factors that promote client's will to live.
12. Observe client for raised spirits, an indication that client has made decision to kill self.	To prevent self-harm that may follow a lifting depression and an energy increase.
13. Respond to feelings of hopelessness.	To reduce hopeless feelings by presenting realistic optimism.

NURSING ACTIONS	RATIONALE
14. Explore client's guilt feelings and identify sources of guilt.	To determine reality of guilt feelings.
15. Encourage forgiveness of self and acceptance of the forgiveness of others (see Guilt, p. 155).	To help client relieve guilt feelings.

Intellectual Dimension

1. Involve client in treatment plan.	To promote client's active participation in making decisions that involve treatment.
2. Assist client in developing a plan for daily activities and encourage active participation.	To help client assume responsibility for activities.
3. If necessary, assign structured tasks, basing the simplicity or complexity of the task on the client's capacity to respond.	To involve client in an activity in which client can succeed and which will lessen client's preoccupation with suicide.
4. Help client identify stressors that precipitated self-destructive behavior.	To help client learn to cope with stressors constructively.
5. Explore with client coping strategies used in past.	To build on effective past coping skills.
6. Teach problem solving (see Appendix C).	To help client become skillful in solving problems with rational thinking.
7. Explore alternative solutions to problem with client.	To increase client's options for solving problems.
8. Ask client how problem(s) can be solved and assist in developing at least three viable options.	To help client broaden thinking about possible solutions to problems.
9. Teach assertiveness skills.	To help client gain confidence in self and meeting own needs.
10. Assist client in evaluating situations in realistic manner.	To prevent client from thinking irrationally and reaching conclusions without sufficient information.
11. Positively reinforce decision making.	To provide feedback for appropriate decision making.
12. Encourage client's realistic expectations.	To promote reality.
13. Teach client to use "I" statements such as "Stop" when hallucinations suggest suicide.	To help client learn to interrupt hallucinations that suggest self-harm.
14. Assist client in clarifying thoughts regarding suicide.	To help client distinguish thoughts from feelings about suicide.
15. Help client determine early symptoms of self-destructive behavior (depression).	To encourage client to seek help before symptoms become severe.
16. Encourage client to make judgments and seek out others to validate them consensually.	To help client learn to share thoughts and feelings with others and receive feedback from them.
17. Help client make lists of things to be done to achieve goals.	To prevent client from becoming overwhelmed with multiple, unrealistic goals, to clarify steps for achieving each goal.
18. Help client determine which goals realistically can be achieved.	To prevent failure and lowered self-esteem.
19. Explore with client how self-destructive behavior works for client (the needs it meets).	To increase client's awareness of behavior.
20. Provide opportunities for client to succeed and provide positive reinforcement.	To enhance self-esteem.
21. Discuss with client effects of threats or attempts on others and explore secondary gains or manipulative efforts.	To increase client's awareness of behavior.
22. Teach client effects of medication and need for special precautions.	To reduce client's anxiety by preparing client for possible side effects.
23. Teach client to ask for help when he needs it.	To lessen passivity.
24. Teach client social skills.	To promote comfort in social situations.

Social Dimension

1. Enhance client's self-concept (see Negative Self-Concept, p. 231).	To promote feelings of confidence and competence and lessen helplessness and feeling that the only solution is suicide.
2. Interrupt negative statements about self.	To limit self-defeating statements.
3. Provide positive reinforcement for responsible actions.	To emphasize and promote appropriate behavior.
4. Identify and make list of available community resources.	To increase client's awareness of community resources available for suicide prevention.
5. Identify with client those persons who can provide support to client.	To help client identify supportive persons available in the environment.

IMPLEMENTATION—cont'd

NURSING ACTIONS	RATIONALE
6. Discuss which resource should be used first.	To help client set priorities when need for help arises.
7. Assist family or significant others in developing plan to support self-destructive client.	To enlarge support system, to provide information to family about ways to help suicidal person.
8. Involve family or significant others in family therapy.	To promote effective client-family interactions and relationships.
9. Teach client and family to communicate openly and in a caring way.	To facilitate members' expression of feelings and acceptance of them by family members.
10. Encourage active participation in group activities.	To promote feelings of belonging and worth.
11. Encourage independent decision making.	To prevent dependence on others.
12. Explore client's dependent behavior.	To increase client's awareness of behavior and plan interventions.
13. Involve family in discharge planning.	To promote family involvement in client's plan for discharge to solicit their cooperation.
14. Encourage client to be sensitive to and do things for others.	To lessen preoccupation with self, to increase feelings of self-esteem.
15. Assist with identification of loss of significant others or fear of loss.	To increase client's awareness of possible reasons for suicide and plan interventions.
16. Assist client in developing a plan to adapt to changes in life resulting from loss.	To involve client in a plan of action that is realistic and achievable.
17. Discuss problems that may be encountered in community following discharge.	To prevent increased anxiety by considering possible problem areas.
18. Reinforce comments and actions that indicate a will to live.	To increase client's involvement with people and activities that bring pleasure and satisfactions.
Spiritual Dimension	
1. Examine with client his meaning and purpose in life.	To determine positive aspects of life.
2. Discuss the fact that courage is required to question meaning of life and explain that such questioning is manifestation of intellectual honesty.	To reinforce client's positive behavior and increase client's valuing of self.
3. Help client discover a cause higher than self.	To lessen client's preoccupation with self.
4. Help client learn to express love for others.	To create in client a love for self that comes with loving others.
5. Promote client's efforts to become other-centered rather than self-centered.	To lessen preoccupation with self.
6. Assist client in assuming responsibility to create a life with meaning.	To prevent feelings of hopelessness and suicidal behaviors, to help client value life.
7. Discuss with client the inevitability of suffering and meeting it with courage.	To help client learn to accept pain—to grow from it instead of succumbing to it.
8. Help client to stop blaming the past and assume responsibility for what is occurring now.	To promote responsibility for self and life.
9. Encourage client to become involved in activities that will stimulate creativity.	To increase feelings of value and worth.
10. Explore possible conflicts between religious beliefs and self-destructive behavior.	To enable client to understand relationship between behavior and religious beliefs.
11. Communicate expressions of hope based on reality of client's improvement.	To promote confidence that client will feel better in time.
12. Encourage expression of religious values and beliefs.	To strengthen beliefs about life.
13. Examine beliefs on life and death; promote a reality-based interpretation of death.	To determine client's beliefs about death.
14. Discuss realities of death.	To prevent unrealistic view of death.
15. Explore with client expectations of life.	To determine whether realistic or not.
16. Explore reason for living.	To promote life.
17. Reinforce comments and actions that indicate a will to live.	To provide client with positive feedback for appropriate behavior.

EVALUATION

Evaluation of the effectiveness of interventions for the suicidal client is based on measurable goals and outcome criteria and a living client. The following behaviors indicate a positive evaluation:

1. States he is not suicidal
2. Indicates by interactions and relationships with others that life has meaning
3. Agrees to contact help if suicidal feelings arise
4. Has a support system readily available

BIBLIOGRAPHY

Alston MH: Occupation and suicide among women, *Issues Ment Health Nurs* 8(2):109, 1986.

Apter A et al: Correlates of risk of suicide in violent and non-violent psychiatric patients, *Am J Psychiatry* 148(7):883, 1991.

Battin MP: *Ethical issues in suicide*, Englewood Cliffs, NJ, 1982, Prentice-Hall.

Battle AO: Group therapy of survivors of suicide, *Crisis* 5(1):45, 1984.

Bednar R: *Psychotherapy with high-risk clients: legal and professional standards*, Pacific Grove, Calif, 1991, Brooks/Cole.

Blumenthal SJ, Kupfer D, editors: *Suicide over the life cycle: risk factors, assessment, and treatment of suicidal patients*, Washington, DC, 1990, American Psychiatric Press.

Branchey L et al: Depression, suicide and aggression in alcoholics and their relationship to plasma amine acids, *Psychiatry Res* 12(3):219, 1984.

Busteen EL, Johnstone C: The development of suicide precautions for an inpatient psychiatric unit. *J Psychosoc Nurs Ment Health Serv* 21(5):15, 1983.

Camus A: *The myth of Sisyphus*, New York, 1959, Vintage Books.

Capodanno AE, Targum SD: Assessment of suicide risk: some limitations in the prediction of infrequent events, *J Psychosoc Nurs Ment Health Serv* 21(5):29, 1983.

Crow TJ et al: Neurotransmitter receptors and monoamine metabolites in the brains of patients with Alzheimer-type dementia and depression and suicide, *Neuropharmacology* 23(12B):1561, 1984.

Durkheim E: *Suicide*, Chicago, 1951, The Free Press of Glencoe.

Farberow NL: *The many faces of suicide: indirect self-destructive behavior*, New York, 1980, McGraw-Hill.

Farberow NL, Shneidman ES, editors: *The cry for help*, New York, 1961, McGraw-Hill.

Fawcett J et al: Time-related predictors of suicide in major affective disorder, *Am J Psychiatry* 147(9):1189, 1990.

Fitzpatrick JJ: Suicidology and suicide prevention: historical perspectives from the nursing literature, *J Psychosoc Nurs Ment Health Serv* 21(5):20, 1983.

Freud S: Mourning and melancholia. In Strachey J, editor: *Standard edition of the complete works of Sigmund Freud*, vol. 14, London, 1957, The Hogarth Press.

Hamilton MJ et al: Thirty-five law student suicides, *J Psychiatry Law* 11(3):335, 1983.

Hartog J, Audy JR, Cohen YA: *The anatomy of loneliness*, New York, 1980, International Universities Press.

Hatton CL, Valente S: *Suicide: assessment and intervention*, ed 2, East Norwalk, Conn, 1984, Appleton-Century-Crofts.

Hendin H: Psychodynamics of suicide, with particular reference to the young, *Am J Psychiatry* 148(9):1150, 1991.

Hippie JL: Intervention with the alcoholic client who is suicidal, *Alcohol Treatment Q* 1(4):99, 1984.

Hogarty SS, Rodaitis CM: A suicide precautions policy for the general hospital, *J Nurs Admin* 17(10):36, 1987.

Ishii K: Backgrounds of higher suicide rates among "name" university students: a retroactive study of the past 25 years, *Suicide Life Threat Behav* 15(1):56, 1985.

Kelly GL: Childhood depression and suicide, *Nurs Clin North Am* 26(3):545, 1991.

Leenaars AA: Suicide notes and their implication for intervention, *Crisis* 12(1):1, 1991.

Lester D: The study of suicidal lives, *Suicide Life Threat Behav* 21(2):164, 1991.

Litman RE: Predicting and preventing hospital and clinic suicides, *Suicide Life Threat Behav* 21(1):56, 1991.

Maris RS: *Pathways to suicide: a survey of self-destructive behaviors*, Baltimore, 1981, The Johns Hopkins University Press.

Marra R, Orru M: Social images of suicide, *Brit J Soc* 42(2):273, 1991.

McIntosh JL: Suicide among elderly: levels and trends, *Am J Orthopsychiatry* 55(2):288, 1985.

Menninger C: *Man against himself*, New York, 1938, Harcourt Brace.

Motto JA: An integrated approach to estimating suicide risk, *Suicide Life Threat Behav* 21(1):74, 1991.

Pallikkathayil L, Flood M: Adolescent suicide. Prevention, intervention, and postintervention, *Nurs Clin North Am* 26(3):623, 1991.

Pallikkathayil L, Morgan SA: Emergency department nurses' encounters with suicide attempters: a qualitative investigation, *Schol Inq Nurs Pract* 2(3):237, 1988.

Pfeffer CR: Suicidal fantasies in normal children, *J Nerv Ment Dis* 173(2):78, 1985.

Rogers TM, Masterton G, McGuire R: Parasuicide and the lunar cycle, *Psyc Med* 21(2):393, 1991.

Smith JC: Comparison of suicides among Anglos and Hispanics in 5 southwestern states, *Suicide Life Threat Behav* 15(1):14, 1985.

Travis R: Suicide and economic development among the Inupiat Eskimo, *White Cloud J* 3(3):14, 1984.

Tushan JJ, Thase ME: Suicides in jails and prison, *J Psychosoc Nurs Ment Health Serv* 21(5):29, 1983.

Youssef FA: The impact of group reminiscence counseling on a depressed elderly population, *Nurse Practit* 15(4):32, 1990.

Suspiciousness

Suspiciousness is a psychological state in which a person's basic assumptions regarding interactions with others and with the environment are characterized by mistrust and doubt. Paranoia, a behavior commonly associated with suspiciousness, is a pathological suspiciousness in which feelings of mistrust are indiscriminately generalized from interactions with others and with the environment. Paranoia fails to take into account the nature and context of the relationship.

Suspiciousness may be regarded on a continuum from totally trustful to totally mistrustful. Individuals found on either end of the continuum encounter problems, one for being too trusting, the other for being too mistrustful. Suspiciousness has some utilitarian function in society because some individuals do violate the rights of others, generating a degree of mistrust in the population.

Suspiciousness may be displayed when it seems that everything goes wrong and the person tends to blame others for difficulties and to perceive people as ruthless, selfish, and uncaring. Such people go through life feeling unappreciated, frustrated, and keenly aware of real or imaginary injustices.

More pronounced forms of suspiciousness move the individual toward paranoia. The person is unprepared for life and tends to trust and mistrust inappropriately and tends to overreact when others are perceived as betraying trust. Paranoia usually develops gradually. Social, occupational, and marital failures and perceived betrayals result in elaborate defensive structures that logically explain the person's lack of success. The paranoid person is at first confused and bewildered by failures and by his persecution by others. Then, through a process known as *paranoid illumination* he finally discovers the answer—a group of people both real and imaginary have banned together to plot against him.

Ideas of persecution are predominant in many paranoid persons. However, many develop delusions of grandeur or false beliefs, which serve to elevate their status or importance in their imaginary world.

Related DMS-III-R disorders

Schizophrenia, paranoid type
Delusional (paranoid) disorders
Schizophreniform disorder
Paranoid personality disorder
Organic mental disorders
Psychoactive substance-use disorders

Other related conditions

Hearing loss in the elderly
Immigrant status
Refugee status
Prisoner of war status
Induction into military service
Leaving home for the first time

PRINCIPLES

▶ Physical Dimension

1. Chemical imbalances of the nervous system may result in mistrust.
2. Genetics may contribute to pathological suspiciousness.
3. Failure to respect the individual's inherited personality characteristics promotes insecurity and suspiciousness.
4. Physical abuse and trauma may cause some mistrust of others (for example, victims of rape may mistrust men).
5. Loss of hearing can contribute to increased suspiciousness.

The original content for this section was contributed by Lisa Tidrow Martone, R.N., M.N.Sc.

► Emotional Dimension

1. Fear is first experienced during the trauma of birth.
2. Life's frustrations may result in withdrawal and rumination and eventual ego disintegration and regression to an immature repressive defense structure.
3. Unconscious drives, desires, or wishes cause tension, anxiety, and guilt, which are denied and attributed (projected) to others.
4. Emotional tension (anxiety) may interfere with rational thinking and behavior.
5. An individual's psychological equilibrium is influenced by his perceptions.
6. The suspicious person does not trust self.
7. The suspicious person needs outlets for anger and aggression.
8. Overwhelmed by anxiety, an individual may respond with paranoid thinking and delusions.

► Intellectual Dimension

1. Double-bind communication may result in suspiciousness.
2. Conflicting messages received in childhood may result in suspiciousness by preventing the child from developing a sense of self.
3. Cognitive functioning is influenced by physiological status, environmental status, and emotional status. It becomes distorted in persons who do not develop trust.
4. The cognitive process of perception is influenced by the individual's current needs and interests and fund of knowledge. Consequently, the mistrusting person's needs, interests, and knowledge result in vigilance and suspiciousness.
5. A disruption in the quality and quantity of incoming stimuli can affect an individual's thought processes and result in suspiciousness.
6. Development of cognitive ability follows a systematic pattern of maturational experiences and varied perceptual stimulation.
7. Paranoid delusions represent sexual conflicts concerning persons of the same sex projected onto some other person perceived as threatening.

► Social Dimension

1. Lack of security and trust may contribute to the development of suspiciousness.
2. Failure to consistently meet the needs of the infant results in mistrust.
3. The failure of parent-child bonding may result in mistrust about relationships.
4. The foundation for trust is made during the first 2 years of life.

5. Satisfying relationships with others rely on a feeling that the person will not be harmed as a result of the relationship.
6. Persons feeling threatened in interpersonal situations are unable to feel secure and satisfied until the fear is reduced.
7. The self system serves to protect the individual from anxiety.
   a. The self system excludes information that is incongruent with the self and does not profit from experience.
   b. In mistrust and paranoia, information that may decrease self-esteem is eliminated.
   c. The greater the anxiety, the more inflated the self system becomes.
   d. Security operations of the self system include selective inattention, sublimation, and dissociation, a process for minimizing anxiety by which certain experiences are kept out of consciousness.
   e. Anxiety-producing experiences become projections of blame and persecutions in the paranoid person.
8. The person diagnosed as paranoid was unsuccessful in developing basic trust and trust reactions, particularly with parents.
9. The family background of the paranoid person appears to be authoritarian, suppressive, excessively dominating, and critical.
   a. Family members behave in a superior manner to cover up underlying inferiority feelings.
   b. The child learns to behave in a superior, aloof manner, which prevents him from understanding the motives and points of view of others.
10. Paranoid behavior has different manifestations in different cultures and may be based on reality.
11. Suspiciousness results from an inability to check the validity of observations, to look at the situation from another point of view, or to question conclusions.
12. Suspiciousness may be a realistic response to an environment that isolates the individual because he is different.

► Spiritual Dimension

1. There is a general belief that the world is evil and the motivations of others are not to be trusted.
2. A sense of impending danger or doom is maintained.
3. Each human being needs to feel a sense of adequacy and approval. When reality does not foster such feelings, the person resorts to projection.
4. A sense of trust is developed throughout the growing years, and changing vulnerabilities make new demands on a person's faith and trust in self and others.

ASSESSMENT

▶ Physical Dimension

I. History
A. Personal history
1. Activities of daily living
   a. Nutrition—fails to eat because of fear of being poisoned
   b. Sleep—unable to sleep; awakens frequently or easily because of fear of being harmed
2. Habits—may refuse to take medication because of fear of being harmed or "controlled" by others
3. Destructive behavior
   a. May act on suspicions in a destructive way toward self or others (suicide or homicide)
   b. Misinterprets acts of others and may respond aggressively

B. Review of systems
1. GI—vague gastrointestinal discomfort unsupported by objective data
2. Cardiovascular—symptoms associated with anxiety or fear, including shortness of breath, elevated blood pressure, increased pulse rate, and tenseness or nervousness
3. Verbalizations may be indicative of body image distortion

II. Diagnostic tests
A. Rorschach test
B. Thematic Apperception Test (TAT)
C. Minnesota Multiphasic Personality Inventory (MMPI)
D. Draw-a-person test
E. Sentence completion test

▶ Physical Examination

CLIENT DATA	ANALYSIS	NURSING DIAGNOSIS
Poor personal hygiene (cleanliness neglected; grooming untidy; clothing disheveled)	Excessive anxiety and preoccupation with personal safety contribute to lack of concern for personal appearance.	Dressing/grooming self-care deficit: related to anxiety
Hyperalert (may sit on edge of chair, eyes may dart from place to place, easily startled, reluctant to have someone behind him, answers questions evasively if at all)	Excessive fear of environment (a function of anxiety).	Anxiety, fear: related to perceived threats in the environment
Weight loss	Lack of trust or preoccupation with personal safety may result in not eating.	Altered nutrition, less than body requirements: related to fear that food is poisoned

▶ Emotional Dimension

CLIENT DATA	ANALYSIS	NURSING DIAGNOSIS
Anger and hostility (may become physically violent)	Overly concerned with protecting self from environment; overly sensitive.	Potential for violence directed toward others: related to perceived threats or injustices to self
Fear	Results from lack of security and trust.	Fear: related to perceived threats to self
Fear of homosexuality	Unconsciously denied, paranoid delusions represent sexual conflicts concerning persons of same sex projected onto some other person perceived as threatening. More common in males than females.	Anxiety: related to fear of homosexuality
Insecurity	Overly sensitive. Failure to meet needs of infant results in mistrust and insecurity.	Self-esteem disturbance: chronic, related to insecurity and lack of trust

▶ **Emotional Dimension—cont'd**

CLIENT DATA	ANALYSIS	NURSING DIAGNOSIS
Feeling that others cannot be trusted	Misinterpretation of external reality.	Altered thought processes: related to failure to develop trust
Exaggerated feeling of anxiety	In new situation or new social relationship. Persons feeling threatened in interpersonal situations are unable to feel secure and satisfied until fear is reduced.	Anxiety: severe, surrounding new situations or new relationships related to mistrust and suspiciousness
Pervasive feeling of mistrust	Often toward one person who heretofore was trusted person.	Ineffective individual coping: related to pervasive feelings of mistrust
Feelings of being misjudged, conspired against, spied upon, followed, poisoned, drugged, maliciously maligned, harassed, obstructed in achieving long-term goals	Views others as being against him. Loses ability to evaluate reality.	Ineffective individual coping: related to persecutory feeling

▶ **Intellectual Dimension**

CLIENT DATA	ANALYSIS	NURSING DIAGNOSIS
Ideas or delusions of reference or feelings of persecution	Inability to validate reality and resultant overwhelming anxiety.	Altered thought processes: related to inability to evaluate reality, secondary to feelings of mistrust
Grandiose	Attempts to decrease anxiety by creating consistency between perception and reality. Preoccupation with interpreting external events to fit delusional system. Believes he has superior or unique qualities. Ideas center around his mission or social and political reforms.	Altered thought processes: grandiosity related to attempt to decrease anxiety
Perceptual selectivity	Fear associated with feeling that external environment is persecutory in nature. Suspects that others are working against him and begins to notice slightest signs that validate suspicions.	*Selective attention: related to fear of being harmed
Fund of information diminished	Cognitive functioning is influenced by client's current needs and interests. Affected by anxiety and social isolation.	Altered thought processes: diminished fund of information related to anxiety and isolation
Rigid interpretation of external events	Need to keep world consistent with persecutory thinking contributes to rigid interpretation of reality to decrease anxiety. Incapable of seeing things from another's point of view; categorizes people and events as either good or bad.	Altered thought processes: rigid interpretation of events related to attempt to decrease anxiety
Projection	Projection of feelings of weakness onto others to decrease anxiety and keep world consistent.	Ineffective individual coping: projection, related to feelings of weakness
Denial	Denial of having problems. Defense mechanism to reduce anxiety; security operation of self system to decrease anxiety.	Ineffective denial: related to inability to accept own feelings
Hypersensitive to criticism	Cognitive process of perception is influenced by client's current needs.	Ineffective individual coping: oversensitivity related to low self-esteem

▶ **Social Dimension**

CLIENT DATA	ANALYSIS	NURSING DIAGNOSIS
Masks feelings of inferiority, craves recognition and praise Social failures undermine self-esteem Sees others, not self, as having problems Has superior, self-important attitude Does not seek treatment for self; is brought for care by others	Poor insight and lack of reality testing; inability to see self objectively. Defense patterns protect client from feelings of inferiority and worthlessness.	Self-esteem disturbance: chronic low self-esteem related to feelings of worthlessness
Feels persecuted by others; lacks insight	Failure to consider that personal factors may contribute to difficulties.	Ineffective individual coping: related to lack of insight
Seeks isolation and seclusion, avoids and often alienates others	Increased isolation results in decreased dependency on others and increased sense of power and control.	Social isolation: related to fear and mistrust of situation
Behaves eccentrically; has hostile, dominating attitude	Social relationships entered with attitude that drives others away.	Impaired social interactions: related to hostile and dominating attitude
Expects praise for minor achievements	When praise is not given, withdraws from normal contacts.	Social isolation: related to feelings of not being understood or properly appreciated
Is less able to function in social and marital role	Preoccupation with self-preservation and keeping environment consistent impairs ability to function.	*Altered family role: related to preoccupation with self-preservation and need to keep environment consistent related to mistrust and suspiciousness
Is sexually maladjusted	Reflection of individual's serious difficulties in interpersonal relations.	Sexual dysfunction: related to mistrust and suspicions of others

▶ **Spiritual Dimension**

CLIENT DATA	ANALYSIS	NURSING DIAGNOSIS
Views life as persecuting and unfair	Negative and without hope. Goals and expectations are unrealistically high; unable to compromise goals to meet life's problems.	Spiritual distress: related to inability to live up to an idealized value
Lacks participation in religious activities	Isolated and has own interpretation of religion.	Spiritual distress: related to own interpretation of religion
Believes God speaks through him and God is vengeful	Response to overwhelming anxiety.	Spiritual distress: related to belief in vengeful God
Is unable to enjoy life	Preoccupation with keeping world consistent and anxiety at tolerable levels prevents enjoyment of life.	Spiritual distress: related to inability to enjoy life

PLANNING

▶ **Long-Term Goal**

To increase reality testing by learning how perceptions arouse feelings of mistrust

SHORT-TERM GOALS	OUTCOME CRITERIA
Physical Dimension	
To decrease aggressive acts	1. Verbalizes alternative options to aggression in situations that previously resulted in aggression
	2. Demonstrates new behaviors in situations that previously resulted in aggression (see Anger, p. 28)
Emotional Dimension	
To decrease anxiety	1. Verbalizes that he feels less anxious
	2. Decreases social isolation (see Anxiety, p. 48)
Intellectual Dimension	
To learn skills to validate perceptions	1. Participates in activities that teach problem-solving skills
	2. Practices skills learned in role-play situations
To identify trusting characteristics	1. States characteristics found in trusted friend
	2. Identifies trusting characteristics in others
Social Dimension	
To develop a relationship with at least one other person during hospitalization or treatment	1. Verbalizes concerns or problems with some other person
	2. Seeks out some other person to spend time with
To increase social skills	1. Participates in activities aimed at increasing social skills
	2. Demonstrates appropriate social skills in social situations
To increase self-concept	1. (See Negative Self-Concept, p. 231)
Spiritual Dimension	
To examine current life situation and consider options for changing and enriching it	1. Verbalizes that there are various ways of interpreting events, and that all happenings do not directly affect self
	2. Verbalizes practical options for changing life situation and becoming more trusting

Discharge Planning

The following client behaviors indicate a readiness for discharge:

1. Identifies situations where he feels distrustful
2. Has learned ways of socially validating perceptions
3. Interacts socially with others
4. Has an improved self-concept

IMPLEMENTATION

NURSING ACTIONS	RATIONALE
Physical Dimension	
1. Protect client and others from harm when client loses self-control.	To prevent injury to client or others.
2. Identify behaviors associated with increased anxiety, increased psychomotor activity, angry expressions.	To prevent anxiety from escalating and client's loss of control.
3. Encourage involvement in activities in which client can do well.	To ensure success and increase self-esteem.

IMPLEMENTATION—cont'd

NURSING ACTIONS	RATIONALE
4. Promote participation in therapies that involve a lessening of anxiety (relaxation techniques, sports, and hobbies).	To use energy of anxiety adaptively.
5. Be aware that the use of force or hostility with client may be counterproductive to therapeutic goals.	To increase understanding of client's behavior, to intervene effectively.
6. Use touch judiciously.	To prevent misinterpretation.
7. Be aware of potential for violence.	To increase understanding of client's behavior, to intervene before behavior gets out of control.
8. Help with self-care, as appropriate.	To help client maintain self-respect, to prevent ridicule or humiliation.

Emotional Dimension

1. Establish a working and therapeutic relationship with client, realizing that client is hypersensitive and suspicious and uses projection.	To establish trust, without which little else can be accomplished.
2. Make short, frequent contacts with client, avoid whispering, gently question beliefs, avoid arguing about ideas, inform client of schedule changes, and give information in clear, concise words.	To establish a trusting relationship.
3. Be aware that a suspicious client often responds well to an attitude of showing concern and a mild curiosity about what is happening with him.	To increase understanding of client's behavior and provide a basis for stimulating client to change behavior.
4. Be aware that attacking client's delusional system may result in alienation and further decompensation.	To increase understanding of client's behavior and prevent nurse from attacking delusional system.
5. Be aware that self-disclosure is uncomfortable and self-awareness is very difficult.	To prevent pushing or pressuring client, which may in turn increase anxiety.
6. Help client gain experience in sharing feelings.	To promote sharing with others as a way to validate thoughts and feelings and receive feedback.
7. Give assurance that environment is safe.	To lessen anxiety about environment.
8. Reduce anxiety-producing situations.	To lessen anxiety and help decrease further suspiciousness.

Intellectual Dimension

1. Let client know what is acceptable and unacceptable behavior and consequences of each.	To provide information that helps decrease anxiety, to demonstrate clear communication.
2. Assess client for potential to do harm to self or others. With client, develop steps client can take to keep self under control.	To determine risk of harming self or others, to provide client with skills to maintain control and help client realize that he does have some control over what is happening.
3. Assist client in developing communication skills.	To enable client to validate reality with others.
4. Discuss consequences of failure to validate reality with others.	To prevent misinterpretation of client's reality, to prevent alienation from others.
5. Explore situations in which client often feels suspicious and develop alternative ways to react to situation.	To provide client with options for responding to situations that result in suspiciousness.
6. Assist client in analyzing beliefs by raising doubts about beliefs.	To help client evaluate beliefs more realistically.
7. Help client clarify his thoughts.	To avoid misinterpretation.
8. Use communication that helps client maintain his individuality ("I" instead of "we").	To prevent client from incorporating you into his belief system.
9. Teach skills (problem solving, relaxation) that help client maintain his individuality.	To provide client with skills that reduce anxiety, thereby increasing self-esteem and fostering trust.

Social Dimension

1. Encourage involvement in activities.	To increase interactions with others and promote trust.
2. Encourage involvement in group therapy based on problems of daily living and focus on social interaction skills.	To promote comfortableness with others in validating perceptions and to improve relationships with others.
3. Encourage involvement of client's family or other social network in client's treatment, focusing on issues of daily living.	To help family understand client's treatment and be supportive.

NURSING ACTIONS	RATIONALE
4. Give feedback when client is insulting or threatening to others.	To help client recognize his behavior and its impact on others.
5. Help client identify behavior that results in rejection.	To help client change behavior so that he does not set himself up for rejection.
Spiritual Dimension	
1. Attempt to reframe delusional systems that are so threatening that they are debilitating to client.	To prevent further diminishing client's quality of life.
2. Encourage hope and optimism as is appropriate for client.	To promote client's belief that with treatment life can improve.
3. Assist client in recognizing his humanness, worth, and relatedness to others.	To enable client to value himself, to promote a positive self-concept.

EVALUATION

Measurable goals and outcome criteria provide the basis for evaluating the suspicious client. Nurse observations and family reports provide additional data. The following behaviors indicate a positive evaluation:

1. States situations that result in suspiciousness
2. Validates perceptions with a supportive person
3. Has a positive self-concept

BIBLIOGRAPHY

Bentall RP: Paranoia and social reasoning: an attribution theory analysis, *Br J Clin Psych* 30(Pt 1):13, 1991.

Buller DB, Strzyzewski KD, Comstock J: Interpersonal deception: 1. Deceivers' reactions to receivers' suspicions and probing, *Commun Monogr* 58(1):1, 1991.

Cameron N, Rychlak JF: *Personality development and psychopathology: a dynamic approach,* ed 2, Boston, 1985, Houghton Mifflin Co.

Coleman JC, Butcher JM, Carson RC: *Abnormal psychology and modern life,* ed 6, Glenview, Ill, 1980, Scott, Foresman & Co.

Fraser J: Paranoia: interactional views of evolution and intervention, *J Marital Fam Ther* 9(3):383, 1983.

Garety PA, Hemsley DR, Wessely S: Reasoning in deluded schizophrenic and paranoid patients. Biases in performance on a probabilistic inference task, *J Nerv Mental Dis* 179(4):194, 1991.

Garfield D: Paranoid phenomena and pathological narcissism, *Am J Psychother* 45(2):160, 1991.

Houseman C: The paranoid person: a biopsychosocial perspective, *Arch Psychiatr Nurs* 4(3):176, 1990.

Jacobs LI: Cognitive therapy for schizophrenics in remission, *Cur Psychiatr Ther* 21:93, 1983.

Jette CC: Late-onset paranoid disorder, *Am J Orthopsychiatry* 57(4):485, 1987.

Jordan HW: Involutional paranoid disorder: a forgotten syndrome, *J Nat Med Assoc* 81(9):950, 1989.

Jucovy ME: The effects of the Holocaust on the second generation: psychoanalytic studies, *Am J Soc Psychiatry* 3(1):15, 1983.

Kendler KS: Paranoia (delusional disorder): a valid psychiatric entity? *Trends Neurosci* 7(1):14, 1984.

Kolb LC: *Modern clinical psychiatry,* ed 10, Philadelphia, 1982, WB Saunders.

Lanquetot R: First person account: confessions of the daughter of a schizophrenic, *Schizophr Bull* 10(3):467, 1984.

Lazar BS, Harrow M: Paranoid and nonparanoid schizophrenia: drive dominated thinking and thought pathology as two phases of disorder, *J Clin Psychol* 41(2):145, 1984.

Lowe ME: Smoke gets in your eyes, sometimes, *Arts Psychother* 11(4):267, 1984.

Miller NS, Gold MS, Mahler JC: A study of violent behaviors associated with cocaine use: theoretical and pharmacological implication, *Ann Clin Psychiatry* 2(1):67, 1990.

Molinari V, Chacho R: The classification of paranoid disorders in the elderly: a clinical problem, *Clin Gerontologist* 1(4):31, 1983.

Muir-Cochrane E: Everyone's against me, *Nurs Times* 84(31):40, 1988.

Newhill CE: The role of culture in the development of paranoid symptomatology, *Am J Orthopsychiatry* 60(2):176, 1990.

Phan TT, Reifler BB: Psychiatric disorders among nursing home residents. Depression, anxiety, and paranoia, *Clin Geriatr Med* 4(3):60, 1988.

Shomberg K, Leventhal DB: Conceptualization of paranoid schizophrenia: a deficit-discontinuity view, *Psychother* 21:370, 1984.

Tousley MM: The paranoid fortress of David J., *J Psychosoc Nurs Ment Health Serv* 22(4):8, 1984.

Williams D: Nursing care of the paranoid patient, *Adv Clin Care* 5(6):12, 1990.

Zigler E, Levine J: Hallucinations vs. delusions: a developmental approach, *J Nerv Ment Dis* 171(3):141, 1983.

Withdrawn Behavior

Withdrawn behavior is an attempt to avoid interactions with others, thus avoiding relationships with others. The individual feels that he is deprived of intimate relationships and has no opportunity to share thoughts, feelings, accomplishments, or failures. He has difficulty interacting spontaneously with other people. He appears detached, disinterested, and removed and does not share experiences with others. The withdrawn person feels a need or desire for contact and interaction but is unable to make that contact. The withdrawn behavior may be physical (as when a client remains in bed) or verbal (as in silence or mutism). Withdrawn behavior becomes dysfunctional when interpersonal relationships are impaired or distorted. *Aloneness, loneliness, alienation,* and *isolation* are terms frequently used in relation to withdrawn behavior. The distinguishing feature in *aloneness* is that it is a chosen state of being without company to retreat temporarily from others. *Loneliness,* a related concept, suggests a painful experience frequently hidden, disguised, defended against, or expressed in some other way; it is defined as the inability to do anything while alone. *Alienation* implies becoming unfriendly or indifferent toward someone for whom friendliness and affection existed at a previous time. *Isolation* suggests a separation from another or from a group, such as a family.

Related DSM-III-R disorders

Organic mental disorders
Schizophrenia
Delusional (paranoid) disorders
Mood disorders
Avoidant personality disorder

Other related conditions

Crisis situations
Aging
Guilt
Illness
Physical handicap
Catatonia
Incontinence
Conditions with an odor (colostomy, wounds, ulcerating tumor)
Obesity

PRINCIPLES

▶ Physical Dimension

1. Maternal deprivation may be a cause of withdrawal from others.
2. Unmet needs during the development stages of the life cycle result in withdrawal from others.
3. Pain or suffering may cause a person to withdraw from others.

▶ Emotional Dimension

1. Feelings of shame and guilt may cause a person to withdraw.
2. When lacking in self-confidence and inner strengths a person becomes closed to others and withdraws.
3. Love and affection are missing in withdrawn behavior.
4. Anxiety causes the individual to move toward, against, or away from others.
5. Individuals with low self-esteem minimize their anxiety by social isolation.

▶ Intellectual Dimension

1. Defenses are used to protect the self from the pain of isolation and withdrawal.
2. Lack of self-understanding and insight and an inability to share thoughts and feelings impede the development of satisfactory relationships and may result in withdrawal from others.
3. Individuals with a "failure" identity are lonely people who have difficulty facing the world.
4. The inability to establish and maintain trusting relationships with others promotes distortions in perceptions and reality testing and leads to withdrawn behavior.
5. During childhood, the inability of the child to distinguish between fantasy and fact exposes the child to ridicule and punishment and inhibits the child's freedom and enthusiasm in communicating with others.
6. Individuals may lose the ability to use language to socially interact.

▶ Social Dimension

1. The roots of withdrawn behavior result from early life experiences in which remoteness, indifference, emptiness, and rejection are the principle themes that characterize the child's relationships with others.
2. The need for human relationships is instinctual in each person.
3. A weak ego that can no longer repress its impulses results in hostile or erotic behavior and may cause the individual to retreat from relationships.
4. Infants who demonstrate hesitation to new stimuli are likely to continue this pattern of behavior in relationships with others and to withdraw from others.
5. To prevent withdrawing the individual needs to feel he will not be harmed in a relationship.
6. An individual's relationship with others is influenced by his self-concept and ego functioning.
7. By avoiding others the withdrawn client denies self the opportunity to share experiences with others and to develop satisfying relationships with them.
8. Repeated failures and rejections tend to decrease self-esteem and contribute to withdrawn behavior.
9. Social withdrawal is characteristic of the client with schizophrenia.
10. Social isolation during adolescence interferes with the ability to develop intimate relationships.
11. The isolated adolescent uses reverie (daydreams) for interpersonal experience.

▶ Spiritual Dimension

1. Failure to develop inner resources that help to transcend self-alienation serves as a barrier to relating to others and results in withdrawal.
2. A withdrawn person lacks free will; thus he gives up the responsibility for making choices to behave in new ways that will provide a sense of meaning to life.
3. An individual is free to choose to be withdrawn or isolated with a resulting sacrifice in personal growth and life satisfaction.

ASSESSMENT

▶ Physical Dimension

I. History
  A. Activities of daily living
    1. Nutrition
       a. Anorexia or overeating
       b. Weight loss or gain
       c. Deterioration in physical health
    2. Sleep
       a. Excessive sleep
       b. Stays in bed long periods of time
       c. Frequent naps
    3. Recreation, hobbies, and interests
       a. Lack of interest
       b. Indifference
    4. Physical activities and limitations
       a. Decreased activity
       b. Immobility
       c. Pacing, rocking; repetitive, bizarre activity
    5. Sexual activity
       a. No desire
  B. Habits
    1. Alcohol
       a. Excessive intake
    2. Medication and drugs
       a. Abuse or misuse
  C. Destructive behavior
    1. Increased risk for suicide
  D. Health history
    1. Illness
       a. Depression
       b. Organic mental disorders
       c. Schizophrenia
       d. Any disease (physical) when there is a change from usual good health

▶ **Emotional Dimension**

CLIENT DATA	ANALYSIS	NURSING DIAGNOSIS
Feelings of loneliness, dread, anxiety, abandonment, irritation, uselessness, depression, fear, being unloved and uncared for, aloofness, remoteness, fatigue, apathy, and lethargy	Various negative feelings are expressed by withdrawn client.	Ineffective individual coping: related to feelings of *loneliness,* dread, and other feelings (See Client data)
Absence of spontaneous expression of feelings	Flat affect. Early life experiences of rejection and remoteness prevent spontaneity.	Ineffective individual coping: related to absence of spontaneous expression of feelings

▶ **Intellectual Dimension**

CLIENT DATA	ANALYSIS	NURSING DIAGNOSIS
Unrealistic perceptions	Withdrawal from contact with others results in lack of the feedback important for validating thoughts and decreases capacity for reality testing.	Altered thought processes: unrealistic perceptions related to withdrawn behavior
Distorted perceptions	Client may be retreating to fantasy world with hallucinations. Reverie is substituted for interpersonal experiences.	Altered thought processes: distorted perceptions related to withdrawn behavior
Impaired recent and remote memory	Self-preoccupied, withdraws into self.	*Altered memory: related to withdrawn behavior
Impaired orientation for time and place	Self-preoccupied, with lack of attention to time, place, and person.	Altered thought processes: disorientation related to withdrawn behavior
Poverty of thoughts	Lack of external stimulation. Becomes closed to others.	Altered thought processes: poverty of thoughts related to withdrawn behavior
Inability to make decisions; postponement of decisions	Apathy and lethargy interfere with decision making. May fear ridicule in making decisions that evoke anxiety.	Altered thought processes: inability to make decisions related to withdrawn behavior; postponement of decisions related to withdrawn behavior
Doubts ability to survive	Feelings of uselessness and lack of self-confidence, ambivalence.	Self-esteem disturbance: doubt about ability to survive related to withdrawn behavior
Inability to think abstractly	Thinking is concrete because of regression.	*Altered abstract thinking: related to withdrawn behavior
Delusions	Withdrawing from others provides a safeness for delusional thinking.	Altered thought processes: delusional thinking related to withdrawn behavior
Illogical, bizarre ideas, strange fantasies	Retreat from painful real world.	Altered thought processes: illogical or bizarre ideas or strange fantasies related to withdrawn behavior
Self-preoccupation or narcissism	Inability to move beyond self-concerns.	Altered thought processes: preoccupation with own thoughts related to withdrawn behavior
Regression	Retreat from reality to reduce anxiety. Client becomes more dependent.	Defensive coping: regression related to withdrawn behavior
Loose associations, neologisms, echolalia, and magical thinking	Communication impaired; use of symbolism. Autistic meanings not replaced by consensually validated meanings.	Impaired verbal communication: loose associations, neologisms, echolalia, and magical thinking related to withdrawn behavior
Verbal inaction or muteness	Amount of communication is decreased. Client self-preoccupied.	Impaired verbal communication: verbal inaction or muteness related to withdrawn behavior
Rumination	Repetition of thoughts over and over. Client self-absorbed.	Altered thought processes: repetitive thoughts related to withdrawal behavior

▶ **Social Dimension**

CLIENT DATA	ANALYSIS	NURSING DIAGNOSIS
Views self as unwanted, useless, in the way, having no friends; as some other person, if delusional	Loss of self-esteem and value as a person. Individuals with low self-esteem minimize anxiety with social isolation.	*Altered self-concept: related to misperception of self
Self-esteem decreased	Feels unworthy and incompetent.	Self-esteem disturbance: related to feeling unworthy and incompetent
Lack of trust in others	Pain from rejection and anxiety in relating to others prevents openness with others	Social isolation: related to mistrust of others
Dependent on others	Assistance needed with self-care if client has regressed.	Ineffective individual coping: dependence related to withdrawn behavior
Deterioration of social roles	Reduced work, school, family roles, impaired social skills; denies self opportunities to share experiences with others.	Altered role performance: related to withdrawn behavior
Lack of diversional activities	Inability to initiate activities and lack of pleasure from them. Has difficulty facing real world.	Diversional activity deficit: related to withdrawn behavior
Low socioeconomic conditions	Deprivation, downward mobility, and high stress levels contribute to withdrawn behavior.	Social isolation: related to low socioeconomic conditions
Social drifting	Transient life-style, social ostracism, and rejection can lead to withdrawal.	Social isolation: related to transient life-style

▶ **Spiritual Dimension**

CLIENT DATA	ANALYSIS	NURSING DIAGNOSIS
Apathy	Beliefs reflect a "take what comes" or "what I deserve" attitude.	Spiritual distress: apathy toward life related to withdrawn behavior
May become overly zealous about religion	Use of religion as an escape from pain or reality.	Spiritual distress: religiosity related to withdrawn behavior
Despair	Inability to move beyond self-preoccupation without help; inability to transcend separateness and relate to others.	Spiritual distress: despair related to withdrawn behavior
Wish for death	Relief from "hell on earth."	Spiritual distress: wish for death related to withdrawn behavior

PLANNING

Long-Term Goals

To experience satisfaction from relationships with others
To develop alternatives to withdrawn behavior

SHORT-TERM GOALS	OUTCOME CRITERIA
Physical Dimension	
To participate in activities	1. Attends activity group 2. Participates in activity 3. Assists others in activities
Emotional Dimension	
To feel safe in interpersonal relationships	1. Allows nurse to sit with him for brief periods of time daily 2. Expresses an interest in nurse or other person

PLANNING—cont'd

SHORT-TERM GOALS	OUTCOME CRITERIA
	3. Becomes relaxed, comfortable with nurse or other person
	4. States he doesn't have much to talk about at times
	5. Verbalizes positive statements about nurse or other person
Intellectual Dimension	
To explore reasons for withdrawal	1. Discusses situations and events that trigger withdrawn behavior
	2. Verbalizes feelings produced by situations and events that cause him to withdraw from others
	3. Explores other ways to handle situations and events that cause withdrawn behavior
	4. Participates in own treatment planning
Social Dimension	
To increase interactions with others	1. Sits with others
	2. Initiates a conversation with another person
	3. Participates in group activities
	4. Participates in group therapy
	5. Spends decreased amount of time by self
	6. Spends more time with others
To change perception of self	1. Makes positive statements about self
	2. Participates in activities in which he can experience success
	3. Participates in activities that bring pleasure
	4. Makes positive statements about others
Spiritual Dimension	
To have a zest for life or find some joy in life	1. Shows enthusiasm about life events (a ball game, a new baby, a garden)
	2. Demonstrates less despair about life
	3. Makes no statements about lack of personal value or belief that death would be relief

Discharge Planning

The following client behaviors demonstrate readiness for discharge:
1. Can perform activities of daily living with minimum assistance
2. Has a list and schedule of medications and verbalizes importance of taking them as prescribed
3. Has a supporting person with whom he can express his feelings and thoughts
4. Knows whom to contact (name and telephone number) when symptoms reappear
5. Initiates social interactions

IMPLEMENTATION

NURSING ACTIONS	RATIONALE
Physical Dimension	
1. Provide assistance with personal hygiene and self-care until client is able to do for self.	To help client maintain self-respect, to promote increased self-esteem.
2. Provide client's own clothing.	To reinforce client's self-identity.
3. Promote involvement in physical activities.	To increase client's energy level.
4. Provide plant or pet therapy if appropriate.	To promote expression of tender, loving, nurturing feelings.
5. Limit nap taking during daytime.	To enable client to sleep at night.
6. Encourage client to eat a well-balanced diet daily.	To ensure adequate nutritional intake, to prevent deterioration of physical health.
7. Treat somatic complaints matter-of-factly without undue concern.	To promote physical comfort without providing secondary gains.
8. Limit possibilities for destruction to self or others by providing a safe environment.	To prevent harm to self or others.
9. Promote physical closeness (touch) when appropriate.	To demonstrate warmth, caring.
Emotional Dimension	
1. Facilitate expression of painful feelings that cause client to withdraw with empathy statements.	To help client face painful feelings, rather than avoid them, and learn to handle painful feelings in a mentally healthy way.
2. Promote acceptance of painful feelings.	To help client face reality and move on with life.
3. Provide ways to express painful feelings other than verbally (typing, piano playing, painting, or exercise).	To provide a release from painful feelings when unable to talk about them.
4. Show sincere respect for client (speak to him, call him by name, include him in all appropriate activities).	To help client know he is important, to increase self-esteem.
5. Accept client's rejection without personalizing it.	To increase understanding of client's behavior, to prevent personal feelings from interfering with therapeutic relationship.
6. Demonstrate worthiness and uniqueness of client. Show interest even when client does not respond.	To acknowledge client and communicate his importance to you.
7. Avoid placing client in situations where he will fail.	To prevent decreasing self-esteem and further withdrawal from others.
8. Acknowledge client's difficulties in relating to others.	To empathize with client, to promote a trusting relationship that will help client change behavior.
Intellectual Dimension	
1. Discuss situations and events that cause client to withdraw.	To help client identify sources of painful feelings.
2. Examine rational and irrational aspects of client's thoughts about situations and events that cause client to withdraw.	To distinguish between rational and irrational thoughts and plan for interventions.
3. Plant some seeds of doubt when perceptions are unrealistic.	To help client re-examine perceptions.
4. Discuss client's inability to change situation or events and possibilities for changing attitude about it.	To help client face the facts of the situation, to offer choices about ways to respond to the situation.
5. Identify yourself by name, call client by name, and state day and time and purpose of interaction.	To increase client's orientation and sharpen memory.
6. Provide magazines, radio, newspapers, and television.	To stimulate client's thinking, to prevent brooding and further regression.
7. Relieve client of decision making until client is ready.	To prevent increasing anxiety associated with making decisions and fostering further withdrawal.
8. Use simple, concrete terms.	To promote clear communication.
9. Accept a one-sided conversation.	To communicate acceptance of client.
10. Avoid making demands client cannot meet.	To prevent client from becoming discouraged and belittling self.
11. Take initiative in stimulating client's interests in activities.	To promote client's participation. Withdrawn clients seldom initiate an interaction but will often become involved with encouragement from nurse.

IMPLEMENTATION—cont'd

NURSING ACTIONS	RATIONALE
12. Avoid direct confrontation over conflicts and inconsistencies in behavior.	To prevent disrupting the trusting relationship.
13. Discuss meaning of words with client.	To validate communication, to let client hear from another person the understanding of message.
14. Foster client's motivation and willingness to participate in own treatment planning with positive reinforcement.	To promote responsibility for own mental health.
Social Dimension	
1. Seek out client for interacting several times each day.	To decrease anxiety associated with interacting, to foster a sense of being cared about.
2. Stay with client for periods of time, sitting in silence if client is severely withdrawn.	To acknowledge client as important to you and your availability to help when client is ready.
3. Use an object or activity as a basis for forming a relationship.	To participate in an activity may lead client to opening up.
4. Accept client's fumbling with social amenities.	To acknowledge client's uncomfortableness in social skills.
5. Limit number of persons with whom client comes in contact initially.	To help client learn to relate to a consistent person before enlarging relationships to include others.
6. Assist client with social skills.	To promote self-confidence.
7. Provide a safe (physically and emotionally) environment.	To promote a climate of acceptance and help client feel psychologically safe, as well as physically safe.
8. Prevent client from spending long periods of time in room by self.	To prevent client from becoming comfortable with aloneness.
9. Provide group therapy, activity therapy, occupational therapy, recreational therapy, and plant or pet therapy.	To increase social interactions with others.
10. Help strengthen family relationships.	To help client feel less alienated from them.
11. Provide positive reinforcement for participation in activities.	To encourage continued participation in activities.
12. Initiate conversation in which client can participate.	To promote successful feelings from conversations with others.
13. Focus on real things and the here and now.	To present reality.
14. Provide sensory stimulation.	To increase client's sensory input; to see, to hear, to feel, to smell, to taste more acutely.
15. Refrain from rapid chatter.	To prevent client from failing to listen to you. Make every word count.
16. Give client adequate time to respond.	To prevent client from not responding because of your rapid conversation.
17. Expect client to respond.	To use a positive approach to client often results in a positive response.
18. Promote client's involvement in community activities, for example, church or bingo games.	To help client get pleasures from community.
Spiritual Dimension	
1. Promote a sense of value to life by helping client restore faith and optimism in self.	To help client feel he has worth and importance.
2. Offer realistic hope by enhancing relationships with others.	To prevent further withdrawal and despair.
3. Encourage participation in religious activities (if appropriate).	To foster interactions with others with similar spiritual beliefs.
4. Provide opportunities to enrich life with music, art, poetry, dance, or other aesthetic forms of beauty.	To help client experience pleasures.
5. Help client see self realistically as a person of value by challenging his perception of self and helping him reconstruct it.	To promote a positive self-concept and to teach ways to maintain and reinforce it.

EVALUATION

Measurable goals and outcome criteria provide the basis for evaluating the client who is withdrawn from others and the amount of life disruption his behavior is causing. Nurse observations and family reports provide additional data. The following behaviors indicate a positive evaluation:

1. Performs activities of daily living
2. Takes medications as prescribed
3. Is able to express painful feelings to a supportive person
4. Participates in activities with others
5. Statements indicate a positive self-concept
6. Initiates social interactions
7. Assumes responsibility for reaching out to another person when feeling rejected or defeated or when pleased

BIBLIOGRAPHY

Bloch D: Alienation. In Carlson C, Blackwell B, editors: *Behavioral concepts and nursing interventions,* ed 2, Philadelphia, 1978, JB Lippincott.

Coffman J: Adolescence: informed or alienated, *Fla Nurse* 35(10):1, 1987.

Fecteau G, Duffy M: Social and conversational skills with long-term psychiatric inpatients, *Psych Rep* 59:1327, 1986.

Foxx R et al: Teaching social skills to psychiatric inpatients, *Behav Rest Ther* 23:531, 1985.

Iveson-Iveson J: Reinstating the mentally ill into the community, *Nurs Mirror* 14(24):157, 1983.

Jennings L: Nursing care models for adolescent families: caring for the alienated adolescent mother, ANA Publication Division of *Matern Child Health Nurs Pract* 14:7, 1984.

Lenehan G: A nurse clinic for the homeless, *Am J Nurs* 85:1237, 1985.

Peplau H: Loneliness, *Am J Nurs* 55(12):1476, 1955.

Peplau H: Interpersonal technique: the crux of psychiatric nursing, *Am J Nurs* 62:50, 1962.

Pittman D: Nursing case management: holistic care for the deinstitutionalized chronically mentally ill, *J Psychosoc Nurs Ment Health Ser* 27(11):23, 1989.

Sheehan S: *Is there no place on earth for me?* Boston, 1982, Houghton Mifflin.

Tudor G: A sociopsychiatric approach to intervention in a problem of mutual withdrawal on a mental hospital ward, *Perspect Psychiatr Care* 8(1):11, 1970.

Worley N, Albanese N: Independent living for the chronically mentally ill, *Psychosoc Nurs Ment Health Serv* 27(9):18, 1989.

Yoder S: Alientation as a way of life, *Perspec Psychiatr Care* 15(2):66, 1977.

PART THREE

CASE STUDIES

A collection of case studies is presented in Part Three. The case studies illustrate the multiple problems seen in clients and the interaction of the effects of the client's behavior on the client himself, on his family, and on the community. The format of Part Two is followed, using the nursing process as the foundation for planning and implementing care.

An Angry Adolescent

Aggression

Anger

Feeling no one cares

Acting out behaviors

Disturbed family relationships

Lacks self-respect

Parental loss

Negative role model

Marcus, 15, was admitted to the adolescent unit of a psychiatric hospital for *threatening to shoot* his teacher. He stated he knew where he could get a gun and would not hesitate to use it. He is *angry* about being hospitalized, saying he *can look after himself*. He is *failing in his school* work, has been in several *fights,* and has a history of *running away* from home.

According to his mother, Marcus was causing problems at home. He *fights with his two sisters* and *sexually abused his younger brother*. Marcus himself was *sexually abused by his stepfather,* to whom his mother is no longer married. This is the fourth marriage for Marcus's mother. Marcus *wants to go live with his biological father,* whom he seldom sees and who is known to *abuse alcohol.*

ANALYSIS

Marcus's behavior indicates depression resulting from parental loss and the effects of a troubled home environment: his mother's multiple marriages, his sexual abuse as a young child, his disturbed relationships with his family and peers, his aggressive and threatening behavior, his lack of respect for himself, and his idealized thinking about his biological father, with whom he wants to live.

Marcus needs to learn to manage his anger in socially acceptable ways rather than with aggression. Increasing his self-esteem and self-respect will help him feel better about himself and pave the way for learning to manage the stressors in his life in more acceptable ways. He needs to master the developmental tasks of adolescence. Theory-based interventions include establishing his identity as a unique person (Erikson), relating to the opposite sex (Freud), becoming independent from family, and developing social control over his instincts (Sullivan).

It is essential that the family be involved in Marcus's treatment. His mother needs to understand that Marcus's problems are a product of the family situation and that helping the family improve relationships through better communication, problem solving, and conflict resolution will improve the total family situation.

NURSING DIAGNOSES

Ineffective individual coping: related to inability to express anger in socially acceptable ways.

Ineffective individual coping: acting out behaviors (failing grades, fighting, running away, threatening teacher, sexually abusing brother) related to depression.

Self-esteem disturbance: related to feeling that no one cares about him.

High risk for violence to others: related to threatening teacher.

Impaired social interaction: related to fights with sisters and peers.

Ineffective family coping: disabling, related to neglectful relationships with family members

CARE PLAN

Long-Term Goal

To demonstrate socially acceptable ways for dealing with anger

SHORT-TERM GOALS	OUTCOME CRITERIA	NURSING ACTIONS	RATIONALE
Physical Dimension			
To prevent injury to others	Does not injure others	Observe for indications of anger	Awareness of anger permits early intervention
To decrease physical outbursts of anger	Uses energy of anger in physical activity	Plan a physical exercise program—swimming, walking, running, punching bag—as an alternative to cope with anger and increased level of energy	To reduce energy that accompanies anger
Emotional Dimension			
To express angry feelings	Expresses angry feelings	Help client verbalize anger with therapeutic communication techniques; empathy, reflection, clarification	Promotes feeling safe when expressing angry feelings, helps client know it is OK to get angry, but that how it is managed is important
		Provide group therapy	Gives feedback from others about anger, provides a safe environment for expressing anger
Intellectual Dimension			
To decrease verbal abuse	Decreases verbal abuse	Set limits on verbal abuse	To clarify expectations, to communicate that behavior is not acceptable
	Identifies alternate methods for dealing with anger	Explore with client alternate ways to deal with anger, for example, physical activity, talking with a supportive person	Increases repertoire of effective coping skills
Social Dimension			
To tell another person when angry	States angry feelings to another person	Help client acknowledge and take responsibility for angry feelings	To accept responsibility for own actions. Talking about feeling of anger reduces the intensity of the anger
	Uses "I" statements	Teach ways to tell others when angry	To accept responsibility for own feelings without threatening others
Spiritual Dimension			
To decrease bitterness and disappointments about life situation	Expresses feelings of bitterness and disappointment about life situation	Encourage expression of feelings of bitterness and disappointment about life situation with a supportive person	Awareness of feelings promotes hope that changes can be made

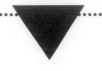

A Client with a Dual Diagnosis: Alcohol Addiction and Posttraumatic Stress Disorder

Noncompliance
Abuses alcohol
Flashbacks of Vietnam

Low self-esteem
Homicidal

Brad is a 42-year-old Vietnam veteran. He *stopped taking his medications* (Prozac and Vistaril) about one week after leaving the hospital. He began *drinking a six pack of beer daily* and progressed to a case a day. He complains of *intrusive thoughts* that are "very bad." He remembers that they were better when on Prozac but was never totally rid of them. Before coming to the hospital, he got his .45 caliber service pistol and went down to the river to *shoot a "gook"* to *make himself feel better.* He then realized that he needed to return to the hospital.

Physical health problems

Brad has had multiple admissions to VA hospitals for both addiction and post-traumatic stress disorder (PTSD). Intrusive thoughts trouble him daily. He came to the hospital for his out-of-control drinking and PTSD issues; *sleep loss; weight loss;* recollections that are vivid, intrusive, and painful to him; and *homicidal thoughts.*

ANALYSIS

Brad's attempts to cope with the intrusive thoughts about Vietnam led to his uncontrolled drinking and potential homicide. In addition, his physical health is threatened by his loss of sleep and weight loss. It will be essential to treat Brad's alcohol problem before attempting to treat his intrusive thoughts about Vietnam. He will be more amenable to psychiatric treatment after his cognitive functions (judgment, reasoning) are restored. In addition, the interaction of the psychiatric medications with alcohol reduces the effects of the psychiatric medications. Brad's strengths include knowing that he needs help controlling his drinking and the intrusive thoughts and that he needs to get back on his medications.

NURSING DIAGNOSES

Sleep pattern disturbance: related to painful intrusive thoughts
Altered nutrition: less than body requirements related to loss of weight
Ineffective individual coping: substance abuse related to inability to manage intrusive thoughts
High risk for violence: directed at others related to homicidal thoughts
Noncompliance: related to not taking his prescribed medications
Altered thought processes: related to intrusive, painful thoughts about Vietnam
Self-esteem disturbance: related to wanting to shoot a "gook" to make himself feel better

348

CARE PLAN

Long-Term Goal

To manage intrusive thoughts without the use of alcohol

SHORT-TERM GOALS	OUTCOME CRITERIA	NURSING ACTIONS	RATIONALE
Physical Dimension			
To withdraw safely from alcohol use	Is detoxified	Assess drinking habits, patterns; determine time and duration of last period of drinking	To be aware of possible onset of DTs
To gain and maintain normal body weight based on body structure and height	Maintains normal body weight	Provide adequate nutrition	To increase general health and well-being and prevent malnutrition
To sleep all night without interruption	Sleeps all night	Assess sleep pattern	To form a baseline for evaluating sleep
		Document sleep patterns	For validating sleep patterns
		Promote sleep-inducing measures, for example, quiet time, warm liquids, reading, music	To foster relaxation and comfort, physical and emotional
To take medications as prescribed	Takes medications	Assess client's self-medication ability	To reduce anxiety and depression and promote self-responsibility for taking medications
		Monitor for side effects of medications	Most side effects can be relieved, to prevent noncompliance
Emotional Dimension			
To express painful feelings associated with Vietnam	Expresses painful feelings	Facilitate expression of feelings with empathy, caring, active listening	Caring behaviors increase trust and promote expression of painful feelings
Intellectual Dimension			
To decrease or eliminate intrusive thoughts	Eliminates intrusive thoughts	Explore with client ways to manage intrusive thoughts without the use of alcohol, for example, music, distractions, social activities, medication	To provide alternatives to drinking for relief of intrusive thoughts and to become less preoccupied with them
		Teach thought stopping	Helps client to assume responsibility for stopping intrusive thoughts
Social Dimension			
To socialize without use of alcohol	Socializes without alcohol	Help client identify two or three social activities to participate in without use of alcohol	To replace alcohol activities with other pleasant social activities
		Explore community resources for leisure time activities	Leisure time activities prevent boredom and tendency to relapse
Spiritual Dimension			
To regain hope for pleasure in life without alcohol or intrusive thoughts	States goals for self that indicate hope	Explore with client goals that indicate hope; establishes supportive relationships, cares for physical health, selects a hobby, attends AA	Replacing self-defeating behaviors with positive activities promotes an enriched quality to life

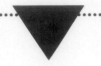

A Substance-Abusing Client

Abuses substances
History of abusing substances
Financially troubled
Illegal activities
No support system
Anxious—can't sleep, weight loss
Low self-esteem
Wants help

Thad, 34 years old, *abuses alcohol and cocaine*. He *started drinking in high school* and has been smoking crack for the past 9 months. He realized that crack was a problem for him about 3 months ago when he began *missing work*. He has *devastated himself financially* by spending all of his paychecks on crack. He then began *selling drugs* to support his cocaine habit. He is divorced and has *no significant others* at the present time. His major symptoms are *difficulty sleeping and anxiety* about the circumstance he finds himself in because of his addiction. He has *lost 31 pounds* over the last 9 months. He thinks life can be better than it is but *feels helpless and inadequate* to do anything about it. He says the *police are aware of his cocaine dealing* and that is a motivating factor in seeking treatment.

ANALYSIS

Thad's addiction is causing multiple problems. He has trouble sleeping and has lost considerable weight. He is severely anxious about his financial situation. His job is in jeopardy. He has no supportive persons since his divorce. He is aware that the police know about his cocaine dealing. His strengths include motivation for treatment, intelligence, past adequate job performance, and a recognition that life can be better than what it is for him.

NURSING DIAGNOSES

Sleep pattern disturbance: related to severe anxiety
Altered nutrition: less than body requirements, related to addicted life-style
Anxiety: severe, related to addictive life-style, lost work time, debts, absence of support system, and fear of police action
Ineffective individual coping: addictive life-style related to inability to manage life stressors
Self-esteem disturbance: related to feeling helpless and inadequate
Impaired social interactions: related to lack of support system
Spiritual distress: related to addictive life-style

CARE PLAN

Long-Term Goals

To verbalize effects of substance abuse on body, mind, family, and job following
implementation of a teaching plan

To verbalize and use effective coping methods instead of using chemical substances in response to stress

SHORT-TERM GOALS	OUTCOME CRITERIA	NURSING ACTIONS	RATIONALE
Physical Dimension			
To sleep 5–7 hours without awakening	Gets 5–7 hours of uninterrupted sleep	Assess sleep patterns, keep a record	Problem must be identified before assistance can be given
		Provide measures that aid sleep	To enhance relaxation and promote sleep
To maintain optimal weight	Gains weight and maintains optimal weight	Ensure adequate caloric intake	Promotes health and general well-being
Emotional Dimension			
To reduce anxiety	Identify signs and symptoms of anxiety	Teach signs and symptoms of anxiety and relationship to behavior	Promotes awareness of feeling and allows client to name feelings and manage them
	Uses stress management to reduce anxiety	Assess level of anxiety	To determine when client teaching can begin
		Teach stress management	To promote self-responsibility
Intellectual Dimension			
To verbalize effects of substance abuse	Verbalizes effects of substance abuse on self and others	Assess level of knowledge of effects of substance abuse on self and others	Baseline assessment is needed before teaching can begin
		Teach effects of substance abuse on self and others	To provide facts about the disease of substance abuse
Social Dimension			
To develop a support system	Identifies supportive persons	Promote interaction with others	To decrease isolation
	Attends AA or NA	Provide schedule for meetings	To promote individual and group support
Spiritual Dimension			
To enrich quality of life	Verbalizes an enriched quality of life	Encourage expression of anger and other feelings in appropriate ways	Lessens isolation and adds to quality of life
To reduce hopelessness	Verbalizations are optimistic and hopeful	Increase self-esteem	Positive feelings about self promote feelings of optimism and hope
		Teach positive self-talk	Promotes kindness to self

A Suicidal Client

Loss of long-term relationship
Depressive symptoms: sad, cries, loss of sleep, early awakening, tired, weight loss, GI symptoms, low energy, poor concentration

Social isolation
Physical health problems
Suicide threat

Janella, 37, has been *depressed* for the past 7 months since the *breakup with her male friend* of 10 years over his unfaithfulness. She lives with her two daughters, ages 8 and 11 years. She states she *feels sad* all the time and *cries* for hours each day. Little things set her off on crying spells. She *sleeps no more than four hours* a night and awakes early unable to go back to sleep. She is *tired* and *sad* on awakening. She *lost 25 pounds* going from 110 to 85 pounds over the past 7 months. When she eats she feels *nauseous and throws up*. She denies self-induced vomiting or deliberate weight loss. She has difficulty working because of her *low energy* and *poor concentration*. She has *withdrawn from friends*. She presently is taking steroids for *medical problems* associated with sarcoidosis. She entered the hospital with a co-worker to whom she *threatened suicide*.

ANALYSIS

Janella is experiencing a severe depression. It is likely that the steroids she is taking contribute to her depressive symptoms. Vegetative symptoms of depression are present, including loss of appetite, weight loss, insomnia, fatigue, low energy, and decreased interest in work, friends, and usual activities. Her energy level may be too low for her to carry out her suicide threat. However,

without a support system, the risk is high and hospitalization was encouraged.

Janella states she lives for her two daughters, to whom she is devoted. She also states that she is willing to participate in therapy to resolve the conflict related to her relationship with her male friend and to work on the somatic complaints associated with sarcoidosis.

NURSING DIAGNOSES

High risk for violence: self-directed, related to threat of suicide associated with depression

Ineffective individual coping: sad and tearful, related to depression associated with relationship conflict

Sleep pattern disturbance: related to depression associated with relationship conflict

Altered protection: related to low energy level associated with depression

Altered nutrition: less than body requirements related to nausea and vomiting associated with depression

Decisional conflict: related to poor concentration associated with depression

Impaired social interaction: related to depression

Noncompliance: high risk, related to depressive side effects of steroid medications

CARE PLAN

Long-Term Goals

To develop coping skills that replace self-destructive behavior
To cope with relationship conflicts without becoming depressed
To maintain physical well-being

SHORT-TERM GOALS	OUTCOME CRITERIA	NURSING ACTIONS	RATIONALE
Physical Dimension			
To not harm self	Does not harm self	Assess for suicide risk	To prevent harm, injury, death
		Have client sign a no-harm contract	Prevents impulsive actions
To maintain adequate self-care, for example, food, fluids, rest, activity, elimination	Maintains adequate self-care	Assist to meet self-care needs	For general health, to increase self-esteem and self-respect
Emotional Dimension			
To identify and express feelings	Identifies and expresses feelings	Facilitate expression of feelings with active listening, empathy, reflection	To build a trust relationship that contributes to hope
Intellectual Dimension			
To verbalize absence of suicide intent	Verbalizes absence of suicide intent	Observe for signs of suicidal intent; sudden change in mood or behavior, focus on death, expression of hopelessness	Suicidal clients often reveal clues prior to attempt
To verbalize other methods to resolve relationship conflicts	Verbalizes other ways to manage relationship conflicts	Explore with client other ways to deal with conflicts—talking with a supportive friend, problem solving, seeking therapy	Client participation promotes sense of control and increases self-esteem
Social Dimension			
To maintain supportive relationships	Maintains supportive relationships	Assist to identify support systems	Sharing concerns with supportive persons is therapeutic
		Provide group therapy	To increase sense of belonging, to learn problem solving
Spiritual Dimension			
To set goals for self that indicate hope	Sets goals for self that indicate hope	Help client set goals for self, for example, go back to work, participate in activities with daughters, see old friends, do fun things	Success in achieving goals contributes to an increase in self-esteem, personal power, and sense of control over life
To develop a will to live	States will to live	Explore with client reasons to live	To strengthen beliefs about life, to promote awareness of positives in life that contribute to hope

A Young Woman With Anorexia

Distorted body image
Childhood relationships
frequently interrupted

Major life change near
puberty
Achievement-oriented family

Fear of obesity
Blames self for mother not
loving her; poor self-esteem

Fear of obesity
Intelligent, good student

Loss of sexual interest
No pleasure in life
Feelings of helplessness, loss
of control
Attempts to gain control
Excessive exerciser
Signs and symptoms of
malnutrition

Ann is a 23-year-old unmarried woman. She is *5'10" and weighs 95 pounds* and considers her weight to be *"just about right."* Ann was *5 years old* when her *parents separated* as a result of her mother's involvement in an extramarital affair. Her parents reconciled, but 2 years later *they divorced* and Ann's father was granted custody of her. *Ann and her father lived with his parents* until she was *12 years old, at which time he remarried.* Although she liked her stepmother and enjoyed being with her, Ann was alone much of the time because both parents had *successful careers,* which demanded much of their time. She combated her loneliness with food and gained weight. Her friends began to tease her about being "fat". She became very *conscious of her weight and began to diet.* Meanwhile her natural mother remarried, but she was never very interested in Ann and *often failed to return her phone calls or answer her letters.* Ann never reconciled herself to her mother's behavior and often asked herself what *she had done to lose her mother's love.* During school and college, Ann *periodically went on strict diets "to keep from getting fat."* She was *an A student in both high school and college.* In college, Ann enjoyed her first long-term sexual relationship with a man. She said, "he made *me feel wanted and desirable.* I'd never felt that way before." Since then, she has been in several sexual relationships but does not *enjoy sex,* is not interested in marriage, and *"finds little pleasure in life."* Ann is currently teaching in a junior high school. She reports that her *work* there *is frustrating and discouraging* and she feels *helpless to change the situation.* "Students are undisciplined, are not interested in learning, and show absolutely no respect to the teachers." Ann's *dieting and laxative use have intensified* since she has started teaching, and *she runs 5 to 10 miles a day* since "the more I run, the more I lose." She *complains of fatigue. Her conjunctiva and mucous membranes are pale, and she has not had a menstrual period in a year.* Ann's physician recommended hospitalization, and Ann agreed that she would gain weight while in the hospital.

ANALYSIS

Ann had a turbulent childhood. Significant relationships in her life were frequently interrupted. Premature separation from significant others, her mother and grandparents, became the norm for Ann and probably affected her sense of trust and autonomy. A major change occurred in Ann's life when her father remarried and she moved from her grandparent's house. This change happened at about the time of puberty, and Ann may have experienced a feeling of loss of control in her life. Her feeling of loss of control in life reappeared when Ann began to teach school. Ann's rejection by her natural mother contributed to Ann's poor self-esteem, and she never felt "wanted" until her college relationship. She reports that she has no pleasure in her life and has lost interest in sexual activity. Ann has a body image disturbance. Normal body weight for her age and height is around 149 pounds. She has become an avid exerciser and has amenorrhea. She is beginning to exhibit the signs and symptoms of malnutrition.

NURSING DIAGNOSES

Altered nutrition: less than body requirements, related to fear of obesity
Altered nutrition: less than body requirements related to excessive exercise
Fatigue: related to malnutrition
*Helplessness: related to fear of losing control
Self-esteem disturbance: chronic, related to mother's rejection
Spiritual distress: related to loss of pleasure in life

---

*PND diagnosis.

CARE PLAN

Long-Term Goals

To maintain nutritional eating habits
To maintain at least 90% of expected weight

SHORT-TERM GOALS	OUTCOME CRITERIA	NURSING ACTIONS	RATIONALE
Physical Dimension			
To increase caloric intake and promote weight gain	Stays within agreed planned caloric intake	Establish an agreed-upon contract for a weight goal and renegotiate as needed	A mutually agreed-upon contract will reduce resistance to treatment and promote client's control and responsibility
		Allow a choice of foods as much as possible	To help client to gain a sense of control in her life
		Serve meals in room initially	To keep other clients from encouraging client to eat and avoid secondary gains associated with not eating
		Present and remove food tray without comment on the amount eaten	To avoid issues of control.
		Remain in room with client for 1 hour with no bathroom privileges following eating	To ensure that client does not hide food or use bathroom to vomit
		Use behavior modification techniques such as granting or restricting privileges based on weight gain or loss	To provide reinforcement for weight gain or loss

CARE PLAN—cont'd

SHORT-TERM GOALS	OUTCOME CRITERIA	NURSING ACTIONS	RATIONALE
To decrease malnutrition	Is more energetic Normal conjunctiva and mucous membranes	Weigh every other day before breakfast in hospital gown and after voiding	To assure consistency since client may attempt to increase weight by wearing heavier clothing or by retaining urine
		Monitor intake and output	To ensure that client is receiving adequate amounts of fluid
		Monitor lab reports and vital signs	To assure electrolyte balance and renal function
		Monitor elimination patterns	To provide bulk and fluid and decrease risk of constipation
		Provide plenty of foods with fiber	Same as above
To decrease excessive exercise	Exercises in moderation	Observe and record Ann's activity	To monitor her exercise She may secretly exercise in her room or in the bathroom in an effort to lose weight
		Develop an individualized exercise program	To help Ann limit excessive exercising
		Refer to occupational therapy	To provide structured activity
Emotional Dimension			
To decrease feelings of helplessness	Idetifies statements that encourage a helpless position	Listen for and assist Ann in identifying helpless statements	To assist Ann in gaining awareness of statements of helplessness
		Assist Ann in identifying factors that contribute to her sense of helplessness	To discuss the relationship between statements of helplessness and feelings of helplessness
	Makes statements that reflect a sense of control	Help Ann identify choices	To encourage Ann to consider a variety of options available to her
		Assist Ann in identifying issues under her control	To encourage her to assume responsibility and control of her life
		Encourage Ann to make decisions and help her determine alternatives and consequences of actions	To increase Ann's sense of control and to help her learn about the consequences of her actions
		Teach problem solving	To provide Ann with a method for making decisions and establishing control in her life
		Provide opportunities for Ann to practice assuming control of her own behaviors	To help Ann learn to take "risks" in a supportive environment
		Provide assertiveness training	To help her learn to ask for what she wants and gain control of her life
Intellectual Dimension			
To establish a more realistic body image	Acknowledges she is underweight	Have client look in a full-size mirror with little or no clothing. Ask her to describe what she sees and how she would like to be	To assist Ann to realistically appraise her body

SHORT-TERM GOALS	OUTCOME CRITERIA	NURSING ACTIONS	RATIONALE
		Discuss irrational and unrealistic perceptions of her body	To cast some doubt on the way she views her body
		Discuss irrational beliefs of needing to be perfect	To find out possible sources of irrational beliefs, to give permission to be less than perfect and still be a worthwhile person
		Assist Ann in developing realistic beliefs about food, weight, and beauty	To lessen the preoccupation with food and weight, and to promote a healthy, productive life-style
Social Dimension To become aware of negative thoughts about self	Recognizes self as what she is and not what she wishes to be	Explore with Ann realistic self-perceptions	To encourage reality testing
	Acknowledges influence of her previous experiences in the formation of her self-esteem	Assist Ann in recognition of idealized and realistic view of self Discuss Ann's perception's of her mother	To promote insight Same as above
	Acknowledges behavior that enhances self-esteem	Assist Ann in identifying how her mother's behavior affected her	To assist Ann in recognizing that her feelings of inadequacy may be related to her mother's treatment of her. To establish a cause-and-effect relationship
		Teach Ann to make positive affirmations about herself	To focus on the positive rather than the negative Promotes self-care
		Have Ann list her positive assets	To increase self-esteem
Spiritual Dimension To find pleasure in life	Learns new skills that are pleasurable	Help Ann to identify potentially pleasurable experiences	To increase pleasure in life and feelings of worth and value
	Does things for others that are self-rewarding	Assist Ann in identifying personal attributes associated with successful living	To encourage behavioral changes that are compatible with Ann's value system
	Achieves success in tasks and initiated activities	Help Ann to direct attention outside of herself and her immediate concerns	To prevent self-absorption
		Help Ann to identify realistic ways to participate in meaningful activities	To provide Ann with the opportunities to make decisions about herself, thus increasing her sense of worth and value
		Encourage activities in which something is creatively produced in an environment where others are sharing a similar experience	Being creative leads to self-actualization and generates a sense of optimism. Sharing the experience with others enhances the positive value

Appendix A
ANA Standards of Psychiatric and Mental Health Nursing Practice

Standard I—Theory

The nurse applies appropriate theory that is scientifically sound as a basis for decisions regarding nursing practice.

Standard II—Data collection

The nurse continuously collects data that are comprehensive, accurate, and systematic.

Standard III—Diagnosis

The nurse utilizes nursing diagnoses *and standard classification of mental disorders to express conclusions supported by recorded assessment data and current scientific premises.*

Standard IV—Planning

The nurse develops a nursing care plan with specific goals and interventions delineating nursing actions unique to each client's needs.

Standard V—Intervention

The nurse intervenes as guided by the nursing care plan to implement nursing actions that promote, maintain, or restore physical and mental health, prevent illness, and effect rehabilitation.

Standard V-A—Psychotherapeutic interventions

The nurse (generalist) uses psychotherapeutic interventions *to assist clients to regain or improve their previous coping abilities and to prevent further disability.*

Standard V-B—Health teaching

The nurse assists clients, families, and groups to achieve satisfying and productive patterns of living through health teaching.

Standard V-C—Self-care activities

The nurse uses the activities of daily living in a goal-directed way to foster adequate self-care and physical and mental well-being of clients.

Standard V-D—Somatic therapies

The nurse uses knowledge of somatic therapies and applies related clinical skills in working with clients.

Standard V-E—Therapeutic environment

The nurse provides, structures, and maintains a therapeutic environment in collaboration with the client and other health care providers.

Standard V-F—Psychotherapy

The nurse (specialist) utilizes advanced clinical expertise in individual, group, and family psychotherapy, *child psychotherapy, and other treatment modalities to function as a psychotherapist and recognizes professional accountability for nursing practice.*

Standard VI—Evaluation

The nurse evaluates client responses to nursing actions in order to revise the data base, nursing diagnoses, and nursing care plan.

Reprinted with permission of the American Nurses' Association, Kansas City, 1982.

Standard VII—Peer review

The nurse participates in peer review and other means of evaluation to assure quality of nursing care provided for clients.

Standard VIII—Continuing education

The nurse assumes responsibility for continuing education and professional development and contributes to the professional growth of others.

Standard IX—Interdisciplinary collaboration

The nurse collaborates with interdisciplinary teams in assessing, planning, implementing, and evaluating programs and other mental health activities.

Standard X—Utilization of community health systems

The nurse (specialist) participates with other members of the community in assessing, planning, implementing, and evaluating mental health services and community systems that include the promotion of the broad continuum of primary, secondary, and tertiary prevention of mental illness.

Standard XI—Research

The nurse contributes to nursing and the mental health field through innovations in theory and practice and participation in research.

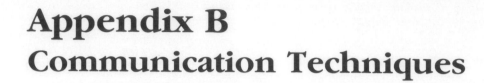

Appendix B
Communication Techniques

VERBAL COMMUNICATION

▶ Therapeutic Techniques

TECHNIQUES	EXAMPLES
1. Using silence	
2. Accepting	Yes. Uh hmm. I follow what you said. Nodding.
3. Giving recognition	Good morning Mr. S. You've tooled a leather wallet. I notice you've changed your hair style.
4. Offering self	I'll sit with you awhile. I'll stay here with you. I'm interested in your comfort.
5. Giving broad openings	What are you thinking about? Where would you like to begin?
6. Offering general leads	Go on. And then? Tell me about it.
7. Placing the event in time or in sequence	What seemed to lead up to . . . ? Was this before or after . . . ? When did this happen?
8. Making observations	You appear tense. You seem uncomfortable when you . . . . I notice that you're biting your lips. I get uncomfortable when you . . . .
9. Encouraging description of perceptions	Tell me when you feel anxious. What is happening? What does the voice seem to be saying?

Therapeutic Techniques—cont'd

TECHNIQUES	EXAMPLES
10. Encouraging comparison	This was something like . . . ? When have you had similar experiences?
11. Restating	**Patient:** I can't sleep. I stay awake all night. **Nurse:** You stay awake all night?
12. Reflecting	**Patient:** Do you think I should tell the doctor . . . ? **Nurse:** You're worried about that. **Patient:** My brother spends all my money and then has the nerve to ask for more. **Nurse:** This causes you to feel angry.
13. Focusing	This point seems worth looking at more closely.
14. Exploring	Tell me more about that. Describe it more fully. What kind of work?
15. Giving information	My name is . . . . Visiting hours are . . . . My purpose in being here is . . . . I'm taking you to the . . . .
16. Seeking clarification	I'm not sure that I follow. What is the main point of what you just said?
17. Presenting reality	I see no one else in the room. That sound was a car backfiring. Your mother is not here; I'm a nurse.
18. Voicing doubt	Isn't that unusual? That's hard to believe.
19. Seeking consensual validation	Tell me whether my understanding of what you said agrees with yours. When you use this word you mean . . . ?
20. Verbalizing the implied	**Patient:** I can't talk to you or to anyone. It's a waste of time. **Nurse:** Is it your feeling that no one understands? **Patient:** My wife pushes me around just like my mother and sister did. **Nurse:** Is it your impression that women are domineering?
21. Encouraging evaluation	What are your feelings in regard to . . . ? In what way does this contribute to your discomfort?
22. Attempting to translate into feelings	**Patient:** I'm dead. **Nurse:** You're suggesting that you feel lifeless? (or) Life seems without meaning? **Patient:** I'm way out in the ocean. **Nurse:** It must be lonely. (or) You seem to feel deserted.
23. Suggesting collaboration	Perhaps you and I can discuss and discover what produces your anxiety.
24. Summarizing	You've said that . . . . During the past hour you and I have discussed . . . .
25. Encouraging formulation of a plan of action	What could you do to let your anger out harmlessly? Next time this comes up, what might you do to handle it?

▶ **Nontherapeutic Techniques**

TECHNIQUES	EXAMPLES
1. Reassuring	I wouldn't worry about.... Everything will be all right. You're coming along fine.
2. Giving approval	That's good. I'm glad that you....
3. Rejecting	Let's not discuss.... I don't want to hear about....
4. Disapproving	That's bad. I'd rather you wouldn't....
5. Agreeing	That's right. I agree
6. Disagreeing	That's wrong. I definitely disagree with.... I don't believe that.
7. Advising	I think you should.... Why don't you...?
8. Probing	Now tell me about.... Tell me your life history.
9. Challenging	But how can you be President of the United States? If you're dead, why is your heart beating?
10. Testing	What day is this? Do you know what kind of a hospital this is? Do you still have the idea that...?
11. Defending	This hospital has a fine reputation. No one here would lie to you. Dr. B. is a very able psychiatrist.
12. Requesting an explanation	Why do you think that? Why do you feel this way? Why did you do that?
13. Indicating the existence of an external source	What makes you say that? Who told you that you were Jesus? What made you do that?
14. Belittling feelings expressed	**Patient:** I have nothing to live for...I wish I was dead. **Nurse:** Everybody gets down in the dumps. (or) I've felt that way sometimes.
15. Making stereotyped comments	Nice weather we're having. I'm fine, and how are you? It's for your own good. Keep your chin up. Just listen to your doctor and take part in activities— you'll be home in no time.
16. Giving literal responses	**Patient:** I'm an Easter egg. **Nurse:** What shade? (or) You don't look like one. **Patient:** They're looking in my head with television. **Nurse:** Try not to watch television. (or) With what channel?
17. Using denial	**Patient:** I'm nothing. **Nurse:** Of course you're something. Everybody is some-body. **Patient:** I'm dead. **Nurse:** Don't be silly.
18. Interpreting	What you really mean is.... You're saying that....
19. Introducing an unrelated topic	**Patient:** I'd like to die. **Nurse:** Did you have visitors this weekend?

NONVERBAL COMMUNICATION

Nonverbal communication is transmitted with or without verbal communication. It is essential that the nurse become aware of her own nonverbal communication in addition to becoming skillful in identifying the client's nonverbal communication. Nonverbal communication provides clues about the validity of the spoken words and congruency with the client's behavior. The phrase "Actions speak louder than words" is generally accurate. A list of ways in which nonverbal communication is conveyed to others follows:

Tone of voice
Voice inflections
Facial expression
Silence
Gestures
Mannerisms
Posture
Rate of speech
Eye contact
A "hurry up" attitude
An "I could care less" attitude
Physical appearance
Touch
Space

Appendix C
Problem Solving

A problem is an obstacle that interferes with the attainment of a goal. It may be a question that requires a solution, a difficulty in interacting with people in everyday situations, or an unmet emotional need. Whatever the problem, problem solving requires a systematic approach, a series of sequential steps, to arrive at a solution. The following steps are involved in problem solving:

1. Define and limit the problem. This requires that the problem be described in language that is clear to both parties. Limit the discussion to one aspect of the problem.

   Client: My father was bedridden for months before he died. Caring for him just wore me and my mother out. Now my mother is sick and between caring for her and the stress of my job, I am just exhausted.

   Nurse: You've identified several things—your mother's illness, the stress of your job, and your exhaustion. Let's limit this to one specific problem.

   Client: Well, I can't make my mother well, and I think my job wouldn't be so stressful if I could just get some time away, get rested and rejuvenated.

   Nurse: So, your problem is your exhaustion. What can you do about your exhaustion?

   Stating the problem in the form of a question often leads the way to finding a solution and moves to the next step in the process.

2. Gather data and analyze the problem. Acquire information about the problem and explore the cause. The client has identified that he has cared for an ill father and mother. He also finds his job stressful. However, identifying the cause of the problem is not sufficient. It is essential to analyze the data. The who, what, when, where, and how aspects of the problem are determined in this step. What is the exact nature of the problem, who is involved, how and when and where does it occur? For example: How long has he cared for his sick parents? Does he provide 24-hour-a-day care? Are relatives available to provide relief? If so, for how long and how often? If not, what financial resources are needed to provide respite care? What events at work are stressful? What does the client do to reduce his stress? Does he have vacation time available? Can he afford to take a vacation? Has he had a physical examination recently?

3. Encourage expression of feelings about the problems. Consider feelings, attitudes, and values that may influence which solution is chosen. The client in this example may consider taking a vacation, but feelings of guilt about leaving an ill mother may preclude this choice.

4. Consider alternative solutions. List all possible solutions to the problem. There is more than one way to solve a problem. When people fail at problem solving, often it is because they do not consider other possible solutions. If the client is unable to take a vacation, perhaps he can arrange to have someone relieve him of caregiving on weekends or every other weekend, or even one night a week. Perhaps other diversional activities could relieve the client's exhaustion. For example, if the client decided he needed a vacation but vacation time was not available, that alternative is not feasible.

5. Consider the consequences of each solution. State the pros and cons of each solution. Some solutions are clearly better than others.

6. Select the best possible solution. Evaluate the solutions that were listed. Determine the consequence of each solution.

7. Plan and implement the solution. Decide how the selected solution can be put into effect, and implement the solution.

8. Evaluate the result. Use the previously determined criteria to evaluate the results. Did the solution solve the problem? Did the solution create another problem? Was the outcome the desired one? Was there a flaw in the plan? Going through the problem-solving process does not guarantee that the problem will be solved. It does demonstrate a process that the client can apply to a variety of life situations.

Appendix D
Defense Mechanisms

MECHANISMS	DEFINITION	EXAMPLE
Compensation	An attempt to make up for real or fancied deficiencies	A high school student does poorly in his studies but becomes a talented artist.
Conversion	Expression of intrapsychic conflict symbolically through physical symptoms	A student develops diarrhea on the day of an important examination.
Denial	Disowning of consciously intolerable ideas and impulses	A client diagnosed with diabetes does not stay on her diet.
Displacement	Redirection of an emotional feeling from one idea, person, or object to another	A principal berates a teacher, and when classes resume the teacher speaks harshly to the students.
Dissociation	Separation and detachment of emotional significance and affect from an idea or situation	A client grins and chuckles when telling about his automobile accident and its tragic consequences.
Fantasy	A conscious creation or distortion of unacceptable fears, wishes, and behaviors.	A client daydreams during an intense group therapy session.
Identification	An attempt to fashion oneself to think, feel, and act like an admired, idealized other	An adolescent dresses like a rock star and mimics his behavior.
Introjection	Unconsciously incorporating loved or hated wishes, values, and attitudes external to oneself	A little girl scolds and spanks her doll like her mother does to her.
Projection	Attributing intolerable wishes, emotional feelings, and motivations to other persons	A teenage girl blames her boyfriend for getting her drunk.
Rationalization	An attempt to make unacceptable feelings and behavior consciously tolerable and acceptable	A student fails an examination and says the lectures were poorly organized and presented unclearly.
Reaction formation	Attitudes, motives, and needs that are directly opposite of those consciously acknowledged	A mother, unaware of her anger toward her children, becomes overly protective.
Regression	Retreat to an earlier and more comfortable level of adjustment	A 4-year-old begins to wet his pants following the birth of his baby brother.
Repression	Involuntary and unconscious forgetting of unbearable ideas and impulses	An accident victim does not remember the details of an accident.
Restitution	Going back or attempting to restore or repair unconscious guilt feelings	The head nurse is short-tempered toward a new nurse and then lets her leave early.
Sublimation	Diversion of consciously unacceptable instinctual drives into personally and socially accepted areas	A highly competitive man becomes a successful business man.
Substitution	Replacement of an unacceptable need, attitude, or emotion with one that is more acceptable	A woman rushes into marriage following a breakup with her boyfriend.
Suppression	The intentional exclusion of material from consciousness	A young woman says she is not ready to talk about her abuse as a child.
Symbolization	Disguising an external object as the outward representation for another internal and hidden idea	A man sends his girlfriend a dozen roses.
Undoing	An attempt to actually or symbolically take away a previously consciously intolerable action or experience	A mother who has just punished her child gives him a cookie.

Appendix E
DSM-III-R Classification: Categories and Codes

DISORDERS USUALLY FIRST EVIDENT IN INFANCY, CHILDHOOD, OR ADOLESCENCE

DEVELOPMENTAL DISORDERS
Note: These are coded on Axis II.

Mental Retardation

317.00	Mild mental retardation
318.00	Moderate mental retardation
318.10	Severe mental retardation
318.20	Profound mental retardation
319.00	Unspecified mental retardation

Pervasive Developmental Disorders

299.00	Autistic disorder
	Specify if childhood onset
299.80	Pervasive developmental disorder NOS

Specific Developmental Disorders

Academic skills disorders

315.10	Developmental arithmetic disorder
315.80	Developmental expressive writing disorder
315.00	Developmental reading disorder

Language and speech disorders

315.39	Developmental articulation disorder
315.31*	Developmental expressive language disorder
315.31*	Developmental receptive language disorder

Motor skills disorder

315.40	Developmental coordination disorder
315.90*	Specific developmental disorder NOS

Other Developmental Disorders

315.90*	Developmental disorder NOS

All official DSM-III-R codes are included in ICD-9-CM. Codes followed by a * are used for more than one DSM-III-R diagnosis or subtype to maintain compatibility with ICD-9-CM.

A long dash following a diagnostic term indicates the need for a fifth digit subtype or other qualifying term.

The term *specify* following the name of some diagnostic categories indicates qualifying terms that clinicians may wish to add in parentheses after the name of the disorder.

NOS = Not otherwise specified

The current severity of a disorder may be specified after the diagnosis as:

mild
moderate — currently meets diagnostic criteria
severe

in partial remission (or residual state)
in complete remission

Disruptive Behavior Disorders

314.01	Attention-deficit hyperactivity disorder
	Conduct disorder
312.20	group type
312.00	solitary aggressive type
312.90	undifferentiated type
313.81	Oppositional defiant disorder

Anxiety Disorders of Childhood or Adolescence

309.21	Separation anxiety disorder
313.21	Avoidant disorder of childhood or adolescence
313.00	Overanxious disorder

Eating Disorders

307.10	Anorexia nervosa
307.51	Bulimia nervosa
307.52	Pica
307.53	Rumination disorder of infancy
307.50	Eating disorder NOS

Gender Identity Disorders

302.60	Gender identity disorder of childhood
302.50	Transsexualism *Specify* sexual history: asexual, homosexual, heterosexual, unspecified
302.85*	Gender identity disorder of adolescence or adulthood, nontranssexual type *Specify* sexual history: asexual, homosexual, heterosexual, unspecified
302.85*	Gender identity disorder NOS

Tic Disorders

307.23	Tourette's disorder
307.22	Chronic motor or vocal tic disorder
307.21	Transient tic disorder *Specify:* single episode or recurrent
307.20	Tic disorder NOS

Elimination Disorders

307.70	Functional encopresis *Specify:* primary or secondary type
307.60	Functional enuresis *Specify:* primary or secondary type *Specify:* nocturnal only, diurnal only, nocturnal and diurnal

Speech Disorders Not Elsewhere Classified

307.00*	Cluttering
307.00*	Stuttering

Other Disorders of Infancy, Childhood, or Adolescence

313.23	Elective mutism
313.82	Identity disorder
313.89	Reactive attachment disorder of infancy or early childhood
307.30	Stereotypy/habit disorder
314.00	Undifferentiated attention-deficit disorder

ORGANIC MENTAL DISORDERS

Dementias Arising in the Senium and Presenium

	Primary degenerative dementia of the Alzheimer type, senile onset
290.30	with delirium
290.20	with delusions
290.21	with depression
290.00*	uncomplicated (Note: code 331.00 Alzheimer's disease on Axis III)

Code in fifth digit:
1 = with delirium, 2 = with delusions,
3 = with depression, 0* = uncomplicated

290.1x	Primary degenerative dementia of the Alzheimer type, presenile onset _____ (Note: code 331.00 Alzheimer's disease on Axis III)
290.4x	Multi-infarct dementia _____
290.00*	Senile dementia NOS *Specify* etiology on Axis III if known
290.10*	Presenile dementia NOS *Specify* etiology on Axis III if known (e.g., Pick's disease, Jakob-Creutzfeldt disease)

Psychoactive Substance-Induced Organic Mental Disorders

	Alcohol
303.00	intoxication
291.40	idiosyncratic intoxication
291.80	uncomplicated alcohol withdrawal
291.00	withdrawal delirium
291.30	hallucinosis
291.10	amnestic disorder
291.20	dementia associated with alcoholism
	Amphetamine or similarly acting sympathomimetic
305.70*	intoxication
292.00*	withdrawal
292.81*	delirium
292.11*	delusional disorder
	Caffeine
305.90*	intoxication
	Cannabis
305.20*	intoxication
292.11*	delusional disorder
	Cocaine
305.60*	intoxication
292.00*	withdrawal
292.81*	delirium
292.11*	delusional disorder
	Hallucinogen
305.30*	hallucinosis
292.11*	delusional disorder
292.84*	mood disorder
292.89*	posthallucinogen perception disorder

Inhalant
305.90*   intoxication

Nicotine
292.00*   withdrawal

Opioid
305.50*   intoxication
292.00*   withdrawal

Phencyclidine (PCP) or similarly acting arylcyclohexylamine
305.90*   intoxication
292.81*   delirium
292.11*   delusional disorder
292.84*   mood disorder
292.90*   organic mental disorder NOS

Sedative, hypnotic, or anxiolytic
305.40*   intoxication
292.00*   uncomplicated sedative, hypnotic, or anxiolytic withdrawal
292.00*   withdrawal delirium
292.83*   amnestic disorder

Other or unspecified psychoactive substance
305.90*   intoxication
292.00*   withdrawal
292.81*   delirium
292.82*   dementia
292.83*   amnestic disorder
292.11*   delusional disorder
292.12   hallucinosis
292.84*   mood disorder
292.89*   anxiety disorder
292.89*   personality disorder
292.90*   organic mental disorder NOS

Organic Mental Disorders Associated with Axis III Physical Disorders or Conditions, or Whose Etiology Is Unknown.

293.00   Delirium
294.10   Dementia
294.00   Amnestic disorder
293.81   Organic delusional disorder
293.82   Organic hallucinosis
293.83   Organic mood disorder
               Specify: manic, depressed, mixed
294.80*   Organic anxiety disorder
310.10   Organic personality disorder
               Specify: if explosive type
294.80*   Organic mental disorder NOS

PSYCHOACTIVE SUBSTANCE USE DISORDERS

Alcohol
303.90   dependence
305.00   abuse

Amphetamine or similarly acting sympatho-mimetic
304.40   dependence
305.70*   abuse

Cannabis
304.30   dependence
305.20*   abuse

Cocaine
304.20   dependence
305.60*   abuse

Hallucinogen
304.50*   dependence
305.30*   abuse

Inhalant
304.60   dependence
305.90*   abuse

Nicotine
305.10   dependence

Opioid
304.00   dependence
305.50*   abuse

Phencyclidine (PCP) or similarly acting arylcyclohexylamine
304.50*   dependence
305.90*   abuse

Sedative, hypnotic, or anxiolytic
304.10   dependence
305.40*   abuse
304.90*   Polysubstance dependence
304.90*   Psychoactive substance dependence NOS
304.90*   Psychoactive substance abuse NOS

SCHIZOPHRENIA

Code in fifth digit: 1 = subchronic, 2 = chronic, 3 = subchronic with acute exacerbation, 4 = chronic with acute exacerbation, 5 = in remission, 0 = unspecified.

Schizophrenia
295.2x   catatonic _____
292.1x   disorganized _____
295.3x   paranoid _____
               Specify if stable type
295.9x   undifferentiated _____
295.6x   residual _____
               Specify: if late onset

DELUSIONAL (PARANOID) DISORDER

297.10 Delusional (paranoid) disorder
Specify: type: erotomanic
grandiose
jealous
persecutory
somatic
unspecified

PSYCHOTIC DISORDERS NOT ELSEWHERE CLASSIFIED

298.80 Brief reactive psychosis
295.40 Schizophreniform disorder
Specify: without good prognostic features or with good prognostic features
295.70 Schizoaffective disorder
Specify: bipolar type or depressive type
297.30 Induced psychotic disorder
298.90 Psychotic disorder NOS
(Atypical psychosis)

MOOD DISORDERS

Code current state of Major Depression and Bipolar Disorder in fifth digit:
1 = mild
2 = moderate
3 = severe, without psychotic features
4 = with psychotic features (*specify* mood-congruent or mood-incongruent)
5 = in partial remission
6 = in full remission
0 = unspecified

For major depressive episodes, *specify* if chronic and *specify* if melancholic type.

For Bipolar Disorder, Bipolar Disorder NOS, Recurrent Major Depression, and Depressive Disorder NOS, *specify* if seasonal pattern.

Bipolar Disorders

	Bipolar Disorder
296.6x	mixed _____
296.4x	manic _____
296.5x	depressed _____
301.13	Cyclothymia
296.70	Bipolar disorder NOS

Depressive Disorders

	Major depression
296.2x	single episode _____
296.3x	recurrent _____

300.40 Dysthymia (or depressive neurosis)
Specify: primary or secondary type
Specify: early or late onset
311.00 Depressive disorder NOS

ANXIETY DISORDERS (or anxiety and phobic neuroses)

Panic disorder
300.21 with agoraphobia
Specify current severity of agoraphobic avoidance
Specify current severity of panic attacks
300.01 without agoraphobia
Specify current severity of panic attacks
300.22 Agoraphobia without history of panic disorder
Specify with or without limited symptom attacks
300.23 Social phobia
Specify if generalized type
300.29 Simple phobia
300.30 Obsessive compulsive disorder (or obsessive compulsive neurosis)
309.89 Post-traumatic stress disorder
Specify if delayed onset
300.02 Generalized anxiety disorder
300.00 Anxiety disorder NOS

SOMATOFORM DISORDERS

300.70* Body dysmorphic disorder
300.11 Conversion disorder (or hysterical neurosis, conversion type)
Specify: single episode or recurrent
300.70* Hypochondriasis (or hypochondriacal neurosis)
300.81 Somatization disorder
307.80 Somatoform pain disorder
300.70* Undifferentiated somatoform disorder
300.70* Somatoform disorder NOS

DISSOCIATIVE DISORDERS (or hysterical neuroses, dissociative type)

300.14 Multiple personality disorder
300.13 Psychogenic fugue
300.12 Psychogenic amnesia
300.60 Depersonalization disorder (or depersonalization neurosis)
300.15 Dissociative disorder NOS

SEXUAL DISORDERS

Paraphilias

302.40	Exhibitionism
302.81	Fetishism
302.89	Frotteurism
302.20	Pedophilia
	Specify: same sex, opposite sex, same and opposite sex
	Specify: if limited to incest
	Specify: exclusive type or nonexclusive type
302.83	Sexual masochism
302.84	Sexual sadism
302.30	Transvestic fetishism
302.82	Voyeurism
302.90*	Paraphilia NOS

Sexual Dysfunctions

Specify: psychogenic only, or psychogenic and biogenic (Note: If biogenic only, code on Axis III)
Specify: lifelong or acquired
Specify: generalized or situational

	Sexual desire disorders
302.71	Hypoactive sexual desire disorder
302.79	Sexual aversion disorder
	Sexual arousal disorders
302.72*	Female sexual arousal disorder
302.72*	Male erectile disorder
	Orgasm disorders
302.73	Inhibited female orgasm
302.74	Inhibited male orgasm
302.75	Premature ejaculation
	Sexual pain disorders
302.76	Dyspareunia
306.51	Vaginismus
302.70	Sexual dysfunction NOS

Other Sexual Disorders

302.90*	Sexual disorder NOS

SLEEP DISORDERS

Dyssomnias

	Insomnia disorder
307.42*	related to another mental disorder (non-organic)
780.50*	related to known organic factor
307.42*	Primary insomnia
	Hypersomnia disorder
307.44	related to another mental disorder (non-organic)
780.50*	related to a known organic factor
780.54	Primary hypersomnia
307.45	Sleep-wake schedule disorder
	Specify: advanced or delayed phase type, disorganized type, frequently changing type
	Other dyssomnias
307.40*	Dyssomnia NOS

Parasomnias

307.47	Dream anxiety disorder (Nightmare disorder)
307.46*	Sleep terror disorder
307.46*	Sleepwalking disorder
307.40*	Parasomnia NOS

FACTITIOUS DISORDERS

	Factitious disorder
301.51	with physical symptoms
300.16	with psychological symptoms
300.19	Factitious disorder NOS

IMPULSE CONTROL DISORDERS NOT ELSEWHERE CLASSIFIED

312.34	Intermittent explosive disorder
312.32	Kleptomania
312.31	Pathological gambling
312.33	Pyromania
312.39*	Trichotillomania
312.39*	Inpulse control disorder NOS

ADJUSTMENT DISORDER

	Adjustment disorder
309.24	with anxious mood
309.00	with depressed mood
309.30	with disturbance of conduct
309.40	with mixed disturbance of emotions and conduct
309.28	with mixed emotional features
309.82	with physical complaints
309.83	with withdrawal
309.23	with work (or academic) inhibition
309.90	Adjustment disorder NOS

PSYCHOLOGICAL FACTORS AFFECTING PHYSICAL CONDITION

316.00	Psychological factors affecting physical condition
	Specify physical condition on Axis III

V CODES FOR CONDITIONS NOT ATTRIBUTABLE TO A MENTAL DISORDER THAT ARE A FOCUS OF ATTENTION OR TREATMENT

V62.30	Academic problem
V71.01	Adult antisocial behavior

V40.00	Borderline intellectual functioning (Note: This is coded on Axis II.)

V71.02	Childhood or adolescent antisocial behavior

PERSONALITY DISORDERS
Note: These are coded on Axis II.

Cluster A

301.00	Paranoid
301.20	Schizoid
301.22	Schizotypal

Cluster B

301.70	Antisocial
301.83	Borderline
301.50	Histrionic
301.81	Narcissistic

Cluster C

301.82	Avoidant
301.60	Dependent
301.40	Obsessive compulsive
301.84	Passive aggressive
301.90	Personality disorder NOS

V65.20	Malingering
V61.10	Marital problem
V15.81	Noncompliance with medical treatment
V62.20	Occupational problem
V61.20	Parent-child problem
V62.81	Other interpersonal problem
V61.80	Other specified family circumstances
V62.89	Phase of life problem or other life circumstance problem
V62.82	Uncomplicated bereavement

ADDITIONAL CODES

300.90	Unspecified mental disorder (nonpsychotic)
V71.09*	No diagnosis or condition on Axis I
799.09*	Diagnosis or condition deferred on Axis I

V71.09*	No diagnosis or condition on Axis II
799.90*	Diagnosis or condition deferred on Axis II

MULTIAXIAL SYSTEM

Axis I	Clinical Syndromes V Codes
Axis II	Developmental Disorders Personality Disorders
Axis III	Physical Disorders and Conditions
Axis IV	Severity of Psychosocial Stressors
Axis V	Global Assessment of Functioning

SEVERITY OF PSYCHOSOCIAL STRESSORS SCALE: ADULTS

Code	Term	Examples of Stressors	
		Acute Events	Enduring Circumstances
1	**None**	No acute events that may be relevant to the disorder	No enduring circumstances that may be relevant to the disorder
2	**Mild**	Broke up with boyfriend or girlfriend; started or graduated from school; child left home	Family arguments; job dissatisfaction; residence in high-crime neighborhood
3	**Moderate**	Marriage; marital separation; loss of job; retirement; miscarriage	Marital discord; serious financial problems; trouble with boss; being a single parent
4	**Severe**	Divorce; birth of first child	Unemployment; poverty
5	**Extreme**	Death of spouse; serious physical illness diagnosed; victim of rape	Serious chronic illness in self or child; ongoing physical or sexual abuse
6	**Catastrophic**	Death of child; suicide of spouse; devastating natural disaster	Captivity as hostage; concentration camp experience
0	**Inadequate Information, or No Change in Condition**		

SEVERITY OF PSYCHOSOCIAL STRESSORS SCALE: CHILDREN AND ADOLESCENTS

Code	Term	Examples of Stressors	
		Acute Events	Enduring Circumstances
1	**None**	No acute events that may be relevant to the disorder	No enduring circumstances that may be relevant to the disorder
2	**Mild**	Broke up with boyfriend or girlfriend; change of school	Overcrowded living quarters; family arguments
3	**Moderate**	Expelled from school; birth of sibling	Chronic disabling illness in parent; chronic parental discord
4	**Severe**	Divorce of parents; unwanted pregnancy; arrest	Harsh or rejecting parents; chronic life-threatening illness in parent; multiple foster home placements
5	**Extreme**	Sexual or physical abuse; death of a parent	Recurrent sexual or physical abuse
6	**Catastrophic**	Death of both parents	Chronic life-threatening illness
0	**Inadequate Information, or No Change in Condition**		

GLOBAL ASSESSMENT OF FUNCTIONING SCALE

Consider psychological, social, and occupational continuum of mental health—illness. Do not include impairment in functioning due to physical (or environmental) limitations.

Note: Use intermediate codes when appropriate, for example, 45, 68, 72.

Code

90
|
81
Absent or minimal symptoms (e.g., mild anxiety before an exam), **good functioning in all areas, interested and involved in a wide range of activities, socially effective, generally satisfied with life, no more than everyday problems or concerns** (e.g., an occasional argument with family members).

80
|
71
If symptoms are present, they are transient and expectable reactions to psychosocial stressors (e.g., difficulty concentrating after family argument); **no more than slight impairment in social, occupational, or school functioning** (e.g., temporarily falling behind in school work).

70
|
61
Some mild symptoms (e.g., depressed mood and mild insomnia) **OR some difficulty in social, occupational, or school functioning** (e.g., occasional truancy, or theft within the household), **but generally functioning pretty well, has some meaningful interpersonal relationships.**

60
|
51
Moderate symptoms (e.g., flat affect and circumstantial speech, occasional panic attacks) **OR moderate difficulty in social, occupational, or school functioning** (e.g., few friends, conflicts with co-workers).

50
|
41
Serious symptoms (e.g., suicidal ideation, severe obsessional rituals, frequent shoplifting) **OR any serious impairment in social, occupational, or school functioning** (e.g., no friends, unable to keep a job).

40
|
31
Some impairment in reality testing or communication (e.g., speech is at times illogical, obscure, or irrelevant) **OR major impairment in several areas, such as work or school, family relations, judgment, thinking, or mood** (e.g., depressed man avoids friends, neglects family, and is unable to work; child frequently beats up younger children, is defiant at home, and is failing at school).

30
|
21
Behavior is considerably influenced by delusions or hallucinations OR serious impairment in communication or judgment (e.g., sometimes incoherent, acts grossly inappropriately, suicidal preoccupation) **OR inability to function in almost all areas** (e.g., stays in bed all day; no job, home, or friends).

20
|
11
Some danger of hurting self or others (e.g., suicide attempts without clear expectation of death, frequently violent, manic excitement) **OR occasionally fails to maintain minimal personal hygiene** (e.g., smears feces) **OR gross impairment in communication** (e.g., largely incoherent or mute).

10
|
1
Persistent danger of severely hurting self or others (e.g., recurrent violence) **OR persistent inability to maintain minimal personal hygiene OR serious suicidal act with clear expectation of death.**

Appendix F
Medication Charts

ANTIPSYCHOTIC MEDICATIONS

GENERIC NAME	TRADE NAME	DOSAGE MG/24 HRS	ADMINISTRATION	INDICATIONS FOR USE*
Phenothiazines				
Chlorpromazine	Thorazine	25–2000	Extended release tablets, oral solution syrup, tablets, IM, suppositories	Psychotic manifestations
Prochlorperazine	Compazine	15–150	Syrup, extended release capsules, tablets	Anxiety and severe restlessness
Thioridazine	Mellaril	75–800	Oral suspension, oral solution, tablets	Nausea and vomiting
Fluphenazine hydrochloride	Prolixin	1–20	Elixir, oral solution, tablets, extended release tablets	Hyperkinesis in children
Fluphenazine decanoate	Prolixin Decanoate	Up to 100 mg q 1–3 weeks	IM	Hiccups
Fluphenazine enanthate	Prolixin Enanthate	Up to 100 mg q 1–3 weeks	IM	
Promazine	Sparine	150–800	Oral solution, syrup, tablets	
Trifluoperazine	Stelazine	4–40	Syrup, tablets	
Mesoridiazine	Serentil	30–400	Oral solution, tablets	
Perphenazine	Trilafon	16–64	Oral solution, tablets, extended release tablets, IM	
Butyrophenone				
Haloperidol	Haldol	2–40	Oral solution, tablets, IM	
Thioxanthenes				
Chlorprothixene	Taractan	25–600	Oral suspension, tablets	
Thiothixene	Navane	6–60	Capsules, oral solution	
Others				
Carbamazepine	Tegretol	50–200	Tablets, chewable tablets	Seizures
Clozapine	Clozaril	300–450	Tablets	

*Applies in general to most antipsychotic medications.
†Life-threatening effects are italicized.

CONTRA-INDICATIONS*	COMMON SIDE EFFECTS/ ADVERSE REACTIONS†	DRUG INTERACTIONS*	NURSING IMPLICATIONS*
Hypersensitivity Glaucoma Convulsive disorders Pregnancy Lactation Elderly clients	RESP: Dyspnea, *laryngospasm, respiratory depression* CNS: Extrapyramidal symptoms—pseudoparkinsonism, akathisia, dystonia, tardive dyskinesia, seizures, headache HEMA: Anemia, leukopenia, leukocytosis, *agranulocytosis* INTEG: Rash, photosensitivity, dermatitis EENT: Blurred vision, glaucoma GI: Dry mouth, nausea, vomiting, anorexia, constipation, diarrhea, jaundice, weight gain GU: Urinary retention, urinary frequency, enuresis, impotence, amenorrhea, gynecomastia CV: Orthostatic hypotension, hypertension, ECG changes, *cardiac arrest, tachycardia*	Alcohol or CNS depressants, especially anesthetics, barbiturates, and narcotics: may potentiate and prolong effects of these medications Amphetamines: effects may be decreased Antacids or antidiarrheal suspensions: may inhibit the absorption of orally administered phenothiazines Anticonvulsants: lower the seizure threshold Epinephrine: hypotension may result Guanethidine: antihypertensive effects may be counteracted Levadopa: antiparkinsonian effects may be inhibited Monoamine oxidase (MAD) inhibitors or tricyclic antidepressants: may prolong and intensify the sedative and antimuscarinic effects of these medications Ototoxic medications: may mask some symptoms of ototoxicity	May require several weeks of therapy to obtain desired effects. Take with food or milk to reduce stomach irritation. Watch for signs of blood dyscrasia, such as sore throat, fever. Watch for extrapyramidal symptoms and report to physician. Monitor intake and output for possible urinary retention and constipation. Assess for menstrual irregularities, breast engorgement, lactation, increased libido in women, decreased libido in men. Assess for visual disturbances. Note changes in carbohydrate metabolism, such as glycosuria, weight loss, polyphagia, increased appetite. Consider medication change if excessive weight gain results. Assess for symptoms of hypersensitivity. Watch for symptoms of cholestatic jaundice. Remain with client until medication is swallowed to prevent hoarding or omission. Take baseline reading of BP and pulse before IM administration.

Continued

ANTIPSYCHOTIC MEDICATIONS—cont'd

GENERIC NAME	TRADE NAME	DOSAGE MG/24 HRS	ADMINISTRATION	INDICATIONS FOR USE

ANTIPARKINSON MEDICATIONS

GENERIC NAME	TRADE NAME	DOSAGE MG/24 HRS	ADMINISTRATION	INDICATIONS FOR USE*
Anticholinergics Trihexyphenidyl	Artane	5–15	Extended release capsules, elixir, tablets	Parkinsonism Drug-induced extrapyramidal reactions
Benztropine	Cogentin	1–6	Tablets, IM	
Procyclidine	Kemadrin	6–15	Tablets	
Antihistamine Diphenhydramine	Benadryl	75–400	Capsules, elixir, syrup, tablets, IM, IV	
Dopamine-Releasing Agent Amantadine	Symmetrel	100–200	Capsules, syrup	

*Applies in general to most antiparkinson medications.
†Life-threatening effects are italicized.

CONTRA-INDICATIONS*	COMMON SIDE EFFECTS/ ADVERSE REACTIONS†	DRUG INTERACTIONS*	NURSING IMPLICATIONS*
			Keep the client recumbent for at least 1 hour after IM administration and monitor BP closely for hypotensive reaction.
			Consider that the antiemetic effects may mask other pathological factors such as toxicity to other drugs, intestinal obstruction, or brain lesions.
			Teach client to prevent exposure to sunlight.
			Caution client not to drive or operate machinery requiring mental alertness for at least 2 weeks after therapy has begun.
			Caution client that medication may turn urine pink or reddish brown.
			Emphasize importance of taking medication after discharge and of returning for follow-up care.

CONTRA-INDICATIONS*	COMMON SIDE EFFECTS/ ADVERSE REACTIONS†	DRUG INTERACTIONS*	NURSING IMPLICATIONS*
Glaucoma Tachycardia Hypertension Cardiac disease Asthma Duodenal ulcer	CNS: Headache, dizziness, drowsiness, fatigue, anxiety, psychosis, depression, hallucinations, tremors, convulsions CV: Orthostatic hypotension, *CHF* INTEG: Photosensitivity, dermatitis EENT: Blurred vision HEMA: *Leukopenia* GI: Nausea, vomiting, constipation, dry mouth GU: Frequency, retention	Alcohol or CNS depressants: may cause increased sedative effects Amantadine, antihistamines, antimuscarinics, haloperidol, monoamine oxidase inhibitors, phenothiazine, or tricyclic antidepressants: may intensify atropine-like effects Antacids or antidiarrheal suspensions: may reduce therapeutic effects of antiparkinsonian medications Chlopromazine: metabolism may be increased resulting in decreased plasma concentration because of reduction in gastrointestinal motility	Take with food to relieve gastric irritation. Offer bits of ice or sugarless chewing gum for relief of dry mouth. Be alert to a history of asthma, glaucoma, or duodenal ulcer, which contradicts use of these medications. Advise client to report side effects early. When changing medication, antiparkinson drugs should not be withdrawn abruptly. Caution client about getting up suddenly from a lying or sitting down position.

ANTIANXIETY MEDICATIONS

GENERIC NAME	TRADE NAME	DOSAGE MG/24 HRS	ADMINISTRATION	INDICATIONS FOR USE*
Meprobamate	Equanil, Miltown	1200–1600	Capsules, extended release capsules, tablets	Anxiety disorders Short-term relief of anxiety Acute alcohol withdrawal Insomnia Skeletal muscle spasm Preanesthetic medication
Chlordiazepoxide	Librium	15–100	Tablets, capsules	
Diazepam	Valium	6–40	Extended release capsules, tablets	
Oxazepam	Serax	30–120	Capsules, tablets	
Hydroxyzine hydrochloride	Atarax	75–400	Syrup, tablets	
Hydroxyzine pamoate	Vistaril	75–400	Capsules, oral suspension	
Alprazolam	Xanax	0.5–4	Tablets	
Clorazepate	Tranxene	7.5–60	Capsules, tablets	
Lorazepam	Ativan	0.5–9	Tablets, IM, IV	

*Applies in general to most antianxiety medications.
†Life-threatening effects are italicized.

CONTRA-INDICATIONS*	COMMON SIDE EFFECTS/ ADVERSE REACTIONS†	DRUG INTERACTIONS*	NURSING IMPLICATIONS*
Hypersensitivity Drug-dependent client Glaucoma Liver dysfunction Kidney dysfunction Psychoses Pregnancy Lactation Elderly clients	CNS: Dizziness, drowsiness, confusion, headache, anxiety, tremors, stimulation, fatigue, depression, insomnia, hallucinations GI: Nausea, vomiting, constipation, dry mouth, anorexia, diarrhea INTEG: Rash, dermatitis, itching CV: Orthostatic hypotension, *ECG changes, tachycardia,* hypotension EENT: Blurred vision, tinnitus, mydriasis	Antacids: may delay, but not reduce absorption of Librium and Valium Carbamazepine: may result in increased metabolism and decreased serum concentrations and half lives of carbamazepines and benzodiazepines Cimetidine: may inhibit hepatic metabolism of benzodiazepines that are metabolized by oxidation CNS depressants such as alcohol, analgesics, general anesthetics, and tricyclic antidepressants: may increase effects of these medications Isoniazid: may inhibit elimination of Valium, resulting in increased plasma concentrations Levodopa: may decrease therapeutic effects of levodopa Phenytoin: metabolism may be decreased, resulting in increased phenytoin serum concentration	Assess for frequent requests for medications or for ingestion of larger than recommended doses. Client may be developing physical and psychological dependence. Watch for ataxia, slurred speech, and vertigo, symptoms of chronic intoxication, and indications that client is taking more than recommended dose. Carefully supervise amount and dose prescribed. Remain with client until medication is swallowed. Inform client that sudden withdrawal may cause recurrence of preexisting symptoms or precipitate a withdrawal syndrome. Assess for withdrawal symptoms such as trouble sleeping, irritability, nervousness, mental confusion, muscle cramps, nausea, vomiting, trembling, and convulsions. Avoid drinking beverages containing caffeine. Caution client that these medications may reduce the ability to handle potentially dangerous equipment, such as cars and machinery. Caution client not to drink alcoholic beverages while taking antianxiety agents because depressant effects of both alcohol and antianxiety agent will be potentiated. Avoid abruptly stopping the medication after prolonged and excessive use.

ANTIDEPRESSANT MEDICATIONS

GENERIC NAME	TRADE NAME	DOSAGE MG/24 HRS	ADMINISTRATION	INDICATIONS FOR USE*
Tricyclics				
Amitriptyline hydrochloride	Elavil	75–300	Tablet, IM	Depression Enuresis Chronic pain
Desipramine hydrochloride	Norpramin	75–200	Tablet, capsule	
Doxepin hydrochloride	Adapin Sinequan	75–300	Capsule, oral solution	
Imipramine hydrochloride	Tofranil	75–300	Tablet, capsule, IM	
Nortriptyline hydrochloride	Aventyl Pamelor	75–100	Capsule, oral solution	
Protriptyline	Vivactil	15–60	Tablet	
Clomipramine Amoxapine	Anafranil Assendin	25–250 75–300	Capsules Tablets	
Tetracyclics Maprotiline	Ludiomil	150–300	Tablet	
Others Trazodone Fluoxetine	Desyrel Prozac	150–600 20–80	Tablet Pulvules	
Monoamine Oxidase Inhibitors Isocarboxazid	Marplan	10–30	Tablet	
Phenelzine sulfate	Nardil	15–90	Tablet	
Tranylcypromine sulfate	Parnate	10–30	Tablet	

*Applies in general to most antidepressant medications.
†Life-threatening effects are italicized.

CONTRA-INDICATIONS*	COMMON SIDE EFFECTS/ADVERSE REACTIONS†	DRUG INTERACTIONS*	NURSING IMPLICATIONS*
	Tricyclics		
Hypersensitivity Liver disease Glaucoma Cardiovascular disease Hypertension Epilepsy Pregnancy Lactation	HEMA: *Agranulocytosis, thrombocytopenia, eosinophilia, leukopenia* CNS: Dizziness, drowsiness, confuson, headache, anxiety, tremors, stimulation, weakness, insomnia, nightmares, EPS (elderly), increased psychiatric symptoms GI: Nausea, vomiting, dry mouth, diarrhea, *paralytic ileus,* increased appetite, cramps, epigastric distress, jaundice, *hepatitis,* stomatitis GU: Retention INTEG: Rash, urticaria, sweating, pruritis, photosensitivity CV: Orthostatic hypotension, *ECG* changes, *tachycardia, hypertension,* palpitations EENT: Blurred vision, tinnitus, mydriasis, ophthalmoplegia	Alcohol: serious potentiation of CNS depressant effects Anticonvulsants: enhance CNS depression, lower convulsive threshold, and decrease effects of the antidepressant medication Antihistaminics or antimuscarinics or CNS depressants: may potentiate effects of these medications Clonidine or guanethidine: antihypertensive effects may be blocked Estrogens or oral contraceptives: may potentiate tricyclic antidepressant side effects and reduce antidepressant effect	Take with food to reduce gastrointestinal irritation. May require up to 2 weeks of therapy to obtain optimal antidepressant effects. Caution if any kind of surgery (including dental surgery) or emergency treatment is required. Avoid taking other medications unless prescribed. Avoid alcoholic beverages. Caution client about driving or doing jobs that require alertness. Caution client about getting up from a lying or sitting position. Withdrawal symptoms of headache, nausea, and malaise may occur if high or prolonged dosage is abruptly discontinued. Potentially suicidal patients should not have access to large amounts of these medications.
	Monoamine Oxidase Inhibitors		
Hypersensitivity Liver disease Cardiovascular disease Hypertension	HEMA: Anemia CNS: Dizziness, drowsiness, confusion, headache, anxiety, tremors, stimulation, weakness, hyperreflexia, mania, insomnia, fatigue GI: Constipation, dry mouth, nausea, vomiting, anorexia, diarrhea, weight gain GU: Change in libido, frequency INTEG: Rash, flushing, increased perspiration, jaundice CV: Orthostatic hypotension, hypertension, dysrhythmias, hypertensive crisis EENT: Blurred vision ENDO: SIADH-like syndrome	Sympathomimetics: may result in severe hypertension Thyroid medication: may enhance possibility of cardiac arrhythmias Alcohol, anesthetics, or CNS depressants: CNS depression may be enhanced Anticonvulsants: may cause a change in pattern of epileptiform seizures Antidepressants, tricyclic: hypertensive crisis, convulsions, and death may occur Antihypertensives or diuretics: may result in enhanced hypotensive effect Caffeine-containing preparations: caffeine consumed in chocolate, cola, tea, or "stay awake" products may produce cardiac arrhythmias Insulin or oral hypoglycemics: may enhance severe hypoglycemic effects Narcotics: may produce hypertension Tyramine: foods such as cheese, sour cream, yogurt, pickled herring, chicken liver, canned figs, raisins, bananas, avocados, soy sauces, yeast extracts, and alcoholic beverages may cause sudden and severe hypertension, which can reach crisis levels	Caution patient on importance of diet, of avoiding foods containing tyramine. May require 1 to 4 weeks of therapy to obtain signs of improvement. Caution client about driving or doing jobs requiring alertness. Caution client about getting up suddenly. Caution client about any kind of surgery (including dental surgery) or emergency treatment. Potentially suicidal patients should not have access to large amounts of these medications. Because insomnia may be produced, this medication is not usually given in the evening. After dosage is stopped, effects of this medication may persist for up to 2 weeks. During this time, food and drug contraindications must be observed.

ANTIMANIAC MEDICATIONS

GENERIC NAME	TRADE NAME	DOSAGE MG/24 HRS	ADMINISTRATION	INDICATIONS FOR USE*
Lithium car-bonate	Lithane Lithonate Eskalith	Up to 1800 mg/day initially Up to 900 mg/day for maintenance, adjusted to main-tain serum level of 0.5–1.5 mEq	Capsule, tablet, extended release tablets, citrate syrup	Control of manic episodes

*Applies in general to most antimanic medications.
†Life-threatening effects are italicized.

CONTRA-INDICATIONS*	COMMON SIDE EFFECTS/ ADVERSE REACTIONS†	DRUG INTERACTIONS*	NURSING IMPLICATIONS*
Cardiovascular disease Renal disease Brain damage Clients receiving diuretics Clients on low sodium diets Pregnancy Lactation	HEMA: Leukocytosis CNS: Dizziness, drowsiness, confusion, headache, twitching, ataxia, seizure, slurred speech, restlessness, stupor, memory loss, clonic movements, tremors GI: Nausea, vomiting, dry mouth, diarrhea, incontinence, abdominal pain, anorexia, cramps, epigastric distress, jaundice, *hepatitis*, stomatitis GU: Polyuria, glycosuria, proteinuria, albuminuria, urinary incontinence, polydipsia, edema INTEG: Drying of hair, alopecia, rash, sweating, pruritis, hyperkeratosis CF: Hypotension, *ECG* changes, dysrhythmias, circulatory collapse EENT: Blurred vision, tinnitis ENDO: Hyponatremia MS: Muscular weakness	Aminophylline, caffeine, dyphylline, sodium bicarbonate, or theophylline: may decrease therapeutic effect of lithium because of its increased urinary excretion Diuretics: may provoke toxicity due to reduced renal clearance Haloperidol: monitor closely for neurotoxicity Indomethacin or methyldopa or tetracycline: possible toxicity produced at low serum concentrations when used concurrently Iodine preparations: may produce hypothyroidism Norepinephrine: pressor effects may be decreased Skeletal muscle relaxants: effects may be potentiated or prolonged Sodium chloride: lithium retention increases as sodium intake decreases; as sodium intake increases, lithium retention decreases; low sodium diet is best avoided during lithium therapy	May require from 1 to 3 weeks before improvement begins. Encourage adequate fluid, sodium, and potassium intake. Take with food or milk to reduce gastrointestinal symptoms. Caution client about exercise, saunas, or hot weather. Caution against drinking large amounts of coffee, tea, or colas because of diuretic action. Serum blood levels should be determined 1 to 2 times per week during initiation of therapy and monthly thereafter on blood samples taken 8 to 12 hours after dose.

Appendix G
Extrapyramidal Effects (EPS) of Psychotropic Medications

Acute Dystonic Reaction

Occurs suddenly (frightening spasms of major muscle groups of the neck, back, eyes)

Bizarre facial and head movements

Oculogyric crisis (eyes fixed in one position, usually sideways or upwards)

Torticollis (contractions of the neck muscles twisting the head to one side)

Opisthotonus (protrusion of the tongue, or spasms of the back muscles)

Time of risk

1 to 5 days, possibly following first dose

Psychotropic-Induced Parkinsonism

Akinesia (slowness in movements)

Bilateral fine tremors

Tremor hands (pill rolling)

Muscular rigidity, masklike face,

Shuffling gait

Time of risk

7 to 30 days

Akathisia

Pacing, inner restlessness

Unable to sit still or sleep

Difficulty concentrating,

Weight shifting from one foot to another

Time of risk

5 to 60 days

Neuroleptic Malignant Syndrome

Extreme emergency—20% mortality rate

High fever, tachycardia, unstable B/P (hypotension, hypertension)

Muscle rigidity, dystonia, coarse tremor

Stupor, incontinence

Leukocytosis

Time of risk

From hours to months after drug treatment begins

Develops explosively over 1–3 days

More likely to occur with high-potency drugs

Tardive Dyskinesia

May be irreversible

Involuntary sucking, chewing, smacking, licking, blinking, grimacing, pursing movements of tongue and mouth

Choreiform movements of limbs and trunk

Tongue protrusion, foot tapping

Time of risk

Usually occurs after long-term use, but can occur after short-term use

Appendix H
NANDA-Accepted Diagnoses

Activity intolerance
Activity intolerance, high risk for
Adjustment, impaired
Airway clearance, ineffective
Anxiety
Aspiration, high risk for
Body image disturbance
Body temperature, altered, high risk for
Breastfeeding, effective
Breastfeeding, ineffective
Breastfeeding, interrupted
Breathing pattern, ineffective
Cardiac output, decreased
Caregiver role strain
Caregiver role strain, high risk for
Communication, impaired verbal
Constipation
Constipation, colonic
Constipation, perceived
Coping, defensive
Coping, family: potential for growth
Coping, ineffective family: compromised
Coping, ineffective family: disabling
Coping, ineffective individual
Decisional conflict (specify)
Denial, ineffective
Diarrhea
Disuse syndrome, high risk for
Diversional activity deficit
Dysreflexia
Family processes, altered
Fatigue
Fear
Fluid volume deficit (1)
Fluid volume deficit (2)

Fluid volume deficit, high risk for
Fluid volume excess
Gas exchange, impaired
Grieving, anticipatory
Grieving, dysfunctional
Growth and development, altered
Health maintenance, altered
Health-seeking behaviors (specify)
Home maintenance management, impaired
Hopelessness
Hyperthermia
Hypothermia
Incontinence, bowel
Incontinence, functional
Incontinence, reflex
Incontinence, stress
Incontinence, total
Incontinence, urge
Infant feeding pattern, ineffective
Infection, high risk for
Injury, high risk for
Knowledge deficit (specify)
Mobility, impaired physical
Noncompliance (specify)
Nutrition, altered: less than body requirements
Nutrition, altered: more than body requirements
Nutrition, altered: high risk for more than body requirements
Oral mucous membrane, altered
Pain
Pain, chronic
Parental role conflict
Parenting, altered
Parenting, altered, high risk for
Peripheral neurovascular dysfunction, high risk for
Personal identity disturbance
Poisoning, high risk for
Post-trauma response

From the Proceedings of the Tenth National Conference of the North American Nursing Diagnosis Association, 1992.

Powerlessness
Protection, altered
Rape-trauma syndrome
Rape-trauma syndrome: compound reaction
Rape-trauma syndrome: silent reaction
Role performance, altered
Self-care deficit, bathing/hygiene
Self-care deficit, dressing/grooming
Self-care deficit, feeding
Self-care deficit, toileting
Self-esteem disturbance
Self-esteem, chronic low
Self-esteem, situational low
Self-mutilation, high risk for
Sensory/perceptual alterations (specify) (visual, auditory, kinesthetic, gustatory, tactile, olfactory)
Sexual dysfunction
Sexuality patterns, altered
Skin integrity, impaired
Skin integrity, impaired, high risk for
Sleep pattern disturbance

Social interaction, impaired
Social isolation
Spiritual distress (distress of the human spirit)
Stress syndrome, relocation
Suffocation, high risk for
Swallowing, impaired
Therapeutic regimen (individual), ineffective management of
Thermoregulation, ineffective
Thought processes, altered
Tissue integrity, impaired
Tissue perfusion, altered (specify type) (renal, cerebral, cardiopulmonary, gastrointestinal, peripheral)
Trauma, high risk for
Unilateral neglect
Urinary elimination, altered patterns of
Urinary retention
Ventilation, inability to sustain spontaneous
Ventilatory weaning response, dysfunctional (DVWR)
Violence, high risk for self-directed or directed at others

Appendix I
Psychiatric Mental Health Nursing Diagnoses

CLASSIFICATION OF HUMAN RESPONSES OF CONCERN FOR PSYCHIATRIC MENTAL HEALTH NURSING PRACTICE

1. **HUMAN RESPONSE PATTERNS IN ACTIVITY PROCESSES**

1.1 Motor behavior
- 1.1.1   Potential for alteration
  - *1.1.1.1   Activity intolerance
  - 1.1.1.2
- 1.1.2   Altered motor behavior
  - *1.1.2.1   Activity intolerance
  - 1.1.2.2   Bizarre motor behavior
  - 1.1.2.3   Catatonia
  - 1.1.2.4   Disorganized motor behavior
  - *1.1.2.5   Fatigue
  - 1.1.2.6   Hyperactivity
  - 1.1.2.7   Hypoactivity
  - 1.1.2.8   Psychomotor agitation
  - 1.1.2.9   Psychomotor retardation
  - 1.1.2.10   Restlessness
- 1.1.99   Motor behavior not otherwise specified (NOS)

1.2 Recreation patterns
- 1.2.1   Potential for alteration
  - 1.2.1.1
  - 1.2.1.2
- 1.2.2   Altered recreation patterns
  - 1.2.2.1   Age-inappropriate recreation
  - 1.2.2.2   Antisocial recreation
  - 1.2.2.3   Bizarre recreation
  - *1.2.2.4   Diversional activity deficit
- 1.2.99   Recreation patterns NOS

1.3 Self-care
- 1.3.1   Potential for alteration in self-care
- *1.3.2   Altered health maintenance
- 1.3.3   Altered self-care
  - *1.3.3.1   Altered nutrition
    - 1.3.3.1.1   Binge-purge syndrome
    - 1.3.3.1.2   Nonnutritive ingestion
    - 1.3.3.1.3   Pica
    - 1.3.3.1.4   Unusual food ingestion
    - 1.3.3.1.5   Refusal to eat
    - 1.3.3.1.6   Rumination
  - *1.3.3.2   Altered feeding
    - *1.3.3.2.1   Ineffective breastfeeding
  - *1.3.3.3   Self-care deficit: dressing/grooming
  - *1.3.3.4   Altered health maintenance
  - *1.3.3.5   Health-seeking behaviors
    - *1.3.3.5.1   Knowledge deficit
    - *1.3.3.5.2   Noncompliance
  - *1.3.3.6   Self-care deficit: bathing/hygiene
  - 1.3.3.7   Altered participation in health care
  - *1.3.3.8   Self-care deficit: toileting
- *1.3.4   Impaired adjustment
- *1.3.5   Knowledge deficit
- *1.3.6   Noncompliance
- 1.3.99   Self-care patterns NOS

1.4 Sleep/arousal patterns
- 1.4.1   Potential for alteration
- *1.4.2   Sleep pattern disturbance
  - 1.4.2.1   Decreased need for sleep
  - 1.4.2.2   Hypersomnia
  - 1.4.2.3   Insomnia
  - 1.4.2.4   Nightmares/terrors
  - 1.4.2.5   Somnolence
  - 1.4.2.6   Somnambulism
- 1.4.99   Sleep/arousal patterns NOS

Modified from O'Toole A, Loomis M: *Revision of the phenomena of concern for psychiatric mental health nursing,* Arch Psych Nurs 3(5):288, 1989.
*Approved NANDA diagnosis.

2. **HUMAN RESPONSE PATTERNS IN COGNITION PROCESSES**

2.1 **Decision making**
   2.1.1   Potential for alteration
   2.1.2   Altered decision making
   2.1.3   Decisional conflict
   2.1.99   Decision-making patterns NOS

2.2 **Judgment**
   2.2.1   Potential for alteration
   2.2.2   Altered judgment
   2.2.99   Judgment patterns NOS

2.3 **Knowledge**
   2.3.1   Potential for alteration
  *2.3.2   Knowledge deficit
      2.3.2.1   Agnosia
      2.3.2.2   Altered intellectual functioning
   2.3.99   Knowledge patterns NOS

2.4 **Learning**
   2.4.1   Potential for alteration
   2.4.2   Altered learning processes
   2.4.99   Learning patterns NOS

2.5 **Memory**
   2.5.1   Potential for alteration
   2.5.2   Altered memory
      2.5.2.1   Amnesia
      2.5.2.2   Distorted memory
      2.5.2.3   Long-term memory loss
      2.5.2.4   Memory deficit
      2.5.2.5   Short-term memory loss
   2.5.99   Memory patterns NOS

2.6 **Thought processes**
   2.6.1   Potential for alteration
  *2.6.2   Altered thought processes
      2.6.2.1   Altered abstract thinking
      2.6.2.2   Altered concentration
      2.6.2.3   Altered problem solving
      2.6.2.4   Confusion/disorientation
      2.6.2.5   Delirium
      2.6.2.6   Delusions
      2.6.2.7   Ideas of reference
      2.6.2.8   Magical thinking
      2.6.2.9   Obsessions
      2.6.2.10   Suspiciousness
      2.6.2.11   Thought insertion
   2.6.99   Thought processes NOS

3. **HUMAN RESPONSE PATTERNS IN ECOLOGICAL PROCESSES**

3.1 **Community maintenance**
   3.1.1   Potential for alteration
   3.1.2   Altered community maintenance
      3.1.2.1   Community safety hazards
      3.1.2.2   Community sanitation hazards
   3.1.99   Community maintenance patterns NOS

3.2 **Environmental integrity**
   3.2.1   Potential for alteration
   3.2.2   Altered environmental integrity
   3.2.99   Environmental integrity patterns NOS

3.3 **Home maintenance**
   3.3.1   Potential for alteration
  *3.3.2   Home maintenance management, impaired
      3.3.2.1   Home safety hazards
      3.3.2.2   Home sanitation hazards
   3.3.99   Home maintenance patterns NOS

4. **HUMAN RESPONSE PATTERNS IN EMOTIONAL PROCESSES**

4.1 **Feeling states**
   4.1.1   Potential for alteration
      4.1.1.1   Anticipatory grieving
   4.1.2   Altered feeling state
      4.1.2.1   Anger
    *4.1.2.2   Anxiety
      4.1.2.3   Elation
      4.1.2.4   Envy
    *4.1.2.5   Fear
    *4.1.2.6   Grief
      4.1.2.7   Guilt
      4.1.2.8   Sadness
      4.1.2.9   Shame
   4.1.3   Affect incongruous in situation
   4.1.4   Flat affect
   4.1.99   Feeling states NOS

4.2 **Feeling processes**
   4.2.1   Potential for alteration
   4.2.2   Altered feeling processes
      4.2.2.1   Lability
      4.2.2.2   Mood swings
   4.2.99   Feeling processes NOS

5. **HUMAN RESPONSE PATTERNS IN INTERPERSONAL PROCESSES**

5.1 **Abuse response patterns**
   5.1.1   Potential for alteration
   5.1.2   Altered abuse response
    *5.1.2.1   Post-trauma response
    *5.1.2.2   Rape trauma syndrome
    *5.1.2.3   Rape trauma syndrome: compound reaction
    *5.1.2.4   Rape trauma syndrome: silent reaction
   5.1.99   Abuse response patterns NOS

5.2 **Communication processes**
   5.2.1   Potential for alteration
  *5.2.2   Altered verbal communication
      5.2.2.1   Altered nonverbal communication
    *5.2.2.2   Altered verbal communication
        5.2.2.2.1   Aphasia
        5.2.2.2.2   Bizarre content
        5.2.2.2.3   Confabulation
        5.2.2.2.4   Ecolalia
        5.2.2.2.5   Incoherent
        5.2.2.2.6   Mute
        5.2.2.2.7   Neologisms
        5.2.2.2.8   Nonsense/word salad
        5.2.2.2.9   Stuttering
   5.2.99   Communication processes NOS

5.3 Conduct/impulse processes
5.3.1   Potential for alteration
     *5.3.1.1   High risk for violence
     5.3.1.2   Suicidal ideation
5.3.2   Altered conduct/impulse processes
     5.3.2.1   Accident prone
     5.3.2.2   Aggressive/violent behavior toward environment
     5.3.2.3   Delinquency
     5.3.2.4   Lying
     5.3.2.5   Physical aggression toward others
     5.3.2.6   Physical aggression toward self
          5.3.2.6.1   Suicide attempt(s)
     5.3.2.7   Promiscuity
     5.3.2.8   Running away
     5.3.2.9   Substance abuse
     5.3.2.10 Truancy
     5.3.2.11 Vandalism
     5.3.2.12 Verbal aggression toward others
5.3.99 Conduct/impulse processes NOS

5.4 Family processes
5.4.1   Potential for alteration
     *5.4.1.1   High risk for altered parenting
     *5.4.1.2   Coping, family: potential for growth
*5.4.2 Altered family processes
     5.4.2.1   Ineffective family coping
          *5.4.2.1.1   Compromised
          *5.4.2.1.2   Disabling
5.4.99 Family processes NOS

5.5 Role performance
5.5.1   Potential for alteration
*5.5.2 Altered role performance
     5.5.2.1   Altered family role
          5.5.2.1.1   Parental role conflict
          5.5.2.1.2   Parental role deficit
     5.5.2.2   Altered play role
     5.5.2.3   Altered student role
     5.5.2.4   Altered work role
*5.5.3 Ineffective individual coping
     *5.5.3.1   Defensive coping
     *5.5.3.2   Ineffective denial
5.5.99 Role performance patterns NOS

5.6 Sexuality
5.6.1   Potential for alteration
5.6.2   Altered sexual behavior leading to intercourse
5.6.3   Altered sexual conception actions
5.6.4   Altered sexual development
5.6.5   Altered sexual intercourse
5.6.6   Altered sexual relationships
*5.6.7 Altered sexuality patterns
5.6.8   Altered variation of sexual expression
*5.6.9 Sexual dysfunction
5.6.99 Sexuality processes NOS

5.7 Social interaction
5.7.1   Potential for alteration
*5.7.2 Impaired social interaction
     5.7.2.1   Bizarre behaviors
     5.7.2.2   Compulsive behaviors
     5.7.2.3   Disorganized social behaviors
     5.7.2.4   Social intrusiveness
     *5.7.2.5   Social isolation
     5.7.2.6   Unpredictable behaviors
5.7.99 Social interaction patterns NOS

6. HUMAN RESPONSE PATTERNS IN PERCEPTION PROCESSES

6.1 Attention
6.1.1   Potential for alteration
6.1.2   Altered attention
     6.1.2.1   Hyperalertness
     6.1.2.2   Inattention
     6.1.2.3   Selective attention
6.1.99 Attention patterns NOS

6.2 Comfort
6.2.1   Potential for alteration
*6.2.2 Pain
     6.2.2.1   Discomfort
     6.2.2.2   Distress
     *6.2.2.3   Pain
          6.2.2.3.1   Acute pain
          *6.2.2.3.2   Chronic pain
6.2.99 Comfort patterns NOS

6.3 Self-concept
6.3.1   Potential for alteration
6.3.2   Altered self-concept
     *6.3.2.1   Body-image disturbance
     *6.3.2.2   Personal identity disturbance
     *6.3.2.3   Self-esteem disturbance
          *6.3.2.3.1   Chronic low self-esteem
          *6.3.2.3.2   Situational low self-esteem
     6.3.2.4   Altered sexual identity
          6.3.2.4.1   Altered gender identity
6.3.3   Undeveloped self-concept
6.3.99 Self-concept patterns NOS

6.4 Sensory perception
6.4.1   Potential for alteration
*6.4.2 Sensory perceptual alterations
     6.4.2.1   Hallucinations
          *6.4.2.1.1   Auditory
          *6.4.2.1.2   Gustatory
          *6.4.2.1.3   Kinesthetic
          *6.4.2.1.4   Olfactory
          *6.4.2.1.5   Tactile
          *6.4.2.1.6   Visual
     6.4.2.2   Illusions
6.4.99 Sensory perception processes NOS

7. HUMAN RESPONSE PATTERNS IN PHYSIOLOGICAL PROCESSES

7.1 Circulation
7.1.1   Potential for alteration
     7.1.1.1   Fluid volume deficit
7.1.2   Altered circulation
     7.1.2.1   Altered cardiac circulation
          *7.1.2.1.1   Decreased cardiac output
     7.1.2.2   Altered vascular circulation
          *7.1.2.2.1   Fluid volume deficit

7.10 Physical regulation processes
7.10.1   Potential for alteration
    *7.10.1.1   High risk for altered body
                 temperature
    *7.10.1.2   High risk for infection
7.10.2   Altered physical regulation processes
    7.10.2.1   Altered immune response
        7.10.2.1.1   Infection
    7.10.2.2   Altered body temperature
        *7.10.2.2.1   Hyperthermia
        *7.10.2.2.2   Hypothermia
        *7.10.2.2.3   Ineffective
                       thermoregulation
7.10.99   Physical regulation processes NOS

**8.   HUMAN RESPONSE PATTERNS IN
       VALUATION PROCESSES**
8.1   Meaningfulness
8.1.1   Potential for alteration
    8.1.2.1   Helplessness
    *8.1.2.2   Hopelessness
    8.1.2.3   Loneliness
    *8.1.2.4   Powerlessness
8.1.99   Meaningfulness patterns NOS

8.2   Spirituality
8.2.1   Potential for alteration
8.2.2   Altered spirituality
    8.2.2.1   Spiritual despair
    *8.2.2.2   Spiritual distress
8.2.99   Spirituality patterns NOS
8.3   Values
8.3.1   Potential for alteration
8.3.2   Altered values
    8.3.2.1   Conflict with social order
    8.3.2.2   Inability to internalize values
    8.3.2.3   Unclear values
8.3.99   Value patterns NOS

Appendix J
Treatment Modalities

Assertiveness Training
Definition

A type of behavior therapy in which the client learns to communicate both positive and negative feelings in an open, honest, direct, and appropriate way. It is important to differentiate passive, assertive, and aggressive behavior so that the client can make an informed choice about the appropriate action to take.

Major concepts

A key concept in learning assertive behavior is choice. The client is free to choose what he will do. The client has the right to make a request, and others have the right to refuse the request. Rights have accompanying responsibilities. A client cannot change others, but he can change his own behaviors so that self-esteem and self-respect are enhanced.

Goals of therapy

To have self-respect because integrity has been upheld by standing up for a person's own rights without abusing other's rights

Other goals include clarifying what a person wants and deciding if those wants are feasible

Goals need to be realistic and achievable within a short period of time

Role of the nurse

To teach the differences between passive, assertive, and aggressive behavior

To target the behavior the client wants to change and to set up a plan of action, implement the action, and give positive reinforcement for the successful achievement of a targeted behavior

To help the client learn positive self-reinforcement

Behavior Modification Therapy
Definition

A treatment approach in which undesirable behavior is changed to desirable behavior by rewarding desirable responses and not rewarding or punishing undesirable behavior.

Major concepts

Behavior modification is based on the following principle: behavior that has rewarding consequences is learned and strengthened, and behavior that has negative consequences is weakened or extinguished. Environmental events are the determinants of behavior and are the source of rewards and punishment. Intrapsychic conflict or past traumatic events are not a concern of behavioral therapy.

Behavior modification has proven to be useful in the treatment of a wide range of maladaptive behaviors and to be effective with all ages.

Goal of therapy

The goal of behavioral therapy is to modify behavior by manipulating environmental contingencies by the use of reward or punishment. This is done by identifying the behavior (symptom) to be changed, by recording the frequency of the behavior and the sequence of events involved in producing and maintaining the behavior, and by deciding how to change the events with the use of reinforcements to decrease undesirable behavior and increase desirable behavior.

Role of the nurse

To identify the behavior (symptom) to be changed, modified, or developed

To determine in which settings the behavior is elicited

To determine how the behavior is maintained

To identify things that can be used as reinforcers (reward) and things that can be used as negative reinforcers (punishment)

To establish situations in which the behavior may be changed through a system of reward or punishment

Crisis Intervention
Definition

A type of short-term therapy whereby the nurse actively enters into the life situation of a person, family, or group who is undergoing a crisis to decrease the impact of the crisis event and to assist the individual in mobilizing his resources, regaining equilibrium, and, if possible, moving to a higher level of functioning. Crises may be of a situational or maturational nature and occur when the individual faces an obstacle to important life goals. For a time that obstacle seems insurmountable with the use of usual coping skills.

Major concepts

The client is an active participant in the intervention process. He assists in clarifying the problem, verbalizes feelings and thoughts about the situation, identifies goals and options for reaching goals, and decides on a plan and a timetable to carry out the plan.

Three interrelated balancing factors contribute to the production and the outcome of a crisis: (1) the perception of the problem, (2) situational supports, and (3) coping skills.

Crisis situations are short in duration, lasting no more than 4 to 6 weeks. The focus of the intervention is on the immediate problem.

Goal of therapy

To help the client resolve the problem and return to his precrisis level of functioning or to a higher level of functioning in a short period of time.

Role of the nurse

To assess the situation quickly and accurately and to assist the client in a tentative formulation of his problem. At times the nurse needs to make life or death decisions within a short time; thus quickness and accuracy are crucial for effective functioning.

Family Therapy
Definition

A type of therapy that involves treatment of the entire family unit for symptoms that are problematic. Symptoms of family disruption are often displayed in the behavior of one family member. Symptoms do not represent intrapsychic processes but are a signal of family system distress.

Major concepts

The focus is on the "here and now"; that is, present feelings and behavior rather than past feelings and behavior. Families are helped to enact, in the therapists' presence, how they usually resolve conflicts, support each other, enter into alliances and coalitions, and relieve stress. Dysfunctional communication is investigated, and meanings are clarified. Dysfunctional behavior is relabeled or reframed. One intervention is the technique of paradoxical intervention, which is used to help families resistive to change. Another technique is family sculpting, a process in which relationships between family members are recreated to symbolize the emotional position of each family member. It is used to engage children who express themselves quite naturally, nonverbally.

Goals of therapy

To remove family system pathological factors and to improve the functioning of the family as an interdependent group. The goals are accomplished according to the theoretical orientation of the therapist—behavioral, communication, interactional, or structural.

Role of the nurse

The nurse functions in the role of family therapist using a varied approach and a particular theoretical base. Basic to working with families is focusing on members' interactions with each other, confronting members with their behavior, and analyzing the family unit as an interconnecting system.

Group Therapy
Definition

A type of treatment that involves a group of people meeting at planned times with a qualified therapist to focus on awareness and understanding of oneself, improving interpersonal relationships, and making behavioral changes. Gestalt, encounter, and couples groups are examples of group therapy.

Major concepts

Since the problems of most persons involve their feelings and behavior toward others, it is believed that in a group setting the client will be able to develop an awareness of how his thoughts, feelings, and behavior affect others. Through group feedback and support the client can change his behavior and establish more effective interpersonal relationships.

Goals of therapy

The goals of group therapy are determined by the needs of the group. Goals may include a reconstruction of the personality as in psychoanalytical and transactional analysis groups, awareness of feelings and behavior in self and others as in gestalt groups, or improved communication and interpersonal relationships as in couples groups.

Role of the nurse

To make administrative arrangements for holding group meetings

To select and orient group members and establish group cohesion

To manage group conflicts

To help members meet their identified needs

Hypnosis
Definition

Hypnosis is an altered state of consciousness whereby clients are helped to use their own mental associations, memories, and life potentials to achieve their therapeutic goals. It is a technique used in helping clients discover the critical experiences in their background that have been responsible for their present distress. These experiences are then reframed. Reframing is changing the frame in which a person perceives events in order to change the meaning. When the meaning changes, the person's responses and behavior change.

Major concepts

The trance state is a naturally occurring phenomenon. It provides an opportunity for the therapist and client to make maximum use of their responses and focus intently on mastering psychological and physical distress. The effectiveness of hypnosis is enhanced by helping the client develop a new perspective on his problems. The intense concentration and willingness to suspend critical judgments that are characteristic of the trance state can facilitate the process.

Hypnosis may be induced by a skilled therapist, or it may be self-induced through a prelearned method. Problems such as hiccups, vomiting, blocked communication, and recall of repressed traumatic events can be helped through hypnosis.

Goals of therapy

To relieve pain

To reduce anxiety

To change undesirable behavior/habits (smoking, excessive eating, phobias)

To change physiological mechanisms (blood pressure)

To increase recall

Role of the nurse

To assess the client's ability to use hypnosis in a therapeutic way

To have a thorough knowledge of the client

To induce client into a trancelike state with a suggestion or strategy

Following relaxation, to explore a topic that is problematic and causing distress

Individual Therapy
Definition

An intimate professional relationship between a mental health professional and a client, who engage in a series of interactions over a period of time with an agreed upon purpose of change in behavior for the client. The therapist uses the psychological means inherent in a therapeutic professional relationship to influence the client toward a positive change in areas of interpersonal pain or dysfunction. The interactions proceed through three stages: orientation, working, and termination stages.

Major concepts

Major concepts include an awareness of content (what is said) and process (how it is said) and a working knowledge of transference, countertransference, resistance, acting out, and insight.

Goals of therapy

To relieve painful symptoms and to feel increased satisfactions in life

Role of the nurse

To promote positive personality growth and development through the intimate relationship with the client

To facilitate the expression of thoughts and feelings as a way to use more effective behaviors in dealing with stress

Marital or Couples Therapy
Definition

Couples therapy is for married or unmarried couples living together who have difficulties in their relationship and are unable to resolve conflicts and find a satisfactory solution to their problems. Most therapists emphasize mutual needs gratification within the social and sexual aspects of the relationship.

Major concepts

In couples therapy, therapeutic techniques focus on problems specific to a couple's relationship. Couples typically are seen together. Therapy for both partners is considered to be more effective in resolving relationship problems since each contribute to their maintenance. Therapy involves clarifying and improving interactions, examining mutual expectations and needs gratification, and discovering the rules that govern the relationship.

Goals of therapy

To identify marital conflicts

To facilitate open communication patterns

To use problem-solving techniques to resolve conflicts

Role of the nurse

The theoretical framework of the therapist guides her practice and defines her role. Some states require that a marital therapist be licensed and may require at least a master's degree.

Milieu Therapy
Definition

Scientifically planned environment for therapeutic purposes. All personnel have active roles in maintaining a therapeutic social milieu because every interaction with the client is seen as having potentially beneficial outcomes.

Major concepts

The therapeutic milieu counteracts the regressive effects of institutionalization (dependence, adoption of institutional attitudes, loss of contact with the outside world) by the distribution of power, open communication, structured interactions, work-related activities, involvement of family and community, and adaptation of the environment to meet client's developmental needs.

Other assumptions include: clients' personalities have strengths and conflict-free parts, clients have abilities to constructively influence their own treatments and the treatments of others, treatment is dependent on therapeutic staff involvement, and all personnel have the potential for exercising their influence.

Goal of therapy

To increase responsibility for therapy on the part of both client and staff. This is best achieved through a consciously incorporated plan. Ultimately, client autonomy is the goal.

Role of the nurse

The focus is on action and solving problems in everyday experiences. Interpersonal relationships are within a context of goal-directed activities.

Pain Management
Definition

Use of a variety of treatment modalities to meet individual client needs and to help the client discover relief from chronic pain, which has not been successfully managed by traditional medical and surgical techniques.

Major concepts

Clients with chronic pain receive secondary gains from their pain

Clients lack insight regarding the pain; self-disclosure through group therapy helps increase insight

Factual information given through educational sessions increases cognitive understanding of the pain process

Psychological testing provides assistance in vocational planning when pain interferes with work

Litigation counseling assists with workmen's compensation and lawsuits resulting from pain.

Goals of therapy

To develop greater mobility and independence through self-management of specific pain problems

To improve the quality of life by reducing pain and returning to an optimal level of health

Role of the nurse

To offer individual, group, or educational sessions for the purpose of:
    Identifying secondary gains
    Learning alternate ways to meet needs
    Increasing insight about pain
    Establishing emotional contact with others
    Increasing self-disclosure
    Increasing cognitive understanding of pain

Teach relaxation exercise—autogenic training, guided visual imagery, progressive muscular relaxation, biofeedback training, and restricted environmental stimulus technique (REST)

Referring for vocational and litigation counseling

Play Therapy
Definition

Play is viewed as an event occurring naturally throughout a child's development. In therapy the purpose, in addition to having fun, is to serve as a tool for growth and maturation and to help determine the child's behavioral problem and ways it is interfering with development. Drawings, storytelling, puppets, make-believe play (such as toys, dolls and doll houses, soldiers and guns, clay, and other figures), and formal games are used in play therapy.

Major concepts

Play serves a symbolic function and relates to the child's life (fantasy, wishes, dreams, and events). Children under stress (for example, taking a diagnostic test or forthcoming hospitalization) can play the procedure out and relieve the stress. This release play therapy is useful in anticipatory guidance with children. Play is a framework for developing social skills, teaching through play, or developing trust in relationships. Play is useful in reducing hyperactivity and helping the child organize play.

Goals of therapy

To work out problem situations
To learn to trust
To learn to compete, cooperate, and collaborate
To gain mastery over new experiences
To release an uncomfortable emotion
To play creatively

Role of the nurse

To purposefully select toys used in therapy

To communicate therapeutically with the child as a way to help the child develop abilities in interpreting and insight

To introduce toys to facilitate child's development and sense of mastery

To assess misinformation the child has and reduce stress

To promote a positive transference as an educational and therapeutic maneuver

Reality Orientation

Definition

Reality orientation (RO) is a therapeutic approach to increase awareness of person, place, and time in disoriented clients, frequently the elderly.

Major concepts

Reality therapy is ongoing, 24-hour-a-day therapy involving all who come in contact with the client. In addition to orientation to time, place, and person, the client is provided information about activities of daily living. Twenty-four-hour reality orientation may be supplemented with classroom reality orientation. Classes, which are limited to three to five persons, meet daily or weekly and provide basic information about the date and place and provide sensory training.

Goals of therapy

The primary goal of reality orientation is to reduce mild to severe confusion. It is also used to help maintain orientation and to prevent confusion. Reality orientation provides a medium for expression of warmth and concern for the confused individual.

Role of the nurse

To emphasize time, person, and place orientation

To provide an RO board containing information about the date and the place

To provide clocks

To make sure that the person has eyeglasses, dentures, and hearing aids if needed

To allow the person to keep familiar objects

To provide reinforcement to increase motivation

To speak slowly and clearly

To allow time for a response

To provide clues when asking a question

To maintain routines

To have the same person provide daily care

Reality Therapy

Definition

A form of therapy involving a special kind of teaching or training that enables the individual to accept reality and assume responsibility for satisfying his own needs and not depriving others of the ability to fulfill their own needs.

Major concepts

Reality therapy proposes that individuals have two major psychological needs, the need to be loved and the need to feel worthwhile to themselves and others. Irresponsible behavior interferes with the satisfaction of these needs and harms others. The primary task of clients is to learn to accept responsibility for their behavior; irresponsibility is inexcusable.

For the client to change irresponsible behavior, he becomes involved in a genuine and loving relationship with another person; therapy does not progress until then. The client develops this kind of relationship with the therapist so he can begin to face reality.

Present behavior is emphasized. The past cannot be changed nor can past events be used as an excuse for present failures. An increased awareness of current behavior helps the client critically judge its effectiveness and its social acceptability.

Reality therapy has been used successfully with adolescent delinquents and clients with chronic schizophrenia.

Goals of therapy

The client learns how to identify his goals, to make choices, to become responsible, to deal effectively in a warm and loving way with others, and to understand and accept the reality of his existence.

Role of the nurse

To become involved with the client so he can face reality

To reject the client's irresponsible behavior

To offer no excuses for client's behavior

To teach responsible ways to meet needs

Relaxation Therapy

Definition

A group class within a protected environment where participants learn the importance of relaxation, with emphasis on breathing and techniques that enhance relaxation. Under the leadership of the therapist, the participants lie down and focus their awareness for the purpose of obtaining physical and emotional relaxation.

Major concepts

The relaxation response is learned and can be elicited in almost everyone. The techniques are useful as a tool to help clients develop alternative responses to stress. Clients have control over their actions and levels of relaxation.

Goals of therapy

To recognize tension

To improve the ability to relax

To increase insight into control of emotional and physical tension

To focus on stress management in daily living

To improve self-esteem with increased control of emotional and physical stress

To focus on responsibility for self in changing behavior

Role of the nurse

To provide a quiet environment

To promote a mental device that increases awareness of breathing or relaxation, such as a word, a visual image, or a bodily sensation

To promote a passive attitude free from distractions

To promote a comfortable position

To teach that the goal is relaxation, not sleep

Reminiscence Therapy
Definition

A therapeutic approach used with the older adult. Memories of past events and experiences are recalled and reviewed.

Major concepts

Reminiscing is viewed as a particularly adaptive function at the last stage of life. It is a way aged people review their life in an attempt to make order and meaning of past experiences and work toward a new sense of identify. Reminiscence therapy is distinguished from life review, which is a process of resolving past conflicts and disappointments.

Goals of therapy

As a technique used with the cognitively impaired, it helps to maintain the individual's self-esteem and identity and to encourage active participation in interactions with others. Those with little or no cognitive impairment benefit from memory stimulation and have the opportunity to integrate life experiences and to be actively involved in interpersonal relations.

Role of the nurse

To introduce topics or items that encourage reminiscing

To encourage the expression of grief, disappointment, and regret

To select props that will stimulate memories

To provide a comfortable and somewhat stimulating environment

To give praise and recognition for participation

Remotivation Therapy
Definition

A type of therapy used to orient clients to reality for community living. The focus is present-oriented. Remotivation therapy is useful for the long-term, chronically ill, psychiatric client in a nursing home or extended care facility.

Major concepts

A climate of warm friendliness and acceptance is essential. Reading, poetry, and current events form bridges to reality. Props are used to promote discussion of topics. An appreciation of the client's work in the past is emphasized. A climate of appreciation as expressed in enjoyment at getting together prevails.

Goals of therapy

To focus on the world outside

To assist in coping with the present situation

To provide some universality (holidays, homes, dreams)

To stimulate sensory input (feeling, seeing, touching, hearing, tasting)

To stimulate latent abilities

To provide a sense of meaning or purpose

Role of the nurse

To introduce members

To establish rituals

To explain the specific focus of the group

To introduce subject

To elicit members' comments about subject

To summarize what has been learned and shared

Sex Therapy
Definition

Short-term treatment of sexual dysfunctions with a variety of behaviorally oriented treatment modalities.

Major concepts

Sexual dysfunctions arise from misconceptions, performance anxiety, ignorance of sexual techniques, and inhibitions; they are the reasons couples seek therapy. Treatment emphasizes pleasure and the naturalness of sexual behavior. Sexual partners learn to communicate more openly with each other. Sexual dysfunctions do not indicate disorders in individuals but indicate disorders in relationships. Both parties are involved in a relationship in which a sexual dysfunction exists; consequently, both partners are responsible for the solution of their problems.

Goal of therapy

To maintain healthy and growth-promoting sexual functioning

Role of the nurse

Sexual dysfunctions should be treated by a qualified therapist. The nurse plays a crucial role in sex education, assessing and identifying sexual problems that may result from medical-surgical procedures, medication, or physiological or psychological impairment.

Short-Term Therapy
Definition

Brief, time-limited therapy using specific criteria for the selection of clients and focusing on a central issue. Short-term psychotherapy maximizes the therapeutic effects of time by forcing clients to come to grips with the reality of time in their lives. Average length of treatment is six to twelve sessions.

Major concepts

Selection of clients who can benefit from short-term psychotherapy is a major criterion. The client needs to be motivated to change, to be able to state the complaint, to show ego strength, and to have an ability to form meaningful relationships. Most short-term psychotherapy is conducted on an outpatient basis. Venting emotional tension is an important element of therapy and needs to be done in an atmosphere that promotes a sense of hope and an expectation of support.

Goals of therapy

To achieve insight and resolve intrapersonal conflict
To limit the number of goals and address the specific
    problem that prompted the client to seek help

Role of the nurse

Depends on the approach being used. The role may be as a teacher (to present new techniques to solve problems), helper (to recognize the client's pain and suffering and offer active support), or manager (to plan strategies to help the client solve his problems).

Therapeutic Community
Definition

A special kind of milieu therapy in which the total social structure of the treatment unit is involved as part of the treatment process and every social gathering is viewed as potentially therapeutic. The therapeutic community differs from the therapeutic milieu. In the therapeutic community all social and interpersonal interactions are the main therapeutic tool used to bring about change. The therapeutic milieu emphasizes environment manipulation to bring about change.

Major concepts

Four basic beliefs contribute to the philosophy of the therapeutic community: (1) all members participate democratically in the decision-making process, (2) the open expression of emotion is encouraged, (3) a general sharing in activities of daily living occurs, and (4) confrontation about behaviors as observed by others in the environment is encouraged. It is believed that, over time, the process of confrontation will increase awareness and promote more socially acceptable behavior.

Goal of therapy

To facilitate social learning by encouraging staff and
    clients to confront one another about their behavior

Role of the nurse

Requires maturity and a willingness to have own behavior subject to discussion. Also required is a high level of tolerance for socially deviant behavior, a commitment to honesty with staff and clients, an ability to look at one's own interpersonal problems, and an ability to be flexible in areas of high tension and anxiety.

Index